THE SHUNT BOOK

THE SHUNT BOOK

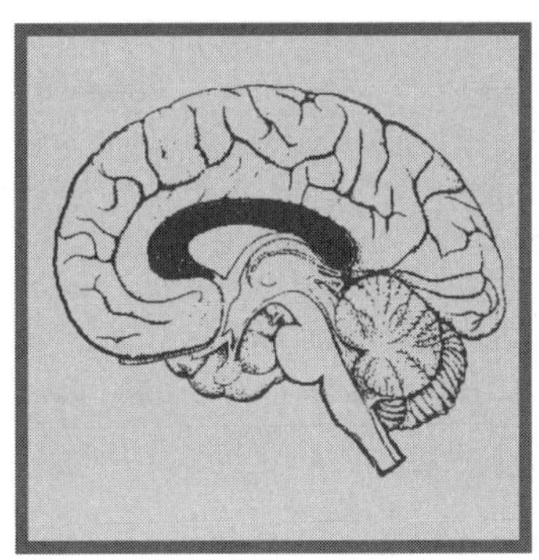

JAMES M. DRAKE, MB BCH

ASSOCIATE PROFESSOR OF SURGERY, UNIVERSITY OF TORONTO
DIVISION OF NEUROLOGICAL SURGERY
HOSPITAL FOR SICK CHILDREN, TORONTO, CANADA

CHRISTIAN SAINTE-ROSE, MD

PROFESSOR OF PEDIATRIC NEUROSURGERY
HOPITAL DES ENFANTS MALADES, PARIS, FRANCE

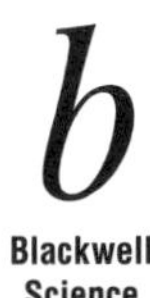

Blackwell
Science

BLACKWELL SCIENCE

Editorial offices:

238 Main Street, Cambridge, Massachusetts 02142, USA
Osney Mead, Oxford OX2 0EL, England
25 John Street, London WC1N 2BL, England
23 Ainslie Place, Edinburgh EH3 6AJ, Scotland
54 University Street, Carlton, Victoria 3053, Australia
Arnette Blackwell SA, 1 rue de Lille, 75007 Paris, France
Blackwell-Wissenschafts-Verlag GmbH, Kurfüstendamm 57, 10707 Berlin, Germany
Blackwell MZV, Feldgasse 13, A-1238 Vienna, Austria

Distributors:

North America	Blackwell Science, Inc. 238 Main Street, Cambridge, Massachusetts 02142 (Telephone orders: 800-215-1000 or 617-876-7000)
Australia	Blackwell Science, Pty Ltd. 54 University Street, Carlton, Victoria 3053 (Telephone orders: 03-347-5552)
Outside North America and Australia	Blackwell Science, Ltd. c/o Marston Book Services, Ltd., P.O. Box 87 Oxford OX2 0DT, England (Telephone orders: 44-865-791155)

Acquisitions: Michael Snider
Development: Gail Segal
Production: Michelle Choate
Manufacturing: Kathleen Grimes
Typeset and designed by Leslie Haimes
Printed and bound by Edwards Brothers, Ann Arbor, MI

Printed in the United States of America

5 4

Library of Congress Cataloging in Publication Data
Drake, James M.
The Shunt Book/James M. Drake, Christian Sainte-Rose.
p. cm.
Includes bibliographical references and index.
ISBN 0-86542-220-6
1. Cerebrospinal fluid shunts. 2. Hydrocephalus - -Surgery.
I. Sainte-Rose, Christian. II. Title
[DNLM: 1. Hydrocephalus--Surgery. 2. Cerebrospinal Fluid Shunts. WL 350 D761s 1994]
RD594.D73 1994
617.4'81059--dc20
DNLM/DLC
for Library of Congress 94-16245
CIP

To Stephanie, Brian, Madeline, Federica, Elise, and George

Contents

Preface

Before shunts became available 35 years ago, hydrocephalus was either fatal, or a severely debilitating neurological condition. With the dramatic improvement in patient outcome that is afforded by shunts, the complications associated with these devices has become manifestly evident. Shunt surgery is the most common operation in most neurological centers, and in pediatric centers, half of the procedures involve shunts. The ratio of shunt insertion to shunt revision is usually 1:1, which is clearly an unacceptable ratio. Part of the attempt to deal with these complications has been the introduction of an overwhelming array of shunt systems, devices, design modifications, etc., all purporting to improve efficacy. It is often very difficult for the surgeon to determine exactly what is inside the shunt system and how it actually works.

This book was written to provide neurosurgeons, neurosurgical residents, nursing staff, and even interested parents or relatives, with information concerning what shunt equipment is available and how it works, as well as what complications might ensue and how we think they can best be avoided. At this time, there is no shunt system or device which has been scientifically proven to be superior to any other. Clinical trials examining the efficacy of various shunt designs are currently underway. In the meantime, we think that an increased awareness of CSF shunts and their complications will allow neurosurgeons to make a more objective assessment of CSF shunt designs and a more rational selection of a particular shunt for an individual patient, be it shunt insertion or revision. We are convinced that this will lead to improved patient outcome.

The authors obviously have their own preferences for the currently available shunt systems. However, we have tried to be as objective as possible, and we are absolutely not recommending any particular shunt design. If some of the discussion in the chapters appears to favor a one design over another, we hope that the readers will use this book's contents to help them make up their own minds.

This book is divided into six chapters. Chapter 1 examines the fascinating history of hydrocephalus and CSF shunts. Chapter 2 tries to explain in the simplest possible terms the way shunts actually work. Chapter 3 describes how shunts are made and tested, which is important given the current attitudes toward implanted devices. Chapter 4 outlines as completely as possible the currently available shunt systems and components. Chapter 5 discusses the incidence, mechanism, and recommendations for avoidance of shunt complications. Finally, in Chapter 6 recommendations are given for how a CSF shunt should be selected and implanted for the individual patient.

James M. Drake

Christian Sainte-Rose

Acknowledgments

The authors would like to acknowledge the assistance of Ron Sierra and Alain Lecuyer of Cordis Corporation and Leanne Lintula of PS Medical Corporation for providing information on shunt materials and manufacture, as well as line diagrams of many of the shunt systems. We also want to thank neurosurgical colleagues Joe Piatt, Paul Chumas, Marcia da Silva, and Giuseppi Cinalli for their research assistance.

NOTICE

The indications and dosages of all drugs in this book have been recommended in the medical literature and conform to the practices of the general medical community. The medications described do not necessarily have specific approval by the Food and Drug Administration for use in the diseases and dosages for which they are recommended. The package insert for each drug should be consulted for use and dosage as approved by the FDA. Because standards of usage change, it is advisable to keep abreast of revised recommendations, particularly those concerning new drugs.

The Shunt Book

Chapter 1

HISTORY OF CEREBROSPINAL FLUID SHUNTS

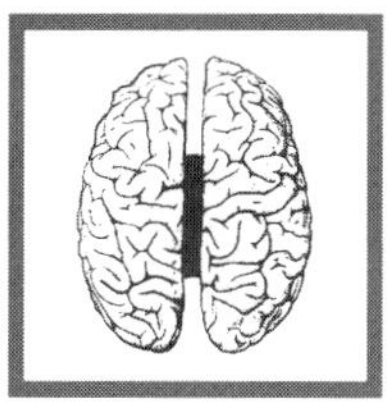

1 History of Cerebrospinal Fluid Shunts

Hydrocephalus has puzzled man since the dawn of civilization. It was only when the pathogenesis of hydrocephalus was understood, the necessity of a valved system realized, and the availability of biocompatible materials was coupled with improved surgical techniques that an effective treatment with CSF shunts was realized in the last half of the twentieth century. The history of the treatment of hydrocephalus parallels the development of medical knowledge, and bespeaks the remarkable ingenuity of the practitioners of the day, armed with little information, much of it incorrect, and facing horrendous failure rates.

EVOLUTION OF THE CONCEPT OF HYDROCEPHALUS

Hippocrates is thought to have recognized that water accumulating in the head caused it to swell, and although he is credited with puncturing the dilated cerebral ventricles, he may have only drained the subdural space (1), underlining the inability of ancient physicians to clearly distinguish between fluid collections inside or outside the brain, or even inside or outside the skull. Galen (130–200 A.D.), who recognized that the ventricles of the brain were in communication, believed that the soul or "animal spirit" contained in the ventricles underwent putrefaction with waste products finding their way through the pituitary body to be discharged from the nose as the "pituita" (2). The Greeks are also reported to have treated hydrocephalus with "lemnisci" — bands of basswood bark twisted about the head and inserted in trephine openings for drainage.

It was not until 500 years later that Vesalius (1514–1564), at the University of Padua, gave a clear description of internal hydrocephalus:

> *The water had not collected between the skull and its outer surrounding membrane, or the skin (where the doctors' books teach that water is deposited in other cases), but in the cavity of the brain itself, and actually in the right and left ventricles of the brain. The cavity and breadth of these had so increased — and the brain itself was so distended — that they contained about nine pounds of water or three Augsburg wine-measures (so help me God) (3).*

However, the diagnosis and treatment of hydrocephalus still remained much of a mystery as indicated in one of the earliest medical books to be printed in the English language, and one of the first books on pediatrics, Thomas Phaire's *The Boke of Chyldren* published in 1545 (4). His treatment, while amusing, was remarkable in that children up to this point were largely regarded as an expendable resource until they had survived the first decade and become useful members of the family.

OF SWELLYING OF THE HEAD

Inflation or swelling of the head, cometh of a wyndye matter, gathered betwene the skynne & the flesh, and sometime between the fleshe and the bones of the sculle, the tokes whereof are manifest ynough to the sight, by the swellyng of puffing vp, & pressed wt the finger, there remayneth a prynte, whiche is a singe of wynde & vicious humours, ye shall heale it thus.

Remedy *First let ye nource auoyde al thinges that engendre wynd, salf or slymy humours, as beanes, peason, eeles, salmon saltfyshe, and lyke: then make a playster to the childes head, after this fashion.*

Take an handfull of fenell, smallache and dylle, and seeth them in water in a close vessell, afterwarde stampe the, and with a litle cummyne, and oyle of bytter almodes, make it vp, and laye it often to the chyldes head, warme. In defaulte of oyle of almons take gosegrease, addyng a ltle vinegre.

And it is good to bath the place with a softe coute, or a sponge in the broth of these herbes: Rue, tyme, maioram, hysope, fenell, dylle, cumyne, sal nitre, myntes, radysh rotes, rocket, or some of them, euer takyng heede that there droppe no porcion of the medicines in the babes eyes, mouthe, or eares.

With the descriptions of the cerebral aqueduct by Franciscus Sylvius (1614–1672), the granular bodies of Pacchioni (1701), the interventricular foramen by Monro (1733–1817), and the pathology of hydrocephalus by Morgagni (1682–1771), the knowledge of the pathogenesis of hydrocephalus was considerably advanced by the end of the eighteenth century (5). Whytt, in an essay on "Observations of Dropsy of the Brain" in 1768, clearly defined internal and external hydrocephalus based on an autopsy series of 20 cases, probably tuberculous meningitis (6). However, he thought the cause of the hydrocephalus was an imbalance of fluid from an exhalant artery over an absorbent vein.

Confusion persisted into the early nineteenth century. Hydrocephalus was thought to be caused by "intermitting, remitting and continual fevers, rheumatism, pulmonary consumption, eruptive fevers and worms"(7). Treatment advocated had not much advanced from the sixteenth century and included bleeding, purging, diuretics, and local cephalic applications, such as cold, blisters, cupping, or inunctions (8). Head wrapping with adhesive plaster or rubber bandages remained popular. Magendie (1738–1855), by describing the outlet of the fourth ventricle that bears his name, ushered in the era of the modern understanding of the concepts of hydrocephalus that was finalized by Key and Retzius (9), who identified the correct pathway of CSF flow by dye injection techniques.

Dandy and Blackfan created hydrocephalus in dogs by obstruction of the foramina of Monro or cerebral aqueduct, and were able to distinguish between obstructive and communicating hydrocephalus (10). They were able to differentiate between the two by intraventricular injection of phenolsulphophthalein and observation of whether or not it appeared in the lumbar CSF.

SURGICAL TREATMENT

OPEN VENTRICULAR DRAINAGE

As mentioned above, ventricular puncture was reportedly practiced by the ancient Greeks. It continued to be used in the eighteenth century, with reports of successful removal of 80 cc of fluid (2). Head wrapping was sometimes combined with the procedure. Injection of astringents, including tincture of iodine and potassium hydriodate, into the ventricles in an attempt to decrease CSF production was also attempted, sometimes with disastrous results. The practice continued into the latter part of the nineteenth century, and included the use of indwelling setons or collared canula for continuous drainage. Repeated lumbar puncture was also introduced. However, it became clear that this procedure usually was ineffective, and death from meningitis was common.

CLOSED CSF DRAINAGE — THE FIRST ATTEMPTS

VENTRICULAR

In order to avoid infection, closed ventricular drainage was attempted near the end of the nineteenth century. The fluid was usually diverted to the subcutaneous or subdural spaces. Miculicz, in 1896, inserted a nail-shaped mass of glass wool into the lateral ventricle with the mass lying under a small osteoplastic flap (1). Gold and glass tubes were also used with poor results (Figure 1-1). Strands of catgut and linen were also passed from the ventricle, usually to the subdural space (Figure 1-2). Sharpe reported in 1917 that of 41 cases treated with linen threads (from the ventricle in non-communicating cases and the subarachnoid spaces in communicating hydrocephalus), 13 patients died within 36 hours, and in 5, there was no improvement; however, 23 improved and 5 were said to have "remarkable benefit" (11). Sporadic success was achieved with a rubber tube passed from the ventricle to the subdural space by Senn and a silver tube from the ventricle to the subcutaneous space by Krause (2). In the first vascular shunts, Payr passed a tube from the ventricle to the longitudinal sinus and to the jugular vein, using hardened calves' veins with a venous sheath. Eight of fifteen patients survived. The modest success of ventricular drainage and better

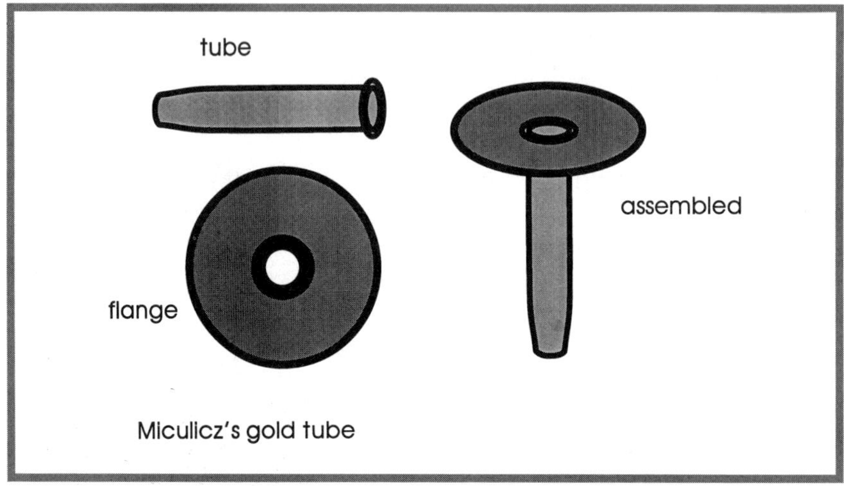

Figure 1-1
Miculicz's gold tube for draining CSF from the ventricles into the space beneath the scalp (1).

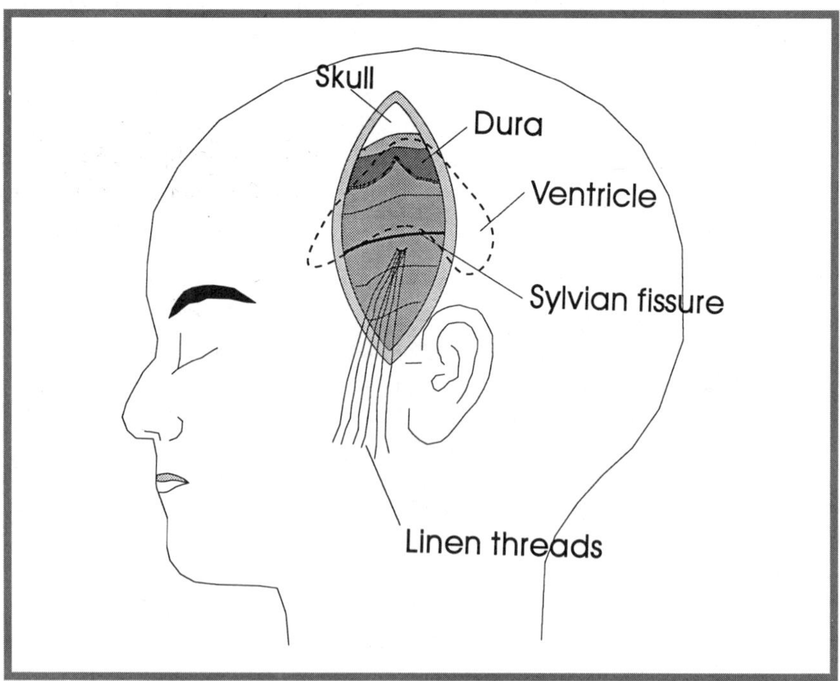

Figure 1-2
Drainage of the CSF from the ventricles into the space beneath the scalp by means of linen threads inserted into the lateral ventricle (11).

understanding of the pathogenesis of hydrocephalus led to two other strategies for treatment, namely, third ventriculostomy and choroid plexus excision.

SPINAL

In 1898, in the first lumboperitoneal shunt, Ferguson removed the arch of the fifth lumbar vertebra, pulled the cord aside, and drilled a hole through the body of the vertebra (12). He passed a loop of silver wire bent inferiorly in the thecal sac, toward the peritoneum. Three cases did poorly. In 1905, Nichol drew the free edge of the omentum into a defect in the spinal dura (13). Cushing anastomosed the spinal subarachnoid space with the peritoneal or retroperitoneal spaces through a combined laminectomy and laparotomy using a silver canula (14). Three patients died of intussusception attributed to the pituitary secretion of the spinal fluid. Heile experimented with several different anastomotic techniques, including intestinal serosa, silk strands, saphenous vein, a rubber catheter, and a direct anastomosis of the kidney pelvis following nephrectomy (15).

THIRD VENTRICULOSTOMY

In 1922, Dandy originally described the procedure that opened the floor of the third ventricle from a subfrontal approach, which required division of an optic nerve (16). He subsequently modified the technique and performed it from a lateral subtemporal approach in which the floor of the third ventricle behind the infundibulum was opened directly into the intrapeduncular cistern. In 1945 (17), he reported his results for 29 patients older than one year at the time of the operation: 24 were cured of their hydrocephalus, 1 died during surgery, 3 died later, and in 1 patient, the procedure could not be performed. The results in 63 children under one year of age were much more dismal: 32 died (10 during surgery, 22 later); 12 of the 21 survivors were cured; the remaining 10 survivors were lost to follow-up. A series of modifications and variations, including the early use of an endoscope by Mixter (18) in 1923, ensued. Third ventriculostomy gradually fell from favor as success with CSF shunts improved but has recently been revived for acquired aqueduct stenosis, as the long-term complications of shunts have become known (19).

CHOROID PLEXECTOMY

The realization that the choroid plexus was the source of CSF production led to coagulation of the plexus through an operating cystoscope by Lespinasse in 1910 (2) and resection of the choroid plexus itself by Hildebrande in 1923. Dandy (20) popularized the technique, and Putnam (21) and Scarff (22) reintroduced endoscopic coagulation to prevent the complications associated with collapse of the ventricles in open approaches. Reviewing the long-term results in his own series and in those reported in the literature in 1963, Scarff found 15% mortality and arrest of hydrocephalus in 71% of cases. Although still advocated periodically, failure to adequately control the hydrocephalus, with unacceptable failure rates, has caused the procedure to be largely abandoned.

CLOSED CSF DRAINAGE — SUCCESS IN THE MODERN ERA

Persistence, the recognition that a one-way valve was required, and new synthetic materials finally resulted in effective CSF diversion. This progress occurred simultaneously and on several fronts. Torkildsen (23) described the lateral ventricle to cisterna magna shunt, and although 6 of his original 13 patients died, subsequent authors described improved success. Matson (24), citing the various failures of CSF diversion "to the subcutaneous tissues, paranasal air sinuses, the pleura, the peritoneum, the thoracic duct, and bloodstream itself, including both the intracranial venous sinuses and veins of the scalp and neck" and relying on previous reports of diversion to the ureter (which seemed equally bad, though he had apparently had better experimental results), introduced the lumbar ureteral shunt (Figure 1-3). In this operation, a polyethylene plastic tube about the size of a #8F catheter was directed downward among the cords of the cauda equina from an L2, L3 laminectomy. The tube was fastened securely to the dura by silk sutures, tunneled through the psoas muscle to the perinephric space, and introduced approximately 6 cm into the ureter, a nephrectomy having been performed already. Matson reasoned that the reason the procedure worked was the natural valve provided by the ureter. Salt loss, requiring supplementation, was a problem in young babies.

Although Matson and Vannevar Bush, working at the Massachusetts

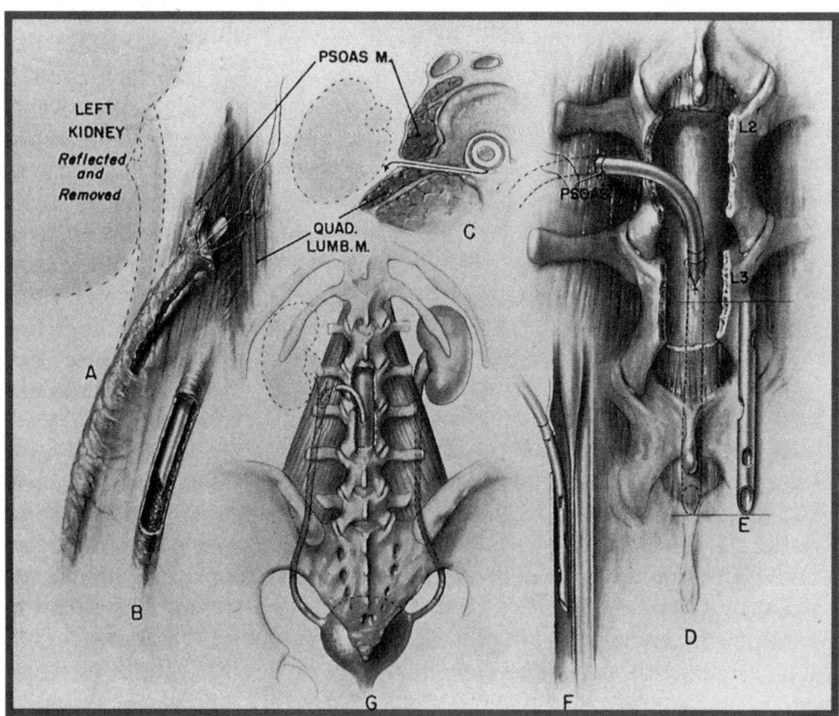

FIGURE 1-3
Lumbar ureteral shunt as described by Matson (31).

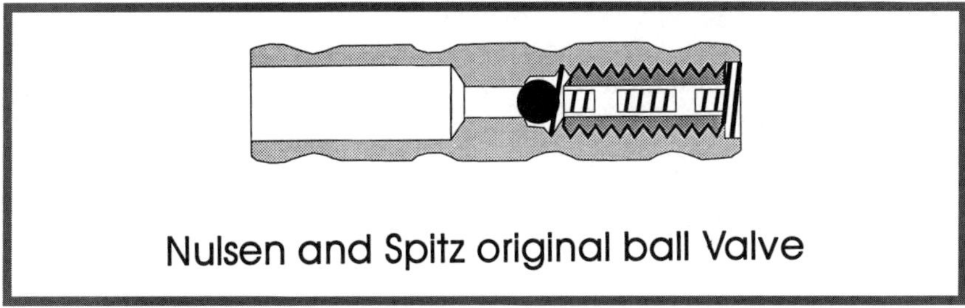

FIGURE 1-4
Nulsen and Spitz's original spring ball valve (25). Diagram shows one half of valve, which contained two spring ball valves in series.

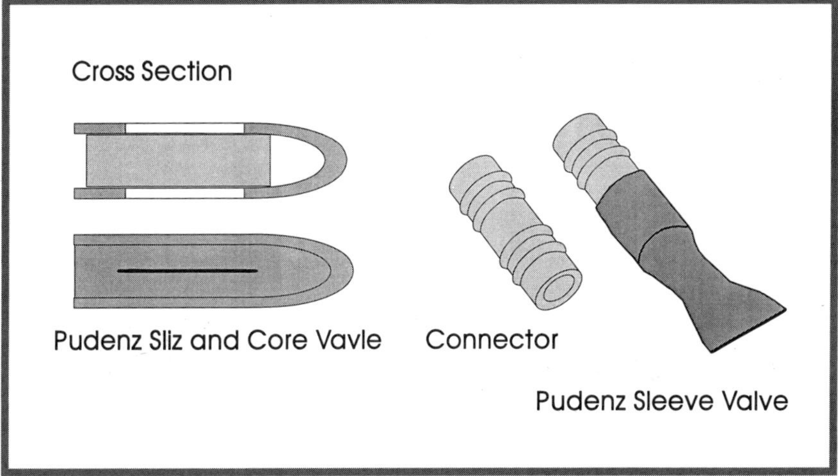

FIGURE 1-5
Pudenz's ventriculoauricular shunt valves (32). Right tetrafluorethylene sleeve valve; left, and silicone slit and core valve.

Institute of Technology, had experimented with a magnetic shunt system, Nulsen and Spitz in 1952 reported the successful use of a ventriculojugular shunt using a spring and stainless steel ball valve (25) (Figure 1-4). The two valves were housed in rubber intravenous tubing, which acted as a flushing device, and connected to polyethylene tubing at either end. (The valve looks remarkably like the currently used Hakim system, Chapter 4) Occlusion of the venous catheter by blood clot was a frequent problem.

The Holter valve was the first shunt to employ silicone, a polymer created from silicone dioxide, found as sand or quartz in the earth's crust, which was used initially as a sealant for ignition systems in World War II aircraft. John Holter was a technician in a machine shop in 1955 when his son was born with a myelomeningocele and developed hydrocephalus (26). Aware of the problems of the spring and ball valves, Holter designed a multiple-slit valve out of silicone for use in his son. Unfortunately, the valve was not ready in time for his son, who received a spring ball valve. The Holter silicone valve was implanted successfully in another child. Holter's son did ultimately receive the valve and did well for 14 months but died from a series of shunt complications and revisions. Holter went on to develop the valve further, and its use became widespread, and is still in use today, Chapter 4.

Almost at the same time, Robert Pudenz, working in the laboratory on many different materials, including silicone, polyethylene, polyvinyl chloride, Teflon, rubber, and stainless steel, came to the conclusion that silicone was the best material and that distal valves should be in place to prevent retrograde filling and thrombosis. He designed two valves, a distal slit and core valve and a sleeve valve (Figure 1-5), both for use as ventriculoauricular shunts (27).

There followed attempts to find a better absorption site other than the vascular system. Ultimately, the complications of vascular shunts became widely known, and based on the work of Ames (28), the peritoneum was settled as the best resorptive site. The progress since that time has been characterized by a proliferation of modifications to these basic first valves as well as some novel devices, such as the antisiphon device (29) and the Orbis Sigma (30), and is outlined in the chapters that follow. The history of CSF shunts has been one of innovation, initial success, and then a dampening of enthusiasm as the unexpected complications became apparent. This is still true today. The quest for the perfect shunt continues.

REFERENCES

1. Davidoff LE. Treatment of hydrocephalus. Arch Surg 1929;18:1737–1762.
2. Fisher RG. Surgery of the congenital anomalies. In: Walker EA, ed. A history of neurological surgery. Baltimore: Williams & Wilkins, 1951:334–347.
3. Torack RM. Historical aspects of normal and abnormal brain fluids. II. Hydrocephalus. Arch Neurol 1982;39:276–279.
4. Phaire T. The boke of chyldren. 1545. Reprint. Edinburgh: E. & S. Livingstone Ltd., 1957:24.
5. Aronyk KE. The history and classification of hydrocephalus. Neurosurg Clin America 1993:4:599–610.
6. Whytt R. Observations on the most frequent species of the hydrocephalus internus. In: The works of Robert Whytt, M.D. 3rd ed. Edinburgh: Balfour, Auld and Smellie, 1768:725–745.
7. Rush B. Medical inquiries and observations. An inquiry into the causes and cure of the internal dropsy of the brain. 3rd ed. Philadelphia: B & T. Kite, M. C. Hopkins, 1809.
8. McCullough DC. A history of the treatment of hydrocephalus. Concepts Neurosurg 1990;3:1–10.
9. Key A, Retzius G. Studien in der Anatomie des Nervensystems und des Bindgewebes. Stockholm: Samson and Wallin, 1876.
10. Dandy WE, Blackfan KD. Internal hydrocephalus. An experimental, clinical, and pathological study. Am J Dis Child 1914;8:406–482.
11. Sharpe W. The operative treatment of hydrocephalus: a preliminary report of forty-one patients. Am J Med Sci 1917;153:563–571.
12. Ferguson AH. Intraperitoneal diversion of the cerebrospinal fluid in cases of hydrocephalus. N Y Med 1898;67:902.
13. Nicholl JH. Case of hydrocephalus in which peritoneo-meningeal drainage has been carried out. Glasgow Med J 1905;63:187–191.
14. Cushing H. The special field of neurological surgery. Cleveland Med J 1905;4:1–25.
15. Heile B. Zur chirugischen behandlung des hydrocephalus internus durch ableitting der cerebrospinal flussikeit nach der bauchhole und nach der pleurakuppe. Arch F Klin Chir. 1914;105:501–516.
16. Dandy WE. An operative procedure for hydrocephalus. Bull Johns Hopkins Hosp 1922;33:189–190.
17. Dandy WE. Diagnosis and treatment of strictures of the aqueduct of Sylvius (causing hydrocephalus). Arch Surg 1945;51:1–14.

18. Mixter WJ. Ventriculoscopy and puncture of the floor of the third ventricle. Boston Med Surg 1923;188:277–278.

19. Drake JM. Ventriculostomy for treatment of hydrocephalus. Neurosurg Clin N Am 1993;4:657–666.

20. Dandy WE. Extirpation of the choroid plexus of the lateral ventricles in communicating hydrocephalus. Ann Surg 1918;68:569–579.

21. Putnam TJ. The surgical treatment of infantile hydrocephalus. Surg Gynecol Obstet 1943;76:171–182.

22. Scarff JE. Treatment of hydrocephalus: an historical and critical review of methods and results. J Neurol Neurosurg Psychiatr 1963;26:1–26.

23. Torkildsen A. A new palliative operation in cases of inoperable occlusion of the sylvian aqueduct. Acta Chir Scand 1939;82:117–124

24. Matson DD. A new operation for the treatment of communicating hydrocephalus. J Neurosurg 1949;6:238–247.

25. Nulsen FE, Spitz EB. Treatment of hydrocephalus by direct shunt from ventricle to jugular vein. Surg Forum 1952;399–403.

26. Wallman LJ. Shunting for hydrocephalus: an oral history. Neurosurg 1982;11:308–313.

27. Pudenz RH, Russell FE, Hurd AH, Sheldon CH. Ventriculo-auriculostomy. A technique for shunting cerebrospinal fluid into the right auricle. J Neurosurg 1957;14:171–179.

28. Ames RH. Ventriculoperitoneal shunts in the management of hydrocephalus. J Neurosurg 1967;27:525–529.

29. Portnoy HD, Schulte RR, Fox JL, Croissant PD, Tripp L. Anti-siphon and reversible occlusion valves for shunting in hydrocephalus and preventing post-shunt subdural hematomas. J Neurosurg 1973;38:729–738.

30. Sainte-Rose C, Hooven MD, Hirsch JF. A new approach to the treatment of hydrocephalus. J Neurosurg 1987;66:213–226.

31. Ingraham FD, Matson DD. Neurosurgery of infancy and childhood. 2nd ed. Springfield: Charles C. Thomas, 1969:222.

32. Pudenz RH. The surgical treatment of hydrocephalus — an historical review. Surg Neurol 1981;15:15–26.

Chapter 2

HOW SHUNTS WORK

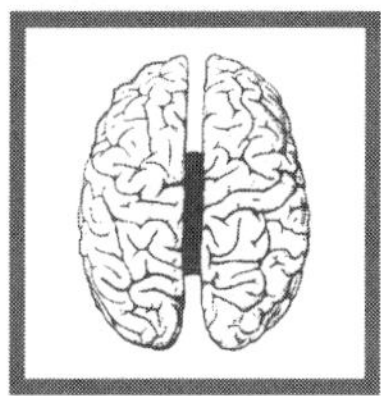

2 CSF Fluid Dynamics

As shunts are devices designed to transport CSF from the secretion or generation site to a reabsorption site and CSF is basically water, some knowledge of fluid dynamics, or *hydrodynamics*, is necessary. This amounts to understanding three important physical concepts — pressure, flow, and resistance. In the following sections, we will attempt to describe these concepts as simply as possible, relating them to hydrocephalus wherever possible.

PRESSURE

Pressure is simply the force per unit area. A solid object (e.g., a brick) exerts a pressure at its base. This pressure is the weight (force) of the brick divided by the surface area of the bottom face of the brick. The weight of solid objects is usually known as they can be readily weighed. A liquid's force can also be thought of as its weight. The weight of a liquid is the volume times the density of the fluid times the force of gravity. If the liquid is contained in a cylindrical vessel, the volume is equal to the cylinder's base surface area multiplied by its height. The pressure at the bottom of a cylinder is the weight divided by the cylinder's base surface area, which becomes the height times the density times the force of gravity (Figure 2-1). These statements are represented in mathematical form as follows (Equation 1):

$$
\begin{aligned}
P &= F/A \\
&= (\rho \times V \times g)/A \\
&= (\rho \times h \times A \times g)/A \\
&= \rho \times h \times g
\end{aligned}
$$

where P = pressure
F = force
ρ = density
V = volume
g = force of gravity
A = surface area
h = liquid height

In simple terms, the higher the column and the greater the density of the fluid, the more pressure at the bottom. As the density of water is essentially constant (and equal to 1 g/ml), the pressure at the bottom of a cylinder is proportional to the height. We employ this principle in the use of manometers, where we measure the pressure at the bottom of the column of fluid by recording the height. There is no requirement that the fluid be cylindrical or in a straight line; the only measurement that is important is the vertical height of

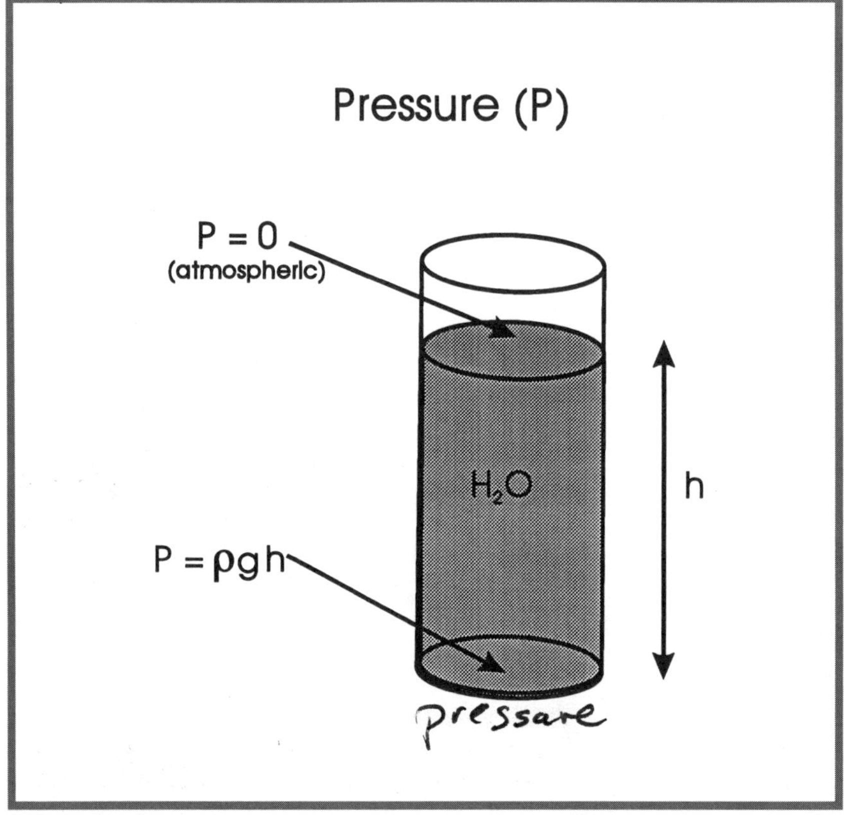

FIGURE 2-1

Column of fluid in container open at the top. Pressure at the top is zero (atmospheric). Pressure at the bottom of the container is due to the weight of the fluid column and is described by Equation 1.

the fluid. This discussion implies that pressure must be measured at some surface, but, of course, pressure exists within fluid itself. At the top of the cylinder, the pressure is zero (or, more correctly, atmospheric, see below).

Most confusion concerning pressure surrounds either the units in which it is measured or that it is related to some other pressure. Different pressure unit equivalents are shown in Table 2-1. We are accustomed to expressing pressure in terms of a barometer, using millimeters of mercury (mm Hg) or millimeters of water (mm H_2O), where 1 mm Hg = 13.65 mm H_2O. One mm H_2O is the pressure required to sustain a column of water 1 mm in height against the force of gravity.

TABLE 2-1 PRESSURE UNITS

MM HG	MM H_2O	PASCAL (N/M^2)	ATMOSPHERE	POUND-FORCE/ SQUARE INCH (PSI)
1.0	13.5951	133.3224	1.315789×10^{-3}	0.0193368
0.0735559	**1.0**	9.80665	9.67841×10^{-3}	1.42233×10^{-3}
7.50062×10^{-3}	0.101972	**1.0**	9.869233×10^{-6}	1.45038×10^{-4}
760.0	1.033227×10^{4}	1.01325×10^{5}	**1.0**	14.69595
51.7149	703.070	6894.76	0.0680460	**1.0**

We usually measure pressure with either a column of fluid or a pressure transducer; the transducer translates pressure into an electrical signal. Unfortunately, we usually fill these pressure transducers with fluid, which have forces unto themselves unrelated to what is going on with the patient. This is why it is so important that a fluid-filled transducer system be at the same height as what is being measured. Otherwise, the pressure at the point being measured will be offset by the difference in height in the column of fluid.

To make matters more confusing, we usually measure pressures in the body relative to atmospheric pressure, which we call zero. This is what we are doing when we "zero" the monitor. In fact atmospheric pressure is anything but zero, and depending on what the weather is doing, it is usually about 30 mm Hg. But, since we live in this pressurized gas-filled compartment and have grown rather accustomed to it and are unaware of this particular pressure, for the purpose of the book, we are going to forget about this and relate all the pressures from now on to atmospheric pressure. When we talk about negative pressure, we mean relative to atmospheric pressure.

As we are 75% water, when standing, we are basically a giant column of fluid with all the accorded pressure changes. This is particularly true in the nervous system, which is bathed in CSF, which behaves just like water. Atmospheric pressure, or zero, is at the level of the right atrium in the lying position and moves to the base of the neck (the jugular venous pulse) in the sitting or lying position. When standing or sitting, intracranial pressure (relative to atmospheric) is slightly negative (1,12). By the same token, pressure in the lumbar sack is quite positive. The pressure in the right atrium is slightly positive, while the pressure in the peritoneal cavity depends on where it is measured, the abdominal contents, the abdominal wall muscular tone, et cetera. The pressure under the diaphragm is less than in the pelvis because of the column of fluid analogy. Overall, peritoneal pressure can be considered basically at atmospheric pressure (2). Intrapleural pressure, however, is consistently negative due to the characteristics of the chest wall.

When describing shunt function, we normally refer to a pressure differential. This is simply the difference in pressure between the two ends of the shunt. It is this pressure differential that is responsible for shunt flow.

FLOW

Flow is the quantity of fluid that passes a point during a particular time period, usually expressed as volume per unit of time, e.g., cubic centimeters/minute (cc/min). Flow can be best conceptualized as a small cylinder of fluid traveling down a tube at constant speed (Figure 2-2A). The flow through a tube is the area of the cylinder times the average velocity of the fluid. Flow may be smooth *(laminar)* or chaotic *(turbulent).* The slow flow of CSF through the constant diameter shunt tubing is probably laminar. Because of friction, this, in fact, produces a velocity profile where the fluid in the center of the tube is traveling the fastest and the fluid near the edges, very slowly (Figure 2-2B). While this would seem to contradict our cylinder traveling down the tube, in fact, if we give the fluid an average velocity and ignore the velocity profile, our concept is preserved. Flow through the narrow orifices of valves is probably turbulent (Figure 2-2C). This adds to the resistance of the valve, which brings up this next important concept.

RESISTANCE

Resistance to the fluid flow in response to a pressure differential is an inherent property. It is expressed as pressure per unit of volume per unit of time, e.g., millimeters of water per cubic centimeter per minute (mm H_2O/cc/min). Resistance is a function of many factors, including diameter of the tubing, geometry of the valve, presence of turbulence, viscosity of the fluid, etc. Fortunately, pressure, flow, and resistance are all inexorably linked by a very simple equation (Equation 2): $Q = DP/R$ (3), where Q is flow, DP is the pressure difference, and R is the resistance (Figure 2-2A). The greater the pressure difference and the lower the resistance, the higher the flow. The resistance of shunt tubing to flow is basically the resistance of a tube to laminar flow, which is described by Poiseuille's law (Equation 3): $R = 8L\mu/\rho g r^4$ (4), where r is the radius of the tube, L is the length of the tube, and μ is the viscosity of the fluid. We can see from this equation that the resistance of silicone shunt tubing is a function of its length and is, in fact, quite low. For flowing CSF at 20 cc/hr, resistance of the tubing 100 cm in length (radius of .6 mm) increases approximately .1 mm Hg per cc/hr of fluid. As can be seen from Equation 3, the resistance of the tubing rises as the fourth power of the radius. The tubing of lumboperitoneal shunts is narrower (radius of .35 mm) and the increase in pressure with increased flow greater, approximately .35 mm Hg per cc/hr of fluid. The resistance of a shunt is perhaps best displayed as a flow pressure curve, as illustrated in Figure 2-3. Flow is normally plotted on the x axis and pressure on the y axis. The resistance is the slope of the line at each point.

VISCOSITY

Viscosity is the resistance that a fluid offers to shear forces. This is best conceptualized as the difference in force required to stir syrup, which has a high viscosity, and to stir water, which has a lower viscosity. Viscosity is important in shunts for two reasons, first it is quite temperature dependent, and second, it

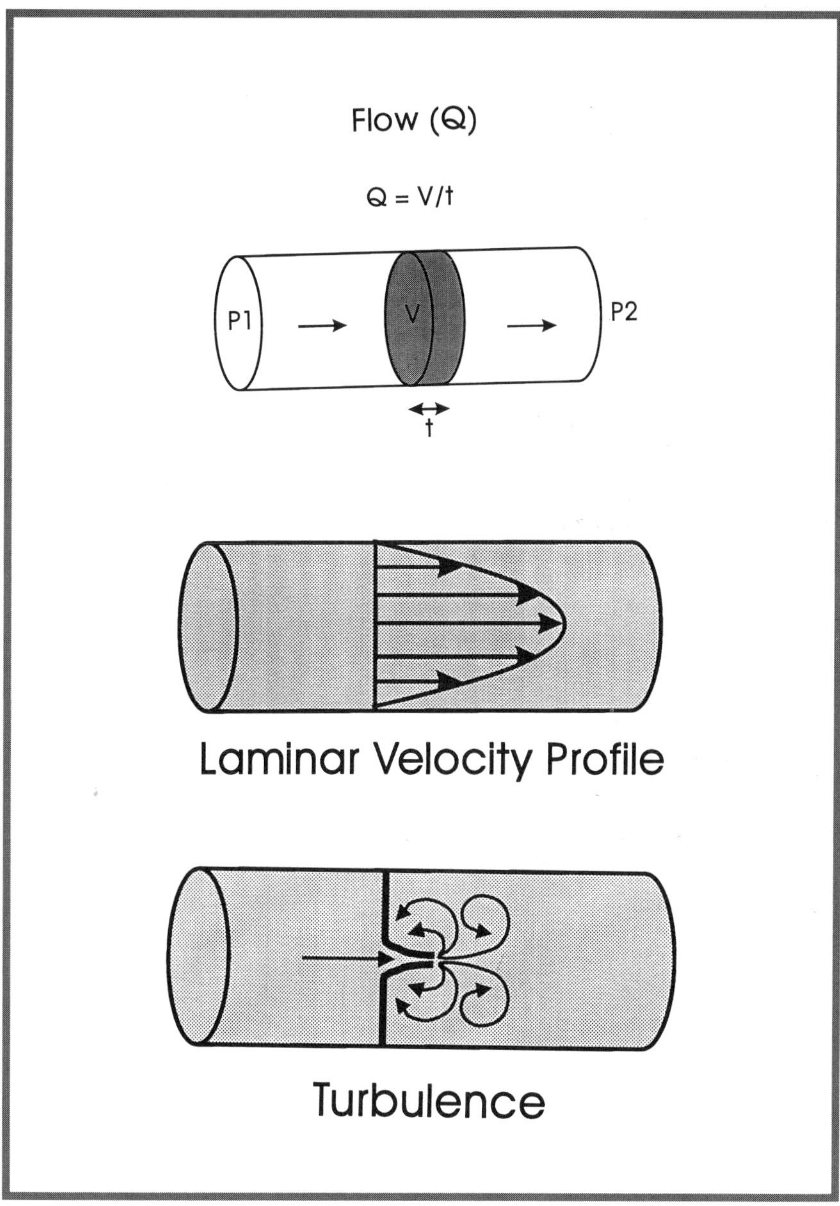

FIGURE 2-2

Flow of fluid through a shunt tube, best visualized as a cylinder moving down the shunt tube at constant velocity, where the flow rate is equal to the pressure difference divided by the total resistance (A). Slow flow in tubes is, in fact, smooth or laminar and has a velocity profile as indicated in (B). The fluid in the center of the tube moves at highest velocity, the fluid near the walls, the slowest. The valve produces turbulence, or a chaotic flow pattern, which increases the resistance (C).

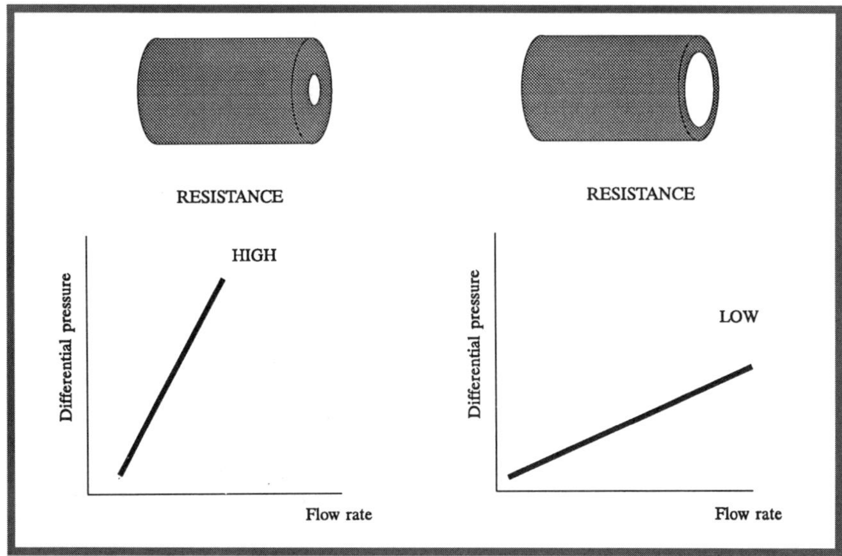

FIGURE 2-3

Resistance is the slope of the differential pressure versus flow curve. Narrowing the diameter of a linear tube increases the resistance, producing an increased slope.

has quite a significant effect in valves with narrow orifices. Table 2-2 shows the changes in viscosity of water with temperature. From Equation 3, resistance is seen to be a linear function of viscosity. If a shunt is tested with water at room temperature (20° C), the flow rate at body temperature (37° C) would actually be 30% higher. This becomes very important with valves such as the Orbis Sigma, or an antisiphon device. It also emphasizes that these devices should be tested at body temperature or, at least, their performance corrected for body temperature.

FLUID DYNAMICS OF PATIENTS

While a thorough discussion of the formation, circulation, and absorption of CSF is beyond the scope of this book, it is necessary to relate the basic principles of fluid dynamics to the human body. The pressure of the CSF is related relative to atmospheric pressure and, at the level of the foramen of Monro in the recumbent position, is normally 120-180 mm H_2O in the adult, and less in infants and children (5). The intracranial pressure (ICP) varies with the arterial pulse and with respiration. The wave form follows the arterial pulse, but with much smaller excursions, with the respiratory excursions superimposed. The constant flow of CSF is from the sites of formation in the choroid plexus and brain to the site of absorption, predominantly in the arachnoid granulations, at a rate of approximately

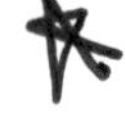

.3 cc/min. Superimposed on this constant flow are transient variations related to the arterial pulse, which is perhaps best visualized in the aqueduct of Sylvius as a to-and-fro motion. The resistance to the constant, or bulk, flow of

CSF is across the arachnoid granulations and is approximately 600 mm H_2O/cc/min. The brain and spinal cord and their coverings have a certain compressibility or elasticity (water is incompressible as far as we are concerned). This means that increases in volume lead to an increase in pressure (and vice versa) (6). This ratio is termed *compliance*. The higher the compliance, the more volume can be injected to obtain a given pressure rise.

TABLE 2-2 VISCOSITY OF WATER

TEMPERATURE (°CENTIGRADE)	VISCOSITY (CENTIPOISE)
15	1.14
20	1.00
25	.89
30	.80
35	.72
40	.65

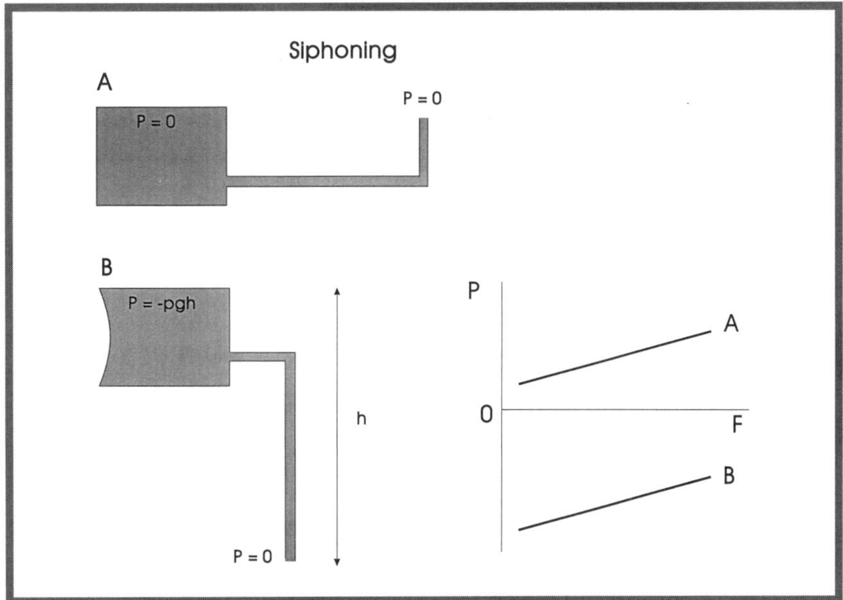

FIGURE 2-4

Closed container with open-ended tube. As the height of fluid in the container and the tube are the same, pressures at both places will be zero. When the end of the tubing is lowered, fluid flow continues until the pressure inside the container is the negative value of the hydrostatic gradient.

SIPHONING

Siphoning is the use of gravity (or hydrostatic forces) to move fluid from a higher to lower location. Those of us practiced at siphoning gas from cars know that to work the tube must be full of fluid and the distal end lower. If the "tank" is open to the atmosphere, then the siphoning continues until the tank is empty or the tube becomes full of air. If the container you are siphoning is sealed, the fluid will flow until the pressure in the container is negative enough to balance the hydrostatic forces. How much fluid will flow depends upon the elastic properties of the container and its contents, or the compliance. In this situation, the lower end of the fluid-filled tube is at atmospheric pressure. The hydrostatic force is equal to the height of the column, and, therefore, the inside of the container will be a negative pressure equal to the hydrostatic force (Figure 2-4). Finally, if you then provide some inflow to the container, e.g., CSF production, then the pressure will remain at the same negative value, but the flow rate will equal the inflow rate into the container, or the CSF production.

A shunt, as a fluid-filled tube subject to the effects of gravity, siphons in the same way. If the patient stands up and the peritoneal catheter is approximately at atmospheric pressure, then CSF will flow out of the head until the volumetric reserve of CSF (relates to brain compliance) is exhausted, then the pressure in the head will be equal to a negative pressure equal to the height of the column of CSF (1,3,7,8) minus the opening pressure of the valve (for reasons we will not go into). If the patient then lies down, the pressure will remain lower than normal until the CSF production replaces the fluid vented during the upright posture. The forces in a column of fluid are extremely important in understanding how shunt systems work. If a small child with a fluid-filled shunt system stands up, there may be typically 30 cm difference in height between the top and bottom of the shunt. This means that there will be a pressure difference between top and bottom of 300 mm H_2O. This pressure difference dwarfs any effects, whether or not a low or medium pressure valve is in place (typical difference 30 mm H_2O) (Figure 2-5).

SHUNT VALVE MECHANICS

In its simplest sense, a valve is a mechanical device that regulates flow. Irrespective of the design of the valve, it will open when the sum of the forces (the difference between the inlet and outlet pressures) acting on it exceed some threshold (9). With CSF shunt valves, this means the difference in pressure between the inlet pressure (ventricular pressure) and outlet pressure (peritoneal pressure). The pressure difference at which a valve opens is called the opening pressure and, naturally enough, the pressure at which it closes, the closing pressure. Opening and closing pressures are sometimes different because valves made of silicone rubber material are deformable, not strictly elastic, sticky, etc., and may behave differently whether opening or closing. This results in an "elbow" at the opening pressure area on a pressure flow graph and a different

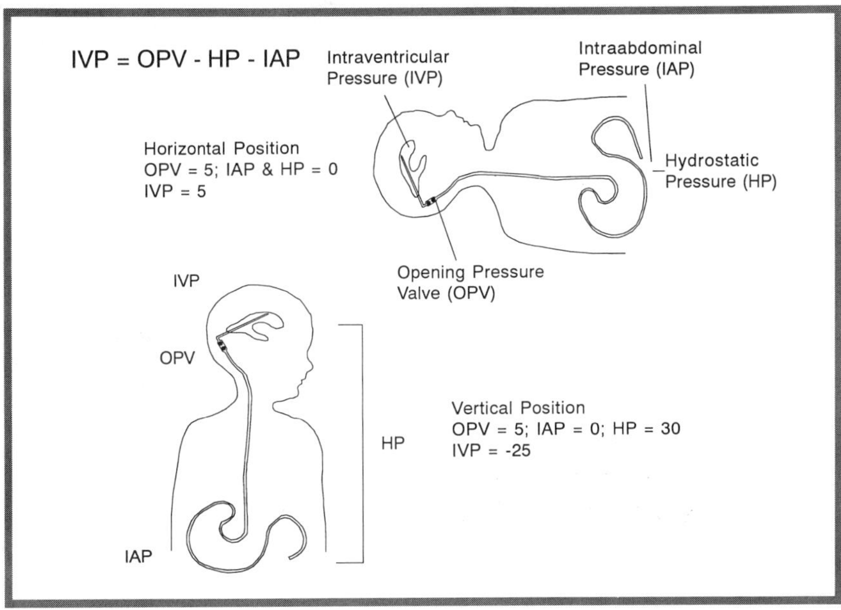

FIGURE 2-5

Fluid dynamics of patients. Valve dynamics predominate in the supine position; hydrostatic effects predominate in the upright position.

pressure profile depending on whether the pressure is increasing or decreasing (hysteresis), as shown in Figure 2-6. The elbow is characterized by an opening pressure that is not the same as the operating pressure, a problem that applies primarily to slit and miter valves. Hysteresis is evident only if a valve is tested in both upward and downward curves. Miter and diaphragm valves readily exhibit this imperfection. Ball-in-cone valves also exhibit this imperfection, but to a lesser degree. Slit, miter, and duckbill valves, with their cohesive surfaces, exhibit a special case of hysteresis, as the sticking between the two sides of the slits causes large deviations between the opening, closing, and operating pressures.

"STANDARD" DIFFERENTIAL PRESSURE VALVES

Standard differential pressure valves can be classified into four categories: silicone rubber slit valves, silicon rubber diaphragm valves, silicon rubber miter valves, and metallic spring ball valves (10,11) (Figure 2-7).

SLIT VALVES

The basic principle of slit valves is a slit in a curved rubber layer. The flow arriving from the concave side, if under sufficient pressure, will open the slit, the size of the opening related to the upstream pressure. This principle is applied in different types of commercial devices, such as proximal valves, the Holter valve and the Holter-Hausner valve (see Chapter 4) and as distal valves, the unishunt distal slit valve or lumboperitoneal shunts. It should be remembered that distal

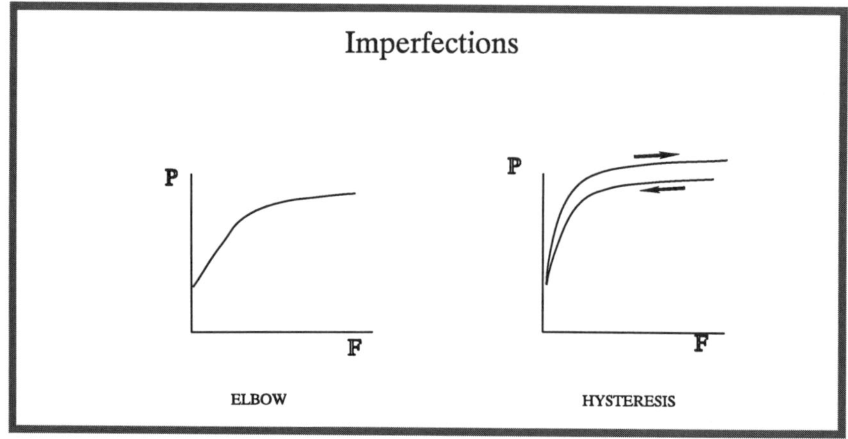

Figure 2-6

Imperfections in actual function of valves. Left, pressure flow elbow; right, hysteresis.

tubing with a closed end and slits provided as distal catheters are pressurized valves in their own right. The hydrodynamics of the valves will depend upon the stiffness and thickness of the rubber and the length of the slits and the number of slits. These basic features are utilized differently by the individual valve designs. Slit valves, when used as proximal valves, are often paired to provide an intervening pumping chamber. In some cases, an internal spring is used to prevent inversion of the slits and reflux. More than one set of slits can be used distally to prevent obstruction from accumulating debris inside the catheter adjacent to the slits (10).

Miter Valves

Miter valves are, in fact, more like "duck bill" valves. The orifice is round at the entrance and converges into two flat horizontally opposed leaflets of silicone. As such, it acts like a "Starling resistor." As with all valves, the leaves part in response to a pressure differential. The pressure characteristics of the miter valve are related to the size and shape, thickness, and length of the leaflets.

Diaphragm Valves

In diaphragm valves, a mobile flexible membrane moves in response to pressure differences. There are several strategies for moving the membrane. In some cases, the membrane is held by a central piston that moves in a sleeve. In other cases, the membrane surrounds the piston, which acts as the occluder. Finally, the membrane can simply be a dome that deforms under pressure. The pressure characteristics of the valves are similarly a function of the stiffness of the silicone rubber as well as the baseline force applied to it.

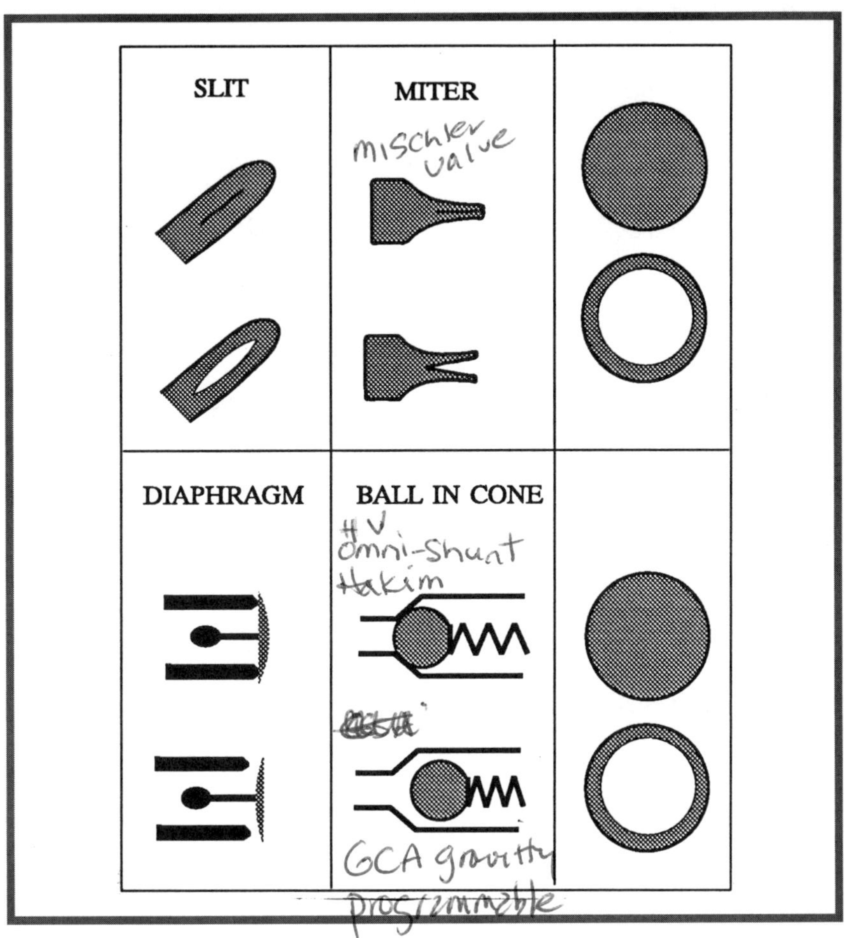

FIGURE 2-7

Schematic diagrams of typical standard differential pressure valves.

SPRING VALVES

Spring valves are characterized by a metallic spring that applies force to a ball made of either metal or industrial corundum (ruby or sapphire) located in an occluding orifice. The spring can apply force along the axis of movement or tangential to it. The springs can be linear, helical, or circular. Finally, the spring can act on a metallic lever, which controls the force on the ball. The opening pressure of the valve is defined by the spring stiffness.

"NONSTANDARD" VALVES

FLOW-REGULATING DEVICES

Flow regulation may be achieved by a solid conical cylinder inserted inside a ring attached to a pressure-sensitive membrane (8). The ring and cylinder are

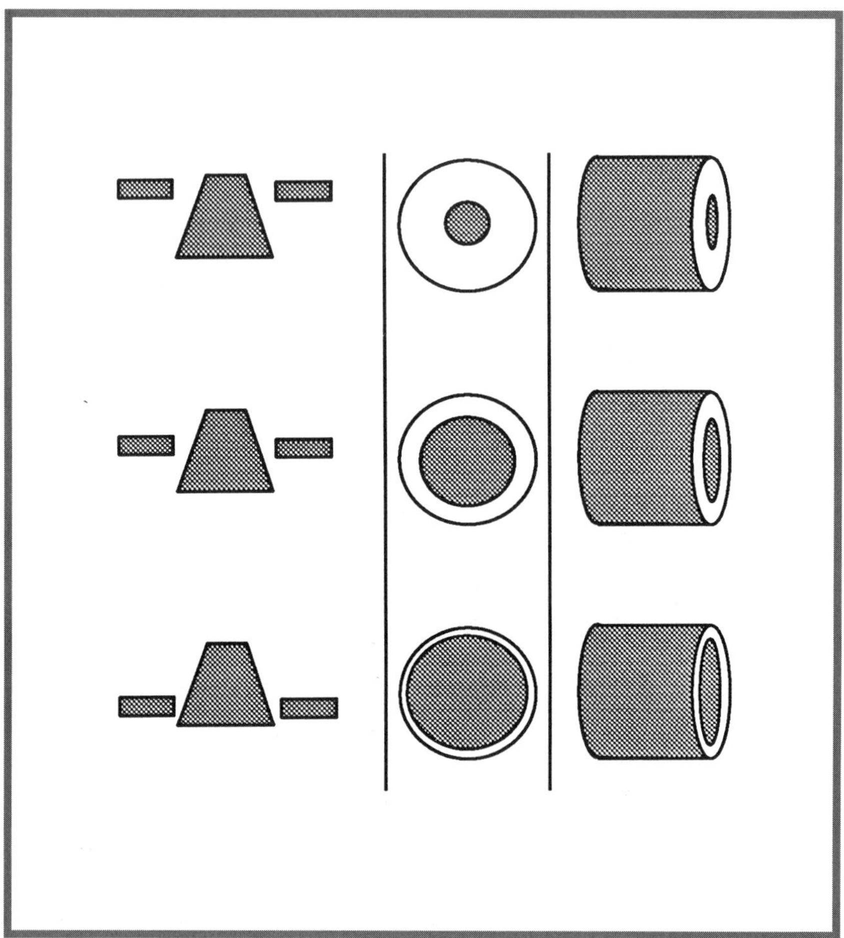

Figure 2-8

Schematic of mechanism of method of achieving flow regulation. As diaphragm descends, the orifice narrows, increasing resistance.

made of corundum. The inner diameter of the ring is slightly greater than the larger outer diameter of the conical cylinder. The space between the inner and outer cylinder can be changed and depends on the position of the cylinder relative to the ring. This function is best explained by Figure 2-8.

By reducing the surface area, the mechanism restricts the amount of liquid that can go through. In the absence of other influencing factors, this would mean a progressive reduction of flow rate. However, the relative motion the outer cylinder can achieve with reduced surface area is compensated by the increase in pressure necessary to displace the outer cylinder. The net result is a constant flow rate irrespective of differential pressure. At very low pressures, the diaphragm functions like a typical diaphragm valve. At very high pressures, the ring moves beyond the central cylinder, as a type of blow-off valve. This gives

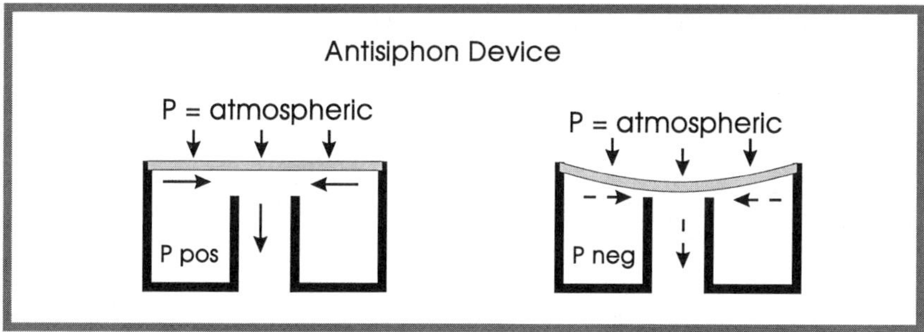

Figure 2-9

Schematic of mechanism of siphon-resistive devices. As pressure inside container falls, atmospheric pressure pushes membrane toward orifice, narrowing it and increasing resistance.

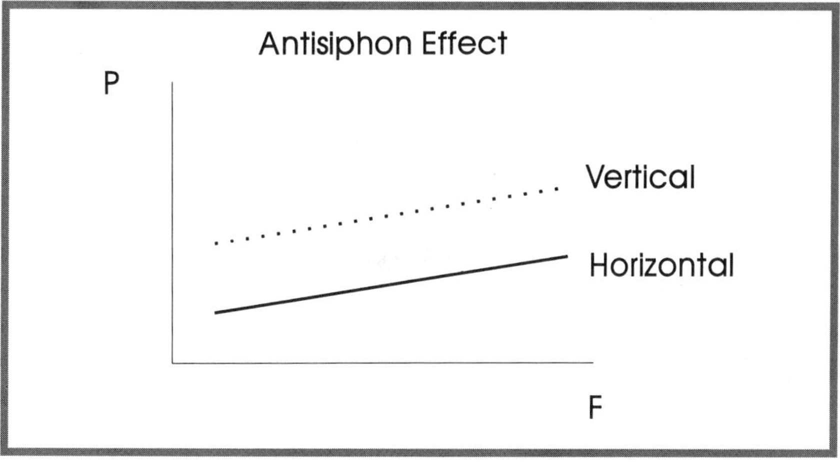

Figure 2-10

Effect of antisiphon device with shunt system in vertical position. Resistance rises, increasing the pressure for a given flow rate.

the valve a sigmoid type of pressure flow curve.

Siphon-Resistive Devices

Antisiphon devices (ASDs) have a mobile membrane that moves in response to a difference in pressure across it (12) (Figure 2-9). The outside pressure is atmospheric (theoretically) and the inside pressure is the pressure in the shunt system distal to the valve. When the pressure inside the shunt is above atmospheric, the mobile membrane moves away from the control orifice and offers very little resistance to flow. When siphoning occurs, the pressure inside the shunt becomes negative. Atmospheric pressure then pushes the membrane against the control orifice, increasing the resistance, preventing further siphoning. Antisiphon devices actually increase the resistance above what it would

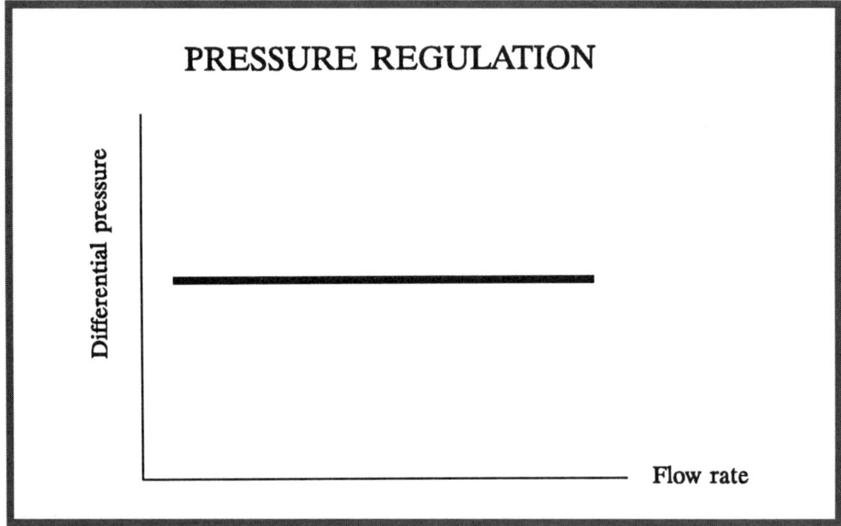

FIGURE 2-11

Differential pressure versus flow curve for "ideal" pressure-regulating system. The curve is horizontal.

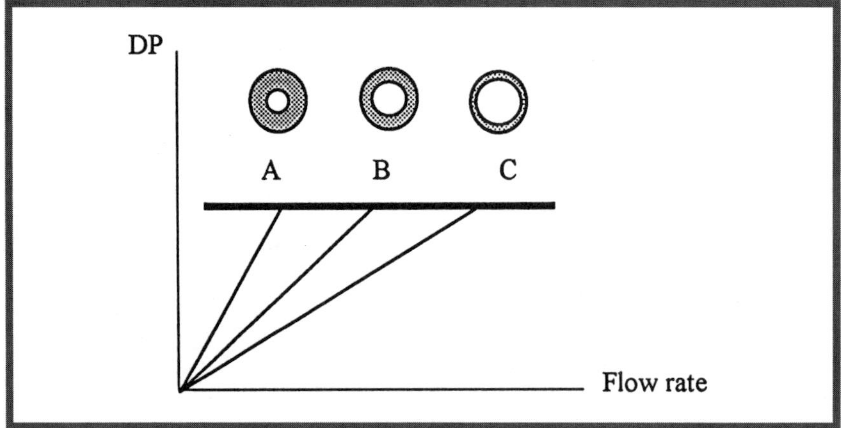

FIGURE 2-12

Effect of increasing orifice diameter in typical pressure-regulating valve. As orifice increases, resistance falls, producing the elbow seen in Figure 2-6.

ordinarily be in the horizontal position (13,14) (Figure 2-10). The extent to which this happens depends on the particular design. On bench testing, the Heyer Shulte ASD and the PS Medical are about the same. The PS Medical delta valve produces less of an increase in pressure in the vertical position. This is achieved by increasing the ratio of the areas of the flexible membrane to the area of the orifice. Positioning the ASD at different locations (or heights) along the course of the shunt will change the negative pressure, measured at the ven-

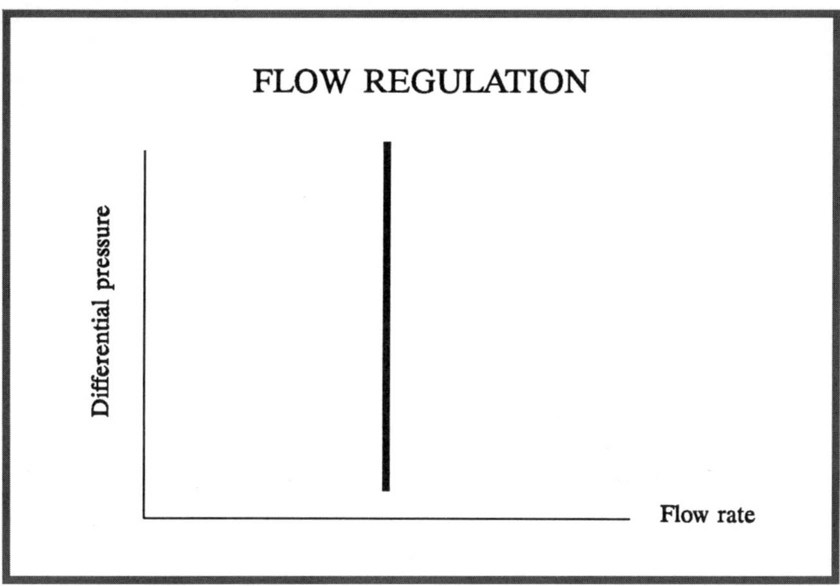

FIGURE 2-13

Differential pressure versus flow curve for "ideal" flow-regulating system. The curve is vertical.

tricle, at which they will begin to act (15). At a lower location, the hydrostatic pressure is less, and, therefore, a greater negative pressure measured at the ventricle is required to cause the device to act. In this way, one can regulate the degree of negative intracranial pressure experienced by an individual patient. Extending this process, ASDs at the distal end of shunts or ASDs attached to lumboperitoneal shunts will not work; they will never see a negative pressure unless the patient spends a lot of time upside down! The route that the shunt system takes from a frontal or occipital burr hole has nothing to do with how an ASD works.

Several comments can be made about these mechanisms. From a strictly mechanical point of view, metallic springs are very stable and predictable. Usually, there is no hysteresis between opening and closing pressures. But, these devices produce artifacts on MRI and CT and are sensitive to strong magnetic fields. By contrast, the fabrication of silicone valves remains an "art form." It is much more difficult to control performance parameters. This means that the construction process is very labor-intensive and technically demanding. Silicone has important hysteresis effects due to its physical properties. Finally, degradation of silicone is known to occur following implantation, and the long-term performance of implanted silicone valves is uncertain.

PRESSURE- AND FLOW-REGULATING MECHANISMS

There is considerable confusion about the difference between flow and pressure-regulating valves. This is in part because some valves that are pressure-regulating, are called "flow control" by the company manufacturer. Simply defined, a pressure regulator is a device that maintains constant differential pressure regardless of the flow, and a flow regulator is a device that maintains a constant flow regardless of the differential pressure.

PRESSURE-REGULATION

The principle of pressure regulation is well known. Numerous examples exist in everyday life, such as the valve on top of a pressure cooker and the regulator used by divers. By definition, pressure-regulating mechanisms try to maintain the same differential pressure, regardless of the flow rate (Figure 2-11).

The pressure-regulating function can be achieved by a variety of mechanisms including the previously discussed differential pressure valves, namely, slit valves, duckbill valves, diaphragm valves, and ball-in-cone valves. Although these mechanisms are physically very different from each other, the net effect is the same. As the differential pressure across the shunt increases, the mechanism opens up, increasing the surface area through which liquid flows, thus allowing more liquid to flow for approximately the same pressure. Points A, B, and C on Figure 2-12 exemplify this phenomenon and correspond to Figure 2-5. Surface area is directly related to hydrodynamic resistance. Pressure regulators are essentially variable resistance mechanisms, where the resistance progressively decreases with increasing differential pressure. The perfect pressure regulator is the device that gives a perfectly horizontal line on a pressure versus flow graph. The mechanisms used for construction of hydrocephalus valves must overcome several functional difficulties, primarily due to the low pressures, very low flow rates, and (small) size of the mechanisms themselves.

FLOW-REGULATION

Contrary to pressure regulation, flow regulation tries to maintain the same flow rate at any differential pressure (Figure 2-13). The way a flow-regulating mechanism goes about its function is also the inverse of a pressure-regulating mechanism. The surface area of the flow-regulating mechanism decreases in a predetermined fashion to produce a constant flow through the valve, regardless of the differential pressure. In other words, a flow regulator attempts to regulate the flow by increasing or lowering its resistance in response to the change in differential pressure, as previously shown in Figure 2-8. In order to effectively regulate flow rate, two parameters must be carefully controlled — the diaphragm's deflection and the way the mechanism's cross-sectional area is progressively reduced. A perfect flow regulator gives a straight vertical line on a pressure versus flow graph. As with pressure control devices, imperfections lead to nonlinear pressure versus flow curves, knee, hysteresis (Figure 2-14), or devices that actually *reduce* or stop flow rate as differential pressure increases (siphon-resistive devices). The knee causes the regulator to allow flow to begin before the process of regulation actually gets underway. Hysteresis results in a difference in increasing and decreasing flow. The most important point to remember is that flow reg-

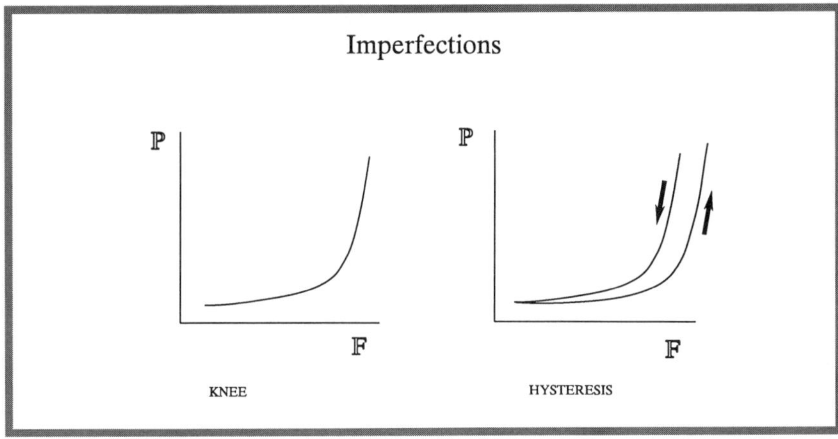

FIGURE 2-14

Typical differential pressure versus flow curve for actual flow-regulating valve showing imperfections.

ulation means a vertical line on a pressure versus flow graph, that is, constant flow rate regardless of differential pressure.

COMBINING VALVES

In a chambered shunt, valves are often combined. If two valves are placed in line in the same shunt system, or in a series, the opening pressures add up so that the total opening pressure is the opening pressure of the first valve plus the opening pressure of the second valve. Similarly, the resistances of the two valves also add up. If two completely separate shunt systems are placed in the same patient, or in parallel, providing the proximal and distal ends are at equivalent levels, then the opening pressure is simply whichever is the lowest. Should both valves be open, then the resistances of the valves are also in parallel, and the total resistance is $1/R_{total} = 1/R1 + 1/R2$ (4).

SHUNT PERFORMANCE CLASSIFICATION

There are no universal standards for shunt valve performance classification. The flow and pressure characteristics of valves are categorized by the manufacturers individually and differently. The terminology usually used is low, medium, and high pressure (extra low and extra high categories exist too). The pressure category is usually a pressure range, varying from one manufacturer to another for a particular flow rate. Some classify according to opening pressure, some according to closing pressure, and others according to pressure at a particular flow rate. This flow rate is usually low, e.g. 5 cc/hr, but some manufacturers give two pressures, one at a low flow rate and one at a high rate. Lumboperitoneal shunts are even more peculiarly described in terms of distal valve slit length. The longer slits offer less resistance to flow and, therefore, are lower pressure. Instructions for use and catalogues often provide a flow pressure range for the valve. Flow pressure curves and pressure ranges for low, medium, and high pressure valves are provided for many of the valves described in Chapter 4. It should be noted that most valves are capable of allowing flow rates far in excess of what would be considered physiological rates.

Several points should be borne in mind when referring to the described categories. First, the performance is not always what the manufacturers claim. Second, deforming a silicone rubber valve, for example, distal slit valve, by opening it up to make sure it is open or flushing a valve prior to implantation may affect its performance for hours. Third, while the low, medium, and other pressure categories are fine when the patient is recumbent, when the patient stands up, hydrostatic pressures of 200 or 300 mm H_2O dwarf any pressure category for standard valves.

REFERENCES

1. Magnaes B. Body position and cerebrospinal fluid pressure. Part 2: Clinical studies on orthostatic pressure and the hydrostatic indifferent point. J Neurosurgery 1976;44:698–705.

2. Yamada S, Ducker TB, Perot PL. Dynamic changes of cerebrospinal fluid in upright and recumbent shunted experimental animals. Child's Brain 1975; 1:187–192.

3. Chapman PH, Cosman ER, Arnold MA. The relationship between ventricular fluid pressure and body position in normal subjects and subjects with shunts: a telemetric study. Neurosurg 1990;26:181–189.

4. da Silva MC, Drake JM. Effect of subcutaneous implantation of anti-siphon devices on CSF function. Pediatr Neurosurg 1990-1991; 16:197–202.

5. Bradley KC. Cerebrospinal fluid pressure. J Neurol Neurosurg Psychiat 1970; 33:387–397.

6. Hakim S, Venegas JG, Burton JD. The physics of the cranial cavity, hydrocephalus, and normal pressure hydrocephalus: mechanical interpretation and mathematical model. Surg Neurol 1976;5:187–210.

7. Foltz EL, Blanks JP. Symptomatic low intracranial pressure in shunted hydrocephalus. J Neurosurg 1988;68:401–408.

8. Sainte-Rose C, Hooven MD, Hirsch JF. A new approach to the treatment of hydrocephalus. J Neurosurg 1987;66:213–226.

9. Fox JL, McCullough DC, Green RC. Effect of cerebrospinal fluid shunts on intracranial pressure and on cerebrospinal fluid dynamics. 2. A new technique of pressure measurements: results and concepts. 3. A concept of hydrocephalus. J Neurol Neurosurg Psych 1973; 36:302–312.

10. Di Rocco C. The treatment of infantile hydrocephalus, Vol. 2. Boca Raton, Florida: CRC Press, Inc., 1987:155–168.

11. Post EM. Currently available shunt systems: a review. Neurosurg 1985;16:257–260.

12. Portnoy HD, Schulte RR, Fox JL, Croissant PD, Tripp L . Anti-siphon and reversible occlusion valves for shunting in hydrocephalus and preventing post-shunt subdural haematomas. J Neurosurg 1973; 38:729–738.

13. Fox JL, Portnoy HD, Shulte RR. Cerebrospinal fluid shunts: an experimental evaluation of flow rates and pressure values in the anti-siphon valve. Surg Neurol 1973;1:299–302.

14. Horton D, Pollay M. Fluid flow performance of a new siphon-control device for ventricular shunts. J Neurosurg 1990;72:926–932.

15. Tokoro K, Chiba Y. Optimum position of the antisiphon device (letter). Neurosurg 1990; 27:332.

Chapter 3

HOW SHUNTS ARE MADE

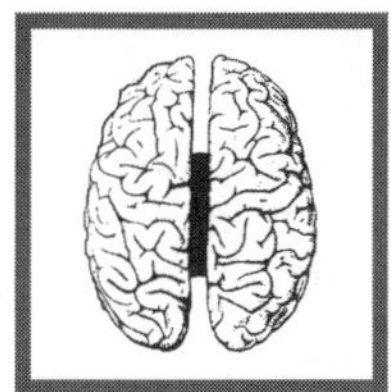

3 HOW SHUNTS ARE MADE

SHUNT MANUFACTURING

Shunt manufacturing remains overall a process of manual component assembly, despite the high level of technology involved in some systems.

The various processes that are used to transform raw materials into shunt components include extrusion or injection molding for catheters, valve chambers, and other plastic components or machining for metals, synthetic ruby, and ceramics.

Each component is submitted to a thorough cleaning process, using hydrochlorinated solvents or detergent solutions. The piece is then rinsed with demineralized water and dried with alcohol or warm air. Sets of clean components are delivered to highly trained production personnel, who assemble them according to validated and approved operation steps. Validated operations are mandatory to guarantee the safety, efficacy, and reproducibility of the manufacturing process. For assembly of the miniature components that compose today's state-of-the-art hydrocephalus valve systems, it is not unusual to have the operators work with microscopes under laminar flow hoods (LFH) in a clean room environment.

Each production batch is assigned a specific lot number and is accompanied through the entire manufacturing process by the related production and traceability documentation. The consistent indexing of all components, subassembly materials, and finished products in lot numbers allows, in the end, for any component, down to the original raw material batch, to be identified from the finished product.

The assembled products are submitted to numerous tests. Each test represents, based on failure mode and effect analysis studies, in vivo situations that could lead to potential problems should the product not meet the test requirements. Functional testing, i.e., determination of the hydrodynamic shunt performance, should be performed on a 100% basis since it is not destructive. Unfortunately, few manufacturers perform 100% functional tests on their valve systems today.

A final quality inspection releases products with full components and operation traceability to the packaging lines. An external cleaning operation is performed again on the finished products to eliminate particulates, e.g., fiber, dust, and so forth, prior to packaging and labeling.

In modern facilities, all these operations of shunt manufacturing take place in a clean room environment (typically class 100,000 as defined per Federal Standard 209-E or better), with respect to all the international standards and guidelines available. Respecting these conditions of cleanliness, product traceability, process validation, and strict quality control constitutes the first step in the observance of good manufacturing practices (GMP). GMP are a set of rules edited by the U.S. Food and Drug Administration (FDA) to regulate the manufacturing of products, such as medical devices, in order to ensure their safety, efficacy, and reliability.

Double blister, or pouch/blister, packaging designs constitute the standard packaging options used for hydrocephalus shunts. They have been found effective in protecting and guaranteeing both the shunt function and sterility.

A labeling operation grouping both the application of labels on the product packaging and the insertion in the product box of all the related documentation, e.g., Instructions for Use, is finally performed. This operation allows for the identification of each production batch. For more sophisticated and critical products, such as valve systems, a serialization of the products is performed by some manufacturers.

A validated sterilization process using ethylene oxide or steam follows the packaging operation. Sterile devices are then released for distribution to the market. A schematic process flow chart is given in Figure 3-1.

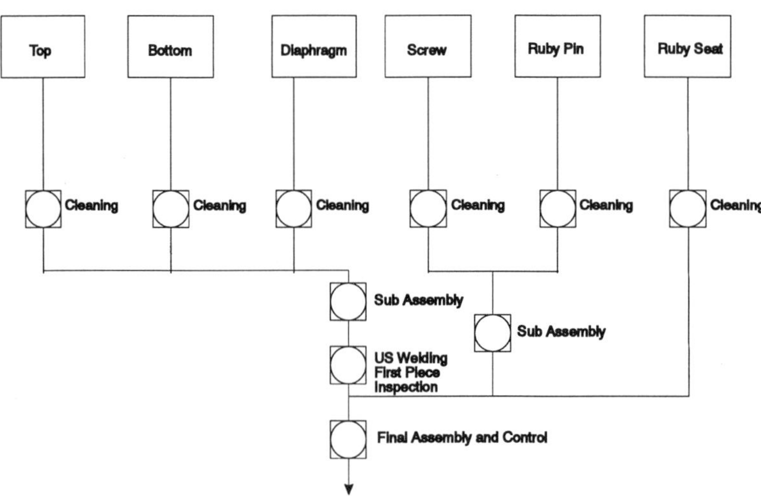

FIGURE 3.1
Schematic process flow chart for validated sterilization.

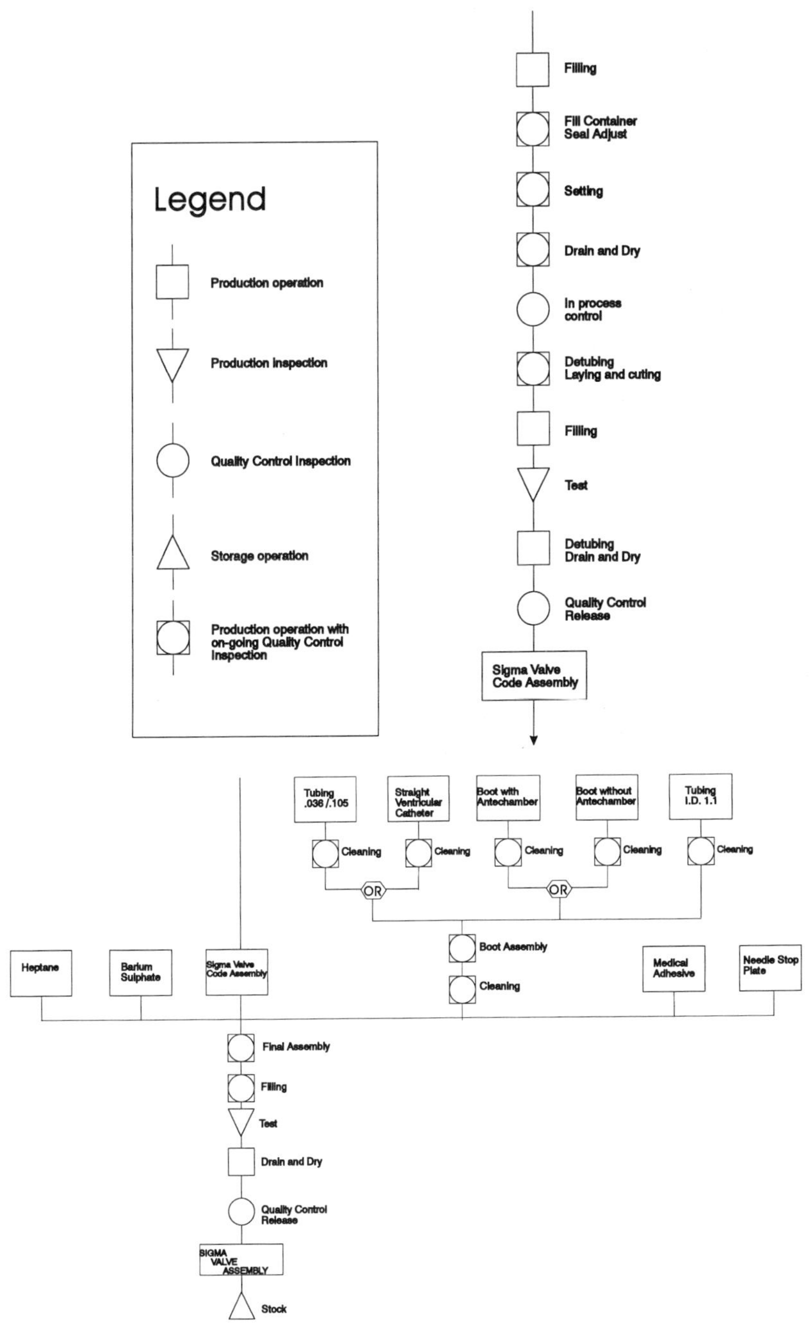
Legend
Production operation
Production inspection
Quality Control Inspection
Storage operation
Production operation with on-going Quality Control Inspection
Filling
Fill Container Seal Adjust
Setting
Drain and Dry
In process control
Detubing Laying and cuting
Filling
Test
Detubing Drain and Dry
Quality Control Release
Sigma Valve Code Assembly
Tubing .036 /.105
Straight Ventricular Catheter
Boot with Antechamber
Boot without Antechamber
Tubing I.D. 1.1
Cleaning
Cleaning
Cleaning
Cleaning
Cleaning
OR
OR
Boot Assembly
Cleaning
Heptane
Barium Sulphate
Sigma Valve Code Assembly
Medical Adhesive
Needle Stop Plate
Final Assembly
Filling
Test
Drain and Dry
Quality Control Release
SIGMA VALVE ASSEMBLY
Stock

SHUNT MATERIALS

The choice of material for any medical device implanted in a patient is influenced by implant parameters: (1) place of contact, (2) contact time, and, (3) performance. Shunts are in contact with the brain for prolonged periods, and their performance affects the well being of the patient. For these reasons they are considered critical and long-term (greater than 30 days) implants (1-3). This substantially affects the choice of materials in the design and construction.

PHYSICAL CHARACTERISTICS

BIOCOMPATIBILITY (1-20)

The essential physical requirement of a shunt is biocompatibility. The requirements for long-term biocompatibility vary, however, there are certain short-term biocompatibility characteristics that can be tested for in order to screen a material, some of which are listed in Table 3-1.

TABLE 3-1 SHORT-TERM BIOCOMPATIBILITY (3)

CRITERIA	TESTS FOR
Cytotoxicity	Cell death, cell growth inhibition, other effect on cells
Sensitization	Allergic or sensitization reactions
Irritation	Irritation potential on specific implantation site
Intracutaneous reactivity	Localized reaction of tissue
Genotoxicity	DNA or gene toxicity
Implantation	Local pathological effects on living tissues (gross and microscopic level)
Hemocompatibility	Effects on blood or blood components

(3) International Standards Organization. ISO/DIS 10993-1.

There are standardized procedures and tests for many of the biocompatibility criteria listed. Meeting these requirements is a first step in determining if a material is suitable for a shunt.

Some common requirements for long-term biocompatibility common to most sources are listed in Table 3.2.Some in vitro tests provide a first step in assuring long-term biocompatibility. Implantation tests provide for placement of the material in question with the appropriate biological structure for prolonged periods of time and examination of the structure thereafter. A variety of in vivo tests may be used to test a material once it has passed the preliminary short- and long-term in vitro biocompatibility tests. This type of testing may be long, expensive, and, depending on the type of implant, an appropriate animal model may not be available. However, there exists a variety of materials that historically have proven their biocompatibility throughout use in human implants. Also, as a general rule, materials with high degrees of chemical inertness are good candidates for long-term implantable materials.

TABLE 3-2 LONG-TERM BIOCMPATIBILITY (3)

CRITERIA	TESTS FOR
Acute system toxicity	Harmful effects of single/multiple exposures due to toxic leachables, degradation products, and pyrogenicity (exposure limited to 24 hours)
Subchronic or subacute toxicity	Same as acute toxicity, but with exposures of more than 24 hours but less than 10% of the test animal's life
Chronic toxicity	Same as acute toxicity, but with exposures of more than 10 % of the test animal's life
Carcinogenicity	Tumorigenic potential of test materials

(3) International Standards Organization. ISO/DIS 10993-1.

MECHANICAL CHARACTERISTICS (6,7,9,10,14,18,21–32)

All shunts share several points in common. They all access and transport CSF, they react to gradients in pressure, and they are implanted subcutaneously. These functions define a device with three different subcomponents, namely, a recovery tube (ventricular or lumbar catheter), a delivery tube (peritoneal or atrial catheter), and a fluid-regulating mechanism (the valve).

The ventricular catheter will be inserted in fluid-filled cavities of reduced size. These cavities are made from soft, sensitive tissues. This application requires a soft material that can be transformed into a shape small enough to access the small cavities. Likewise, the peritoneal catheter will be inserted into similar soft and possibly fluid-filled cavities. Since both catheters will be transporting fluid, the material must have a certain rigidity so that the tubing does not kink. The material should also avoid buildup of substances present in CSF, tissues, or other fluids that surround the catheters. The requirement that the valve be implanted subcutaneously necessitates the use of soft materials, or materials with an appropriate surface finish. The material properties are varied, have different units of measure, and are defined depending on the particular characteristics to be measured. Some of these physical characteristics are listed in Table 3-3. A material can then be evaluated by quantifying its various physical and mechanical properties.

In interpreting these mechanical properties, one must keep in mind that metals behave differently than plastics. While a metal's mechanical properties are largely dependent on its crystalline structure, a plastic will respond due to its viscoelastic behavior. Therefore, some of the mechanical properties and constants used in design formulas for metals may not be directly used for plastics. The designer must then resort to creep analysis in order to properly evaluate a plastic material for a particular application.

TABLE 3-3 MECHANICAL PROPERTIES OF MATERIALS (31,32)

Tensile strength at break (or ultimate tensile strength)	maximum load sustained by a test specimen undergoing tension, divided by its initial cross-sectional area.
Elongation at break	percent change in original test specimen length at failure.
Tensile yield strength	point during the test of a specimen where fur ther increase in elongation (strain) does not produce an increase in load or force (stress).
Tensile/Young's modulus (or modulus of elasticity)	the ratio of stress (force) to strain (elongation) within the elastic/proportional limit.
Compressive modulus	similar to the tensile modulus, but for compressive stresses.
Impact resistance	empirical testing yielding approximate or mean values of a material's resistance to different forms of impact and crack propagation.
Poisson's ratio	ratio of transversal to longitudinal deformation for a test sample under tension
Hardness	resistance to localized penetration, such as scratching or indentation

Reprinted by permission from Agranoff J, ed. Modern plastics encyclopedia . Volume 57. New York: McGraw-Hill, 1980:10A. (32) Baumeister T. Marks, standard handbook for mechanical engineers, 8th ed. New York: McGraw-Hill, 1978.

All shunts perform fluid regulation through mechanical elements that respond to pressure gradients. It is therefore necessary for the valve mechanical elements to be made from a material with a certain elasticity, that will deform within its elastic limit in response to pressure differentials (9,33,34).

MATERIALS

Materials can be natural, man-made, or in between. Primarily due to biocompatibility requirements, materials used in shunt construction must be relatively inert. However, very few of the available materials suitable for long-term implants have found their way into hydrocephalus shunt utilization (Table 3-4).

Elemental metals and their alloys dominate the natural material category. Metals are typically used in applications where rigidity, hardness or strength is required. In the man-made category, only a small number of plastics have been used as shunt materials. Although some types of glass and ceramics are recognized as long-term implant materials, the in-between category contains even fewer choices. The somewhat small number of materials presently used for shunt construction is primarily due to their historical use in human beings. Also, shunt designers have been able to produce a variety of designs while using the same materials of construction. As biomedical technology evolves, more plastics (and other materials) begin to gain "biocompatible" status. Therefore, it is possible that in the near future, a wider choice of materials will be available for shunt construction.

TABLE 3-4 MATERIALS PRESENTLY USED IN SHUNTS

(The following list, although not exhaustive, lists the major materials presently used in shunt construction)

MATERIAL	UTILIZATION
Silicone rubber	- ventricular or lumbar catheters
	- peritoneal or atrial catheters
	- suture clamps
	- access chambers
	- valve external housings
	- valve mechanisms (membrane, slit, duckbill valves)
Stainless steel	- radiopaque marks
	- valve internal housings
	- valve mechanisms (springs, valve seats, gravity-responsive elements)
	- needle stops
	- miscellaneous accessories (connectors, burr hole reservoirs)
Synthetic ruby	- valve mechanisms (components thereof)
Titanium	- needle stops
Plastics (polypropylene, polysulfone, polyethersulfone, nylon)	- valve housing
	- valve seats
	- needle stops
	- miscellaneous accessories (connectors, angling clips, burr hole reservoirs)
Tantalum	- radiopaque marks
Barium sulfate	- general radiopacifier

SILICONE

By far, the material most utilized in shunt construction is silicone rubber. While classified in the plastics category, silicone rubber is a cross-linked plastic or thermoset. This means that, unlike thermoplastics, silicone rubber cannot be melted and reshaped once cross-linked. Silicone rubber has a number of properties that render it very useful as a shunt material. It is widely accepted as biocompatible, primarily due to its long history of use as a long-term implant material. Its physical properties (hardness, flexibility, elasticity, tensile strength) and ease of processing (molding and extrusion) yield a very versatile material that lends itself very well to a variety of designs as well as implantation in contact with soft tissues (brain/subcutaneous tissues).

The term "silicone" describes the organo-silicon oxide polymers as a class and is a popular term for materials referred to in the chemical literature (35) as organopolysiloxanes. These materials are produced in a wide variety of physical forms, whose principal subdivisions are fluids, compounds, resins, and rubber-like products. This last category is the one of interest for shunt manufacturers.

The polysiloxanes used in shunts are well represented by the following general formula:

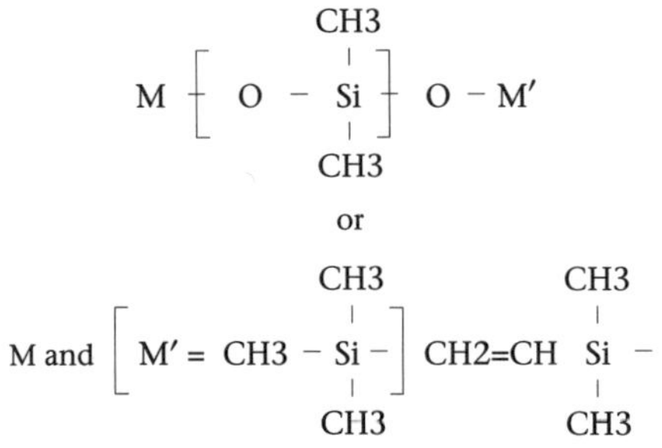

$$M \left[O - \underset{\displaystyle CH3}{\overset{\displaystyle CH3}{\underset{|}{\overset{|}{Si}}}} \right] O - M'$$

or

$$M \text{ and } \left[M' = CH3 - \underset{\displaystyle CH3}{\overset{\displaystyle CH3}{\underset{|}{\overset{|}{Si}}}} - \right] \; CH2{=}CH \; \underset{\displaystyle CH3}{\overset{\displaystyle CH3}{\underset{|}{\overset{|}{Si}}}} -$$

These materials exist in a wide range of molecular weights and viscosities (for example, M can range from 5 to 2,000 for liquid elastomers, and 3,000 to 10,000 for gums). These characteristics are essential for the final processability and mechanical behavior of the elastomer.

Polysiloxanes are obtained after complex reactions between silicon and chloride compounds to obtain chlorosilanes. The bifunctional chlorosilanes are of interest here and will be polymerized through hydrolysis to obtain polymer chains, the length of which (thus, the viscosity and molecular weight) can be adjusted by controlling the equilibrium of the reaction. The inclusion of small quantities of other species than methyl ,e.g., vinyl, modifies or enhances certain desired final properties.

Polymers obtained at the end of this reaction are not yet suitable for shunt component manufacturing. It is necessary to add reinforcing fillers, generally amorphous silica, to increase the final mechanical properties of the polymers (by factors as high as 40). Other adjuvants can also be added to pigment the rubber or give it its radiopacity characteristics. Pigments can be added to color the raw material, either for identification purposes (pressure color bands) or cosmetic reasons. Mineral pigments are more heat stable than organic pigments and are preferred. Carbon graphite is also used as a length marker. Radiopacity, often a desirable characteristic, is commonly obtained with the introduction of Barium sulfate ($BaSO_4$, ~ 10 to 15% in mass), giving the silicone its "white" color. Other radio-opaque fillers, such as Bismuth subcarbonate or tantalum oxide, may be chosen to allow for shunt x-ray imaging. Finally, the three-dimensional stability of the molecular network is obtained by the introduction of curing catalysts that will create chemical crosslinks along the polymer chains. These reactions are initiated during the final polymer transformation. The most common ways to achieve vulcanization are at elevated temperatures or room temperature, depending on the catalyst system used.

Among the catalyst systems used to heat vulcanized silicone rubber, peroxides are the most common. To create free radials, which almost correspond to the rubber transformation temperature, the decomposition temperature varies with the molecules. 2.4 dichlorodibenzoyl peroxide is widely used in medical formulation. Free radicals react with vinyl and methyl side groups of the polymer chain to create a stable network. Reactivity of free radicals varies with the side groups. Post-curing of peroxide-cured silicone is recommended to eliminate byproducts of the reaction. Curing time hardly exceeds five minutes, depending on the temperature and part thickness. Platinum catalyst systems proceed by hydrolysis reaction in the presence of Si-H groups (introduced in the rubber as a low molecular weight silicone molecule), reacting with the termination or side groups of the polymer chains. This additional reaction eliminates the postcuring process, and is also suitable for room temperature vulcanization. Curing time is also in the five minute range. One part room temperature vulcanizing (RTV) compounds often proceeds through hydrolysis reaction using atmospheric water as a reactant. This polycondensation reaction will eliminate byproducts (acid or base) acting as catalysts in this reaction. Proper curing generally is obtained in 24 hours.

As seen above, commercially available silicones are very complex compounds, which enable manufacturers to deliver tailored formulations with specific final properties. On manufacturing sites, the most frequent forms are gums, which can be fully compounded or not. The shunt manufacturer will then use a two roll mill to incorporate its ingredients. It can be injection molded, compression transferred, or extruded. It is available as a mono- or a bi-component product. Liquid silicone rubber, an easily processable material, is generally provided as a two compound material, mixed on a static mixer prior to being injected. High viscosity grades can be extruded. Adhesives (monocomponent, RTV) are frequently used to assemble components when overmolding is unpractical or impossible.

Among the unique properties of cured silicone elastomers, is their exceptional thermal stability (at low and high temperatures), their resistance to oxidation and ozone, their excellent weathering resistance (no hydrolysis), their chemical inertia to many chemicals, their low surface energy, their high gas permeability, and their good electrical properties. But, among all these quite unique properties, it is their very low toxicity level (21) that explains the important role they play in the medical device industry. Because of their low toxicity level, they are often used as a reference material in in vivo evaluation of new materials (22). However, each industrial application has its boundary conditions, which determine a specific chemical formulation, the complexity of which may impair certain biocompatibility aspects.

Table 3-5 lists some of the mechanical properties of the cured elastomers used in shunt manufacturing.

TABLE 3-5 MECHANICAL PROPERTIES OF CURED ELASTOMERS USED IN SHUNT MANUFACTURING

Property	Value
Hardness shore A	30 to 80
Density	1.12
Tensile strength	2 MPa minimum
Elongation	250 % minimum
Tear resistance	50 N/cm
Temperature range	-110° C to 250° C
Compression set	< 20%
Shrinkage	2 to 5%

Due to the organo-mineral character of the strong silicon-oxygen (Si-O) bond, silicones are a unique class of material, whose properties fit very well a large number of medical uses. Some questions have been raised recently on the long-term biocompatibility of implanted silicone (23,33). Although most concerns originated from silicone gels, which are different products from silicone elastomers, a quest for new implantable materials is underway. Silicone elastomers used as shunt components are also known to calcify after several years of implantation. It is important to note that no other materials could today replace silicone elastomers in their wide medical applications.

CONCLUSION

It is worth pointing out that the choice of a material is only the result of a set of conditions imposed by the application and the designer himself. As more is known about biomaterials, as the physiology of hydrocephalus is better understood, and as general technology advances, one can expect to see more sophisticated shunts in years to come. The role of materials is and will be vital in the mission of designing and producing the shunt of the future.

HYDROCEPHALUS SHUNT TESTING

Why test a shunt? As shunt design evolves, different hydrodynamic characteristics are imposed on shunts. Shunt testing permits characterization of a shunt's hydrodynamic properties and assessment of its precision and reliability. This type of testing, followed by evaluation of the shunt's clinical performance, permits further evolution of shunt design.

MEASUREMENT INSTRUMENTS

The pressures needing measurement in shunt testing are very low, given the very low CSF pressure. This creates a challenge as to the choice of a pressure measuring instrument (m.i.) that will accurately and precisely measure pressure in this low range. For the required accuracy/precision, reliability, ease of use, frequency of recording measurements,and price, manometers and piezoresistive transducers are most commonly used in shunt testing.

Water manometers are simple, reliable, and inexpensive. However, they are not very responsive and are difficult to make accurate automatic measurement. Pressure transducers, aside from high accuracy and responsiveness, are easily integrated into automated testing systems.

The typical 0. to 60 ml/hr flowrates are also difficult to measure with common industrial flowmeters. The liquid flow can be weighed at a given time period providing a simple and accurate flow measurement. Alternately, the pressure drop occurs and orifice in the system can be calibrated to provide flow measurement (see Chapter 2).

Time and temperature are measured with standard digital devices (38).

SHUNT TESTING (39–41)

The shunt hydrodynamic characteristics normally measured are opening pressure, closing pressure, pressure-flow response, and retrograde flow. The pressure at which the shunt first lets liquid through is called the opening pressure. Some shunts progressively admit liquid as the pressure increases. These shunts do not have an opening pressure per se, since opening pressure is defined when flow is equal to zero. The notion of opening pressure is, therefore, sometimes redefined to mean the shunt's pressure (as differential pressure is increased) at a predetermined flow rate (usually 5 ml/h). Closing pressure is the exact opposite of opening pressure. Once a shunt has responded to opening pressure by allowing liquid to flow through, it will close off if the differential pressure is lowered below a certain point. This phenomenon is observed during testing as the pressure at which flow becomes zero (as the differential pressure is being lowered) (Figure 3-2)

A shunt's pressure-flow response includes all points between zero and the maximum differential pressure tested for, regardless of whether the curve is upgoing (increasing pressure) or downcoming (decreasing pressure).

Most shunts can be readily filled with water through simple injection or aspiration with a hand-held syringe. However, there are often restrained air bubbles which can affect a shunt's pressure-flow performance. Depending on the shunt design, agents that lower surface tension (surfactants, alcohol) can be used to chase bubbles. If this option is chosen, care must be exercised to completely remove the agents from the shunt itself before testing. Another way to remove air from a shunt is to subject the liquid-filled shunt to a vacuum. By lowering the pressure, any air trapped in the shunt or gases dissolved in the liquid will expand to large bubbles, which will easily exit the shunt. The test liquid and equipment must also be air free. Pure deaerated water should be used in a system with little "dead" space to trap bubbles.

The simplest way to produce a constant differential pressure test system is to use two water-filled beakers, placed at different levels. The shunt is connected to

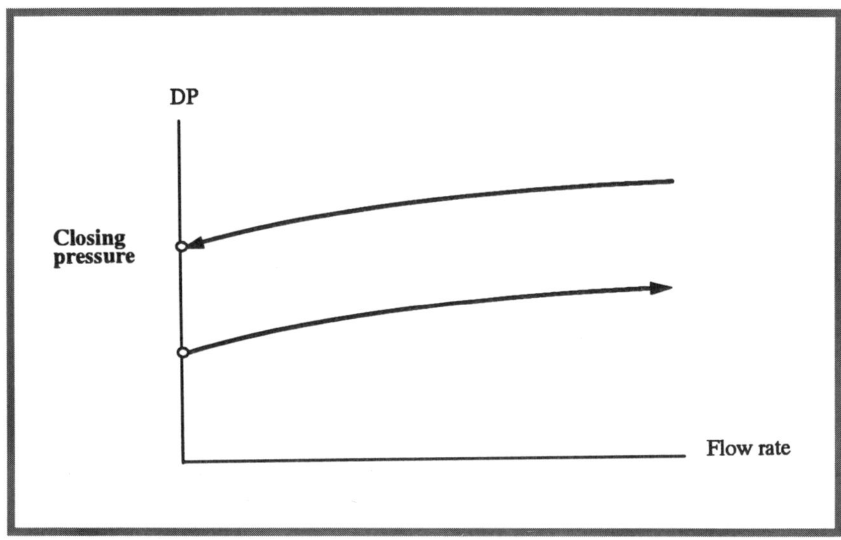

FIGURE 3-2
Pressure-flow diagram.

the two beakers. The difference between the levels of water in the two beakers generates the differential pressure (Figure 3-3A). If the beakers' inner diameters are large enough, the liquid level in the beakers will change slowly and the differential pressure will remain essentially constant. If a tube flowmeter is added upstream of the valve, both flow and pressure measurements will be available (Figure 3-3B). Care must be exerted to calibrate the transducers "zero" at the distal beaker's level.

The upstream beaker may be replaced by a pump as the source of pressure. Constant displacement (syringe and peristaltic) pumps are most commonly used in medical laboratories.

Coordinating the test sequences and recording data is best done by an automated, preferably computerized, system. Such a system requires a microprocessor to coordinate the sequence of operations, a data storage device and media, an analog-to-digital device to transmit the transducers' pressure readings, and a controller to command the pump (Figure 3-4). An accessory (mechanical, electronic or computer controlled) device may be added to produce pressure pulses.

Retrograde testing is performed with the same test equipment used for pressure-flow performance. The test shunt is simply reversed, and flow is measured while pressure is applied. For the shunt to pass the test, no retrograde flow should be observed as pressure rises to a predetermined level.

Shunt testing should be performed at a controlled temperature. It makes sense to test shunts near body temperature, as this simulates physiological conditions. It also makes sense to test shunts with water, as the viscosities of water and CSF are very similar.

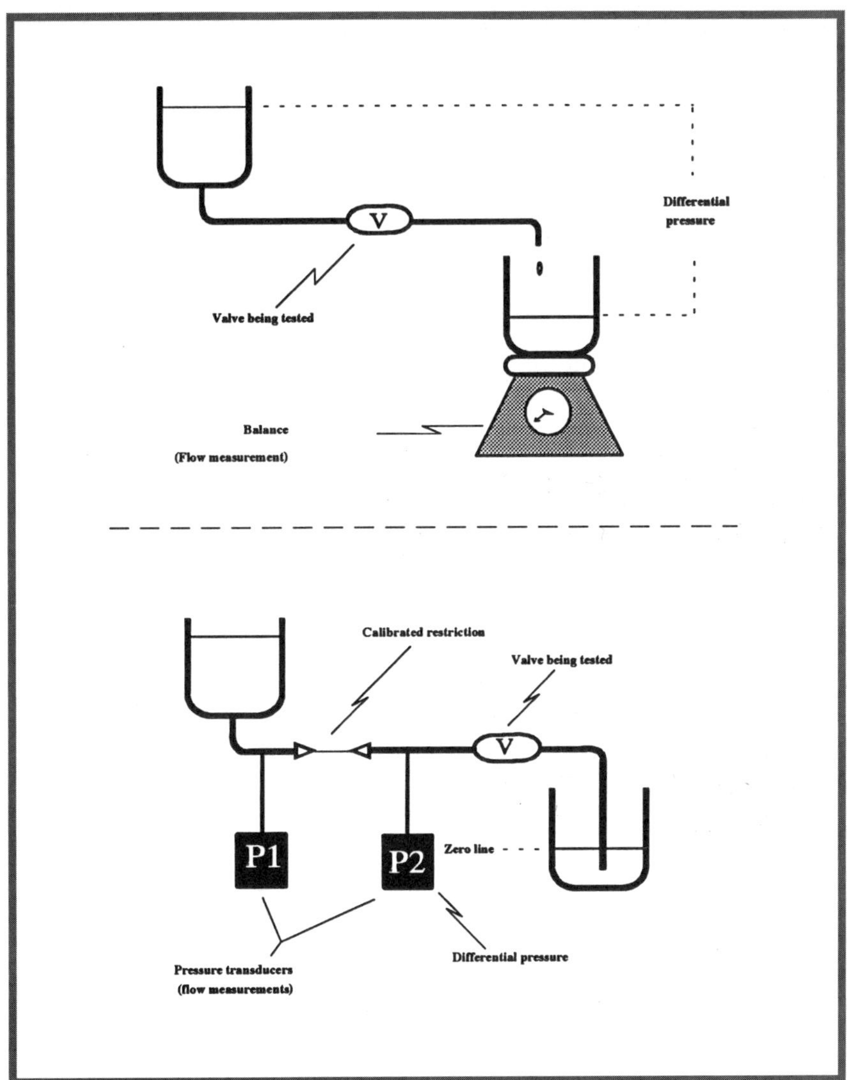

FIGURE 3-3
Simple test rings

Aside from imposing increasing or decreasing differential pressure, some shunts perform differently to changes in position, due to the effects of gravity on internal shunt components, or the effect of the column of water provided by the distal catheter in the vertical position. In order to test these types of shunts, no modifications to the test apparatus are required. However, the distal catheter must be made to lie vertically downward from the shunt, at a predetermined distance. This essentially means placing the distal beaker below the shunt. In addition, for devices that react to gravity, the device itself must be reoriented from the horizontal to the vertical position.

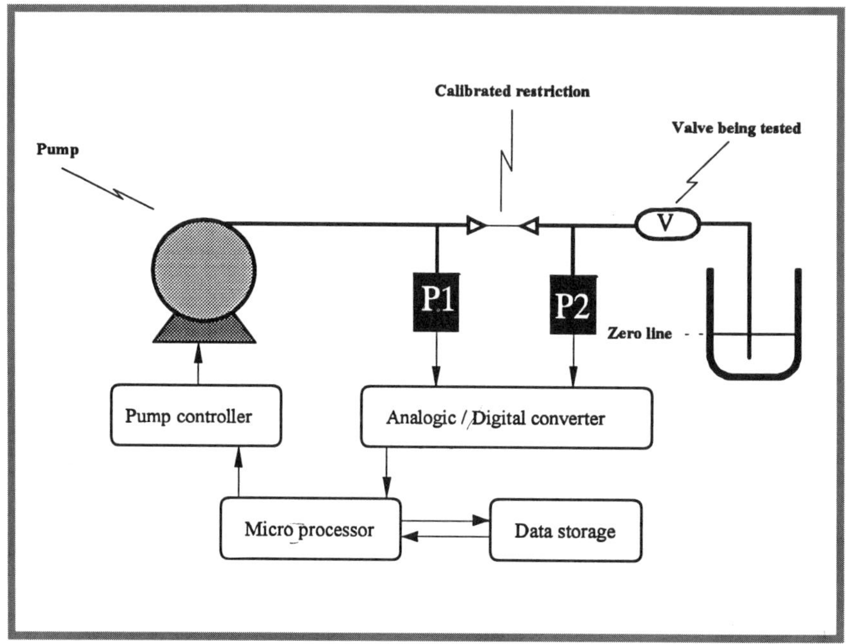

FIGURE 3-4
Computer test rig.

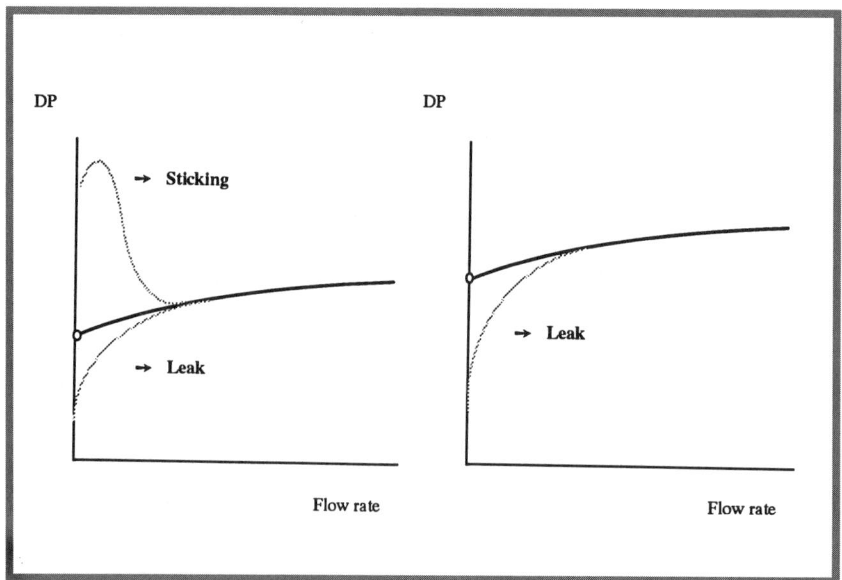

FIGURE 3-5
Opening pressure: As stated earlier, "perfect" opening pressure is a pressure at a flow rate equal to zero. Opening pressure imperfections include leaks, or sticking effects. *Closing pressure*: As with opening pressure, closing pressure may be affected by leaks.

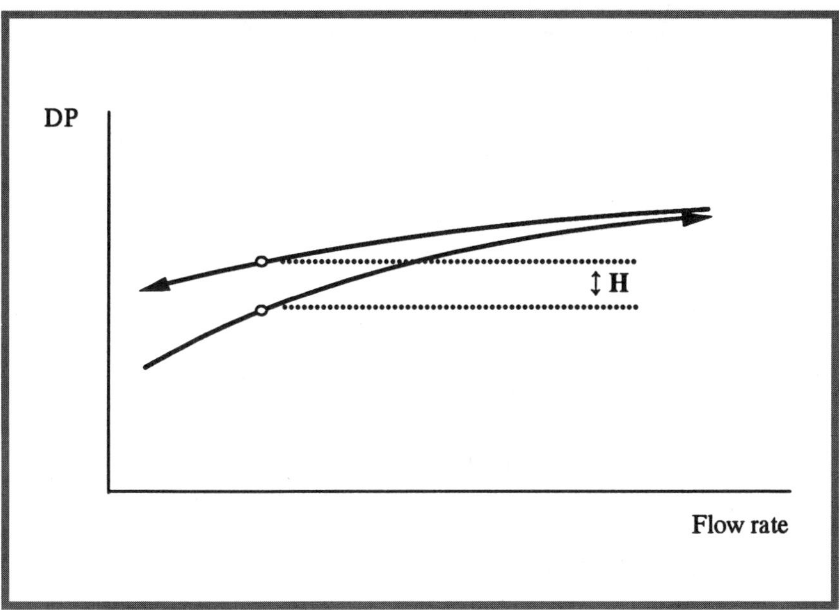

FIGURE 3-6
Hysteresis: this phenomenon is readily apparent when a full pressure-flow excursion in both directions has been performed during shunt testing. Hysteresis is observed when there is a large difference between the upgoing and downcoming curve.

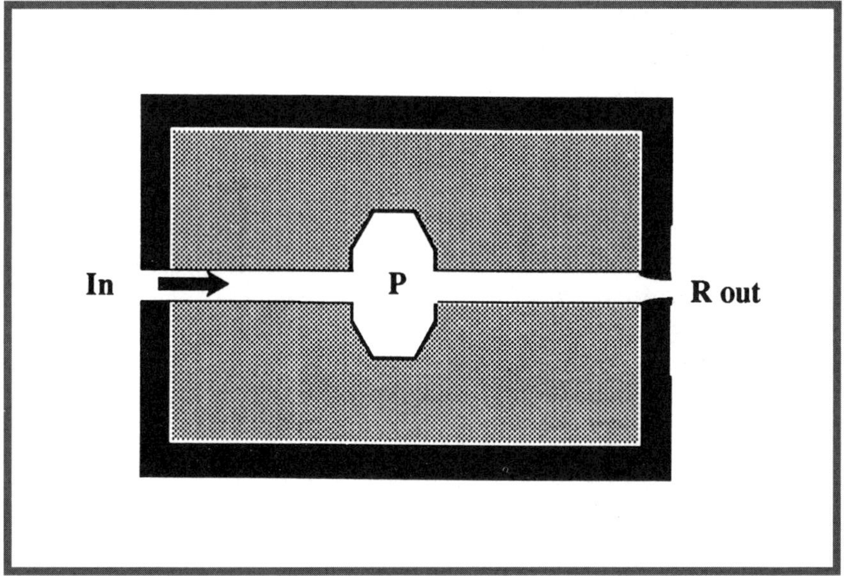

FIGURE 3-7
Conceptualization of the model. A rigid container, a compressible component, and a fluid-containing compartment, into which there is a constant inflow, and an outflow with resistance.

MODELING OF HYDROCEPHALUS FOR CSF SHUNT DESIGN EVALUATION

As it is impossible to measure accurately and continuously the pressure and flow in an implanted shunt, the performance of implanted shunts remains largely a mystery. One way of circumventing this problem is to construct models of the brain and CSF compartment, as well as the various shunt designs, to evaluate and predict the individual shunt performance (42–53). Models can be conceptualized and then constructed either in mechanical form (53) or simulated mathematically on a computer (54). Modeling also helps to conceptualize the process of hydrocephalus and its treatment. In this section, we will begin with the conceptualization of the model, describe a mechanical model, and, finally, illustrate the results of computer modeling.

CONCEPTUALIZATION OF THE MODEL

A simple model of the brain and CSF compartment illustrates some basic hydrodynamic phenomena, is the skull as a rigid outer shell containing a compressible substance. The ventricles are visualized as hollow fluid-filled cavities that connect to an inlet and an outlet (Figure 3-7). The CSF formation, or inflow, is constant (44). The outflow out is dependent on reaching a threshold pressure, or opening pressure, either of the saggital sinus or a shunt valve (48). The outlet has a constant resistance. When represented in a pressure versus flow graph, the equilibrium point of the model is represented by the intersection of the two lines. Since, at equilibrium, whatever comes in must come out, the pressure inside the model must rise until the outflow resistance allows the outflow to be equal to the inflow (55) (Figure 3-8).

If the outflow resistance were to increase, the slope of the outflow line would increase as well. Since the inflow is unaffected by what happens to the model, the inflow line on the graph would not change. Thus, the pressure inside the model would rise until reaching the point where the two lines intersect once more, and the inflow equals the outflow. This represents a new state of equilibrium.

The last parameter that defines this model concerns the compressibility characteristics of the substance between the rigid shell and the cavity, the brain. The substance's compressibility can be defined by a pressure versus volume graph (Figure 3-9). There is considerable evidence that the brain has three phases to its compressibility. At the beginning, it is very incompressible, or inelastic. Due to this very low compliance, the pressure can increase rapidly, while the volume increases very little. Next, during the second phase, the substance becomes very compressible, thus allowing large volume changes, while the pressure changes very slightly. Eventually, as pressure continues to increase, a third phase is reached. This final phase resembles the first phase in that the substances return to a relatively incompressible state. These stages are easy to visualize if represented by a more tangible example, like a reservoir used to hold water for irrigation. The reservoir has a spherical bottom and top. Its middle consists of a cylindrical

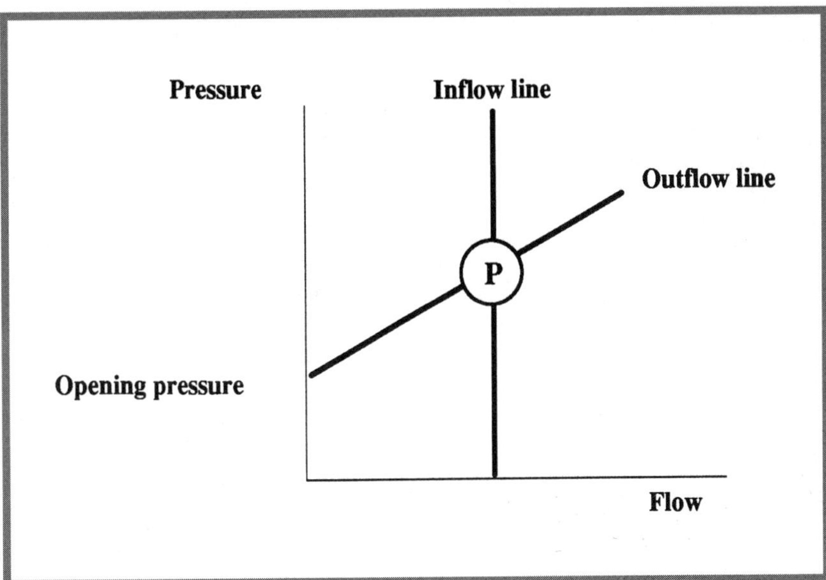

FIGURE 3-8
Equilibrium pressure occurs at the point on the pressure and flow curves where the inflow equals the outflow. The slope of the outflow line is the resistance, which may vary, producing different equilibrium pressures.

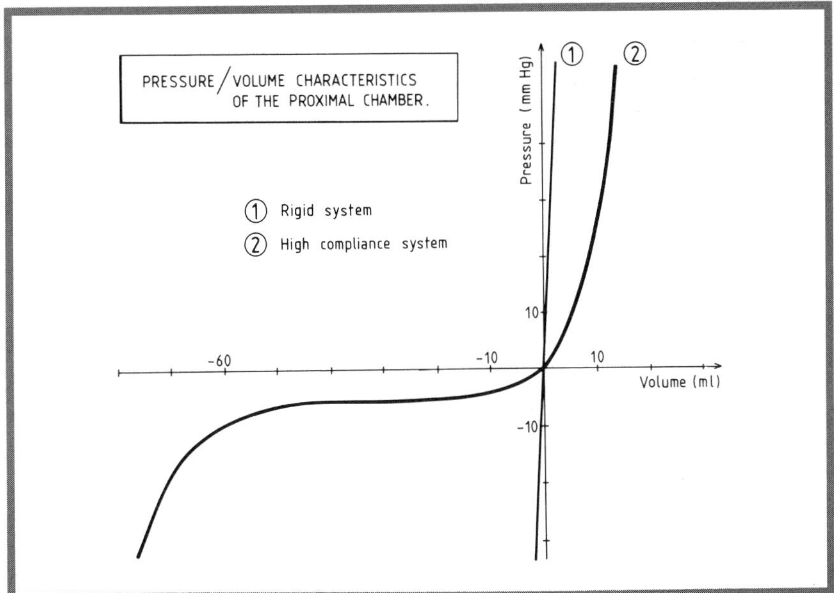

FIGURE 3-9
Compliance curves for a rigid and a compliant proximal chamber. The compliant chamber has a three-stage compliance—low at both extremes of volume, and high in the midportion.

shape. The other top features are exactly as previously described, that is, constant inflow unaffected by the pressures or volumes in the reservoir and the outflow as in the first model. Thanks to the special geometry of this tank, its "compressibility," or compliance, corresponds to the pressure-volume characteristics shown earlier. Due to the spherical/conical bottom, the pressure can increase rapidly without a marked increase in volume. Since the surface area of the reservoir increases as the level increases, the pressure-volume relationship gradually flattens out until it is virtually horizontal. This is due to the very large diameter of the cylindrical section of the reservoir, which allows increases in level only when the volume increases by a very large amount. Eventually, the level reaches the top of the reservoir, which is identical to the bottom, except it is inverted. This geometry allows a transition from high to low compliance. It is now easy to visualize how this reservoir system works. If the outflow resistance is unaffected, it is at its normal value. Liquid coming in equals liquid coming out, and the level in the reservoir represents the pressure necessary to overcome the opening pressure and outflow resistance. If the outflow tube or hose becomes partially or totally obstructed, the value of the resistance and the slope of the outflow line will increase.

How is the level in the irrigation reservoir controlled? One way to control the outflow of the reservoir is with a pressure regulator, which will result in a level (P_n) that corresponds to the opening pressure. As long as the outlet of the pressure regulator is maintained no lower than the bottom of the reservoir, this pressure regulator will work correctly. However, if the outlet is lowered to level 2, the vertical distance between the bottom of the tank and the outlet represents a pressure (P_h), that adds on to the level of the tank to provide the *total* differential pressure across the pressure regulator. Now, the differential pressure becomes the height of water in the reservoir plus the height between its outlet and level 2. This forces the flow rate through the valve to increase tremendously and forces the model into a state of nonequilibrium, since the outflow greatly exceeds the inflow. A new equilibrium is reached when the negative pressure in the rigid tank equals the hydrostatic pressure Ph. If a flow regulator is exchanged for the pressure regulator, special attention must be paid to choosing a flow regulation setting that corresponds to the inflow to the tank. In this case, the model equilibrates at a pressure where the inflow equals the outflow. In doing so, the fluid level will stabilize somewhere in the cylindrical section of the reservoir. When the outflow is lowered to level 2, the outflow increases but slightly. This outflow change causes a slow decrease in liquid level, which more slowly approaches an equilibrium negative pressure. The emptying of the reservoir occurs in three stages. First, the reservoir drains and the level lowers to the middle part of the reservoir. Thanks to its large capacity, the level remains at this part of the reservoir for an extended amount of time. This time depends on the excess amount being drained. When this volumetric reserve is depleted, the level reaches the first part of the reservoir, where the level will lower at a rapid rate until the pressure reaches an equilibrium negative pressure. A situation worse than depleting the reservoir would be to overfill it; therefore, in order to

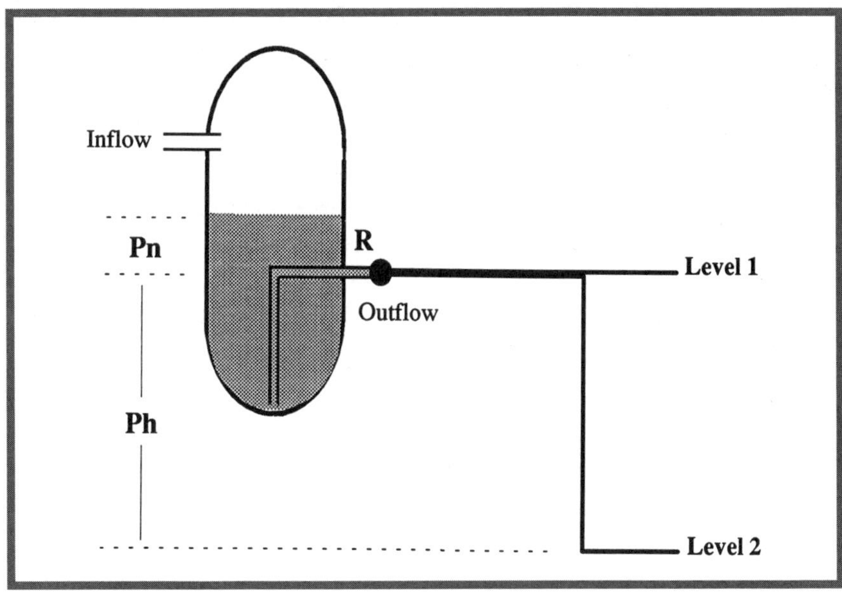

FIGURE 3-10
Schematic model with volume "compliance" and two different outflow levels.

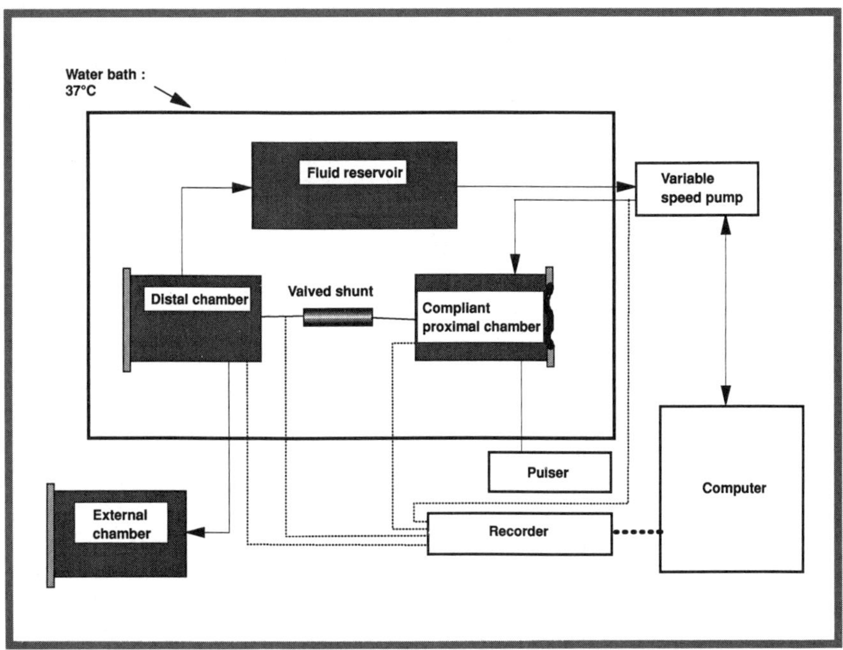

FIGURE 3-11
Schematic diagram of mechanical model for testing CSF shunts.

effectively use a flow-regulating device, the flow must be adjusted at a setting higher than the inflow. In this way, a controlled, but very small, excess amount is drained.

In conclusion, this conceptual model illustrates how equilibruim pressures and volumes can be visualized, and how the effects of pressure on flow regulation can be demonstrated.

Mechanical Models

A mechanical model can be constructed to simulate the concepts described above. In this circumstance, the brain and the CSF compartment are mechanically modeled and the shunts themselves are connected to the outflow port (53). This is illustrated in Figure 3-10. Fluid is pumped into the compliant reservoir by a constant speed pump—a pulsatile component can be added to simulate the cardiac pulsation. The outflow is controlled by various shunts, which act as pressure or flow regulators. The pressure inside the chamber is measured with a transducer. The outflow is measured by weighing the distal chamber. The data is fed to a computer, where the data is stored, flow rates are calculated, etc. The proximal chamber with the compliant membrane has a three-stage compliance curve as suggested in the concept of this model (Figure 3-11). Figure 3-12 shows the pressure in the proximal chamber with a constant flow rate and three different shunt types connected with the catheter initially equal to the inflow level (horizontal) and then at a lower level (vertical) of -25 mm Hg.

With a standard differential pressure valve, the pressure approaches equilibrium in the horizontal position during the first five minutes. When the outlet of the catheter is moved to the vertical position, there is an initial rapid fall in pressure until the container reaches the high compliance portion of the pressure-volume curve, where there is little change in pressure despite the high outflow rate. As the volume is depleted and the "compliance reserve" of the container is reached, the low compliance portion of the negative portion of the pressure-volume curve is reached and the pressure rapidly falls to a new negative equilibrium value.

The flow control valve, the Sigma, behaves quite differently. Although a similar equilibrium pressure is reached in the horizontal position, because of flow limitation the pressure tends to rest in the high compliance portion of the container for much longer and, in fact, for the duration of the experiment. This leads to a reduction in the negative pressure in the vertical position. The differential pressure valve with the antisiphon device approaches the same equilibrium pressure in the horizontal position. In the vertical position, the negative pressure is nullified by the anti-siphon device, and because of the increased resistance of the ASD, a new increased equilibrium positive pressure is reached.

While mechanical models such as these are excellent for testing existing valves, they require the actual valve. It is impossible to test new or modified designs without constructing the actual shunt. Computer modeling has the decided advantage of being able to test theoretical designs prior to manufacture and to predict the performance of valve modifications.

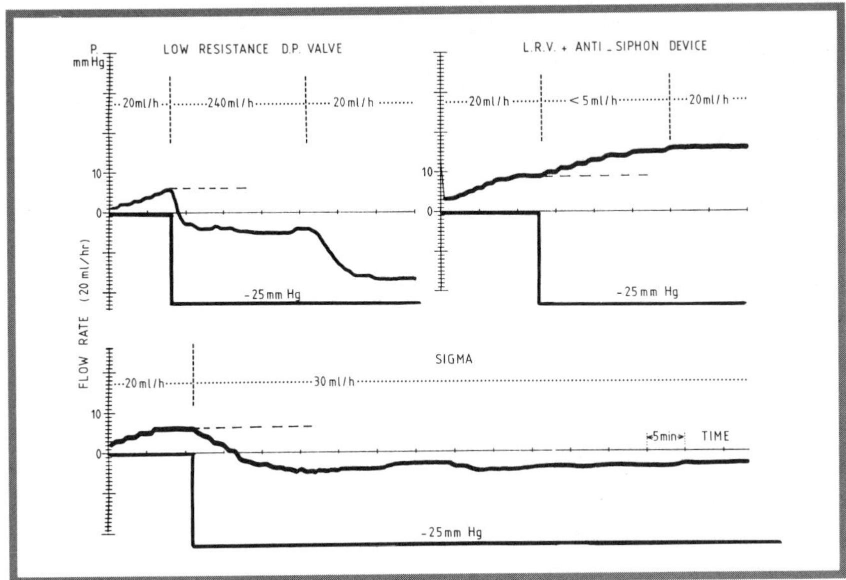

FIGURE 3-12
Results of shunt testing with mechanical model. Pressure is shown as a function of time with a constant inflow rate and the outflow at two different levels, 0 and -25 mm Hg, for a low resistance differential pressure valve, a low resistance valve with an antisiphon device, and a Sigma valve.

COMPUTER MODELING OF HYDROCEPHALUS AND CEREBROSPINAL FLUID SHUNTS

Computer modeling of the CSF compartment and CSF shunts requires a mathematical model of the CSF compartment, mathematical models of CSF shunt design performance, and a computer modeling program to perform the simulation. The simplest approach, and the one for which there is the most data, is the simulation of a model quite similar to the mechanical model described above (42,43,45,48,50,55,56).

MATHEMATICAL MODEL OF THE CSF COMPARTMENT

The mathematical model is constructed by specifying equations that describe the physical processes active in the mechanical model and, by analogy, the real-life situation. The equation for the volume of CSF intracranial compartment as a function of time is the CSF production minus the CSF absorption minus CSF shunt flow. This change is expressed as the derivative of the volume with respect to time (see Table 3-6 for the definitions of terms) or $dV/dt = I_f - I_a - I_s$ (Equation 1).

As in the mechanical model, the CSF production is assumed to be constant and independent of pressure. The model will be made slightly more complicated by including CSF absorption, which is expressed as the function of the saggital sinus pressure and the resistance to absorption. The resistance to absorption is

TABLE 3-6

Abbreviations	Derivative
I_a	CSF absorption rate
I_f	CSF formation rate
I_s	CSF shunt flow rate
k	constant for exponential pressure volume relationship
l	distance between foramen of Monro and siphon reducing device
o	angle betwwen long axis of body and horizon
P	pressure
P_d	pressure distal shunt drainage site
P_h	hydrostatic pressure
P_o	resting or equilibruim pressure
P_{open}	opening pressure of shunt valve
P_{ss}	pressure saggital sinus
P_v	ventricular pressure
R_n	CSF shunt resistance to flow
R_o	resistance to CSF absorption
V	volume

also assumed to be constant and independent of pressure and that absorption is zero for pressure less than the saggital sinus pressure: $I_a = (P - P_{ss})/R_o$ where ($I_a = 0$ and $P < P_{ss}$) (Equation 2).

The compliance of the brain is expressed as the change in volume as a function of pressure: $C(P) = dV/dP$ (Equation 3).

A mathematical model of the CSF compartment that satisfies the three-stage compliance of the mechanical model, is called the positive-negative exponential model (4), where

$P = P_o e^{k\,\Delta V}$ for $V > 0$ (Equation 4)

$P = P_o(2 - e^{k\,\Delta V})$ for $V < 0$ and is shown in Figure 3-13.

To express changes in pressure as a function of time rather than a function of volume, we use the chain rule: $dP/dt = dP/dV\ dV/dt$ (Equation 5).

For the positive-negative exponential model from Equation 4, $dP/dV = P_o k\, e^{k|\Delta V|}$ (Equation 6), where $|\Delta V|$ is the absolute value of ΔV. Rewriting Equation 5 using Equations 1 and 6 leads to the full expression of our model: $dP/dt = P_o k\, e^{k\,|\Delta V|}(I_f - I_a - I_s)$ (Equation 7).

MODELING OF CSF SHUNT FLOW

The performance of CSF shunts can be modeled by writing equations that duplicate the pressure flow characteristics of the devices. As discussed in the shunt testing section, shunts function within a range of opening pressures and closing pressures and exhibit imperfections such as hysteresis, sticking, etc. For the purposes of the mathematical model, we will assume an average behavior devoid of these imperfections. The shunts, then, are described as having an opening and closing pressure that are equal, and a resistance to flow (which may be variable). The pressure acting on the shunt valve includes the ventricular pressure, and hydrostatic pressure related to difference in height between proximal and distal ends, and the pressure in the distal cavity. A reasonable assumption is that the distal pressure is atmospheric pressure. The total pressure acting across the shunt valve is: $P_t = P + P_h - P_d$ (Equation 8). $P_h = \ell \sin \varphi$ where ℓ is a line joining proximal and distal ends and φ is the angle between ℓ and the vertical.

The performance of the different valves can then be described in terms of the total pressure. These are graphically shown in Figure 3.14 for a standard differential pressure valve, an adjustable differential valve, a flow control valve, and a valve containing an antisiphon device. For standard one way valves, $I_s = 0$ for $P_t < P_{open}$ (Equation 9), $I_s = (P_t - P_{open})/R_1$ for $P_t > P_{open}$.

The Cordis Orbis Sigma valve has variable resistance that follows a sigmoid pressure flow curve (hence the name) (53). An idealized and simplified Sigma valve can be described as having three pressure flow levels demarcated by two inflexion points P_1,ℓ_1, and P_2,ℓ_2 (Figure 3-8). For the Sigma, $I_s = 0$ for $P_t < P_{open}$ (Equation 10), $\ell_s = (P_t - P_{open})/R_1$ for $P_{open} < P_t < P_1$, $\ell_s = (P_t - P_1)/R_2 + \ell_1$ f or $P1 < P_t < P_2$, and $\ell_s = (P_t - P_2)/R_3 + \ell_2$ for $P_t > P_2$.

Antisiphon devices (ASD) behave in a rather complicated fashion and are also influenced by the overlying skin. As the patient assumes the upright posture and pressure within the shunt system becomes negative, the resistance in the device rises and the pressure to maintain a particular flow rate actually rises above that required in the horizontal position (56,57). These effects are variable between the particular design types. For a standard valve incorporating an ASD, e.g., the Delta Valve (PS Medical, Goletta CA), we assume a small increment in opening pressure in the vertical position and assume that the hydrostatic effects are otherwise eliminated by simply setting the P_h term to zero. This is for an ASD placed at the level of the foramen of Monro. For ASDs placed lower along the course of the shunt system, P_h is not zero and ℓ is equal to the distance between the foramen of Monro and the ASD.

Modeling Computer Program

While the mathematical equations for the model can be solved exactly, the solutions can be quite complex. It is much simpler to use a variety of computer programs that solve the equations numerically (e.g. the Simulation Control Program [SCoP] produced by the National Biomedical Simulation Resource, Duke University Medical Center, Durham NC). The program requires an IBM PC with at least 640K RAM and a hard disk. It runs in conjunction with Turbo C

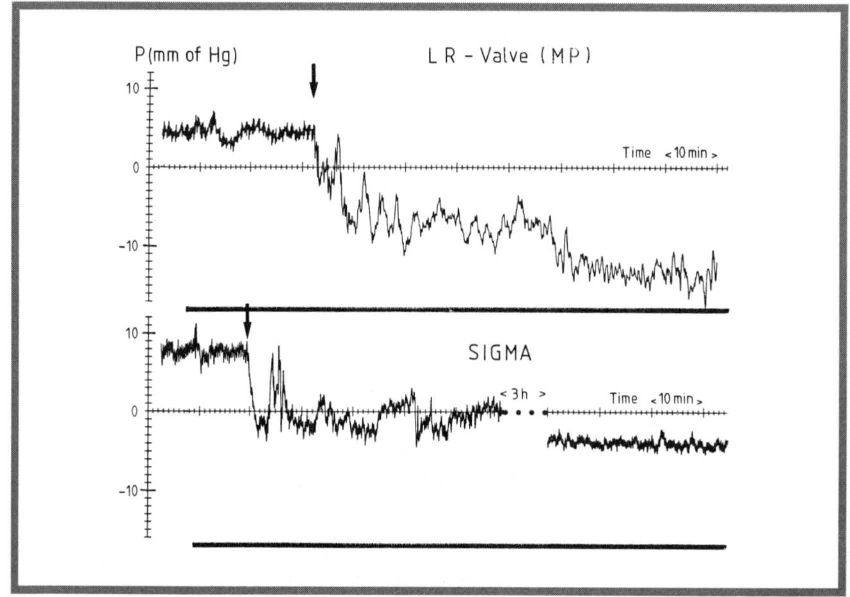

FIGURE 3-13
Pressure in two individual patients with implanted shunts assuming the upright posture. The patient depicted in the top curve has a standard differential valve. The patient in the lower curve has a Sigma valve.

(Microsoft Corporation, Redmond, MA) software. The modeling code syntax is relatively simple. For the simple differential equations, the program uses fourth-order Runge-Kutta integration. Output from the model is graphical to the screen or numerical to the screen or disk. Most model parameters can be changed interactively and in a stepwise fashion. The model can be compared to real data graphically, or model parameters can be fitted to real data.

To verify the accuracy of the model, we compared the numerical output of the model to calculated exact solutions at specific points in time, to bolus and continuous infusions reported by Marmarou (50) and Lofgren (58) and to experimental data concerning shunt pressure and flow in dogs with a shunt that led from the foramen magnum to a drip chamber and then to the right atrium, reported by Yamada (59). In Yamada's experiment, the flow rates and pressures were measured in both the horizontal and upright positions. The correspondence between the computer model and this other experimental data was very good.

The shunts tested with the mechanical model were then simulated using the patient parameters shown in Table 3-7. An adjustable differential pressure valve with the patient in both the horizontal and vertical positions was simulated (Figure 3-15), and corresponds quite reasonably to the results of the mechanical model and to actual pressure measurements in a shunted patient (Figure 3-16). Similarly, the three different valve designs tested in the mechanical model – a

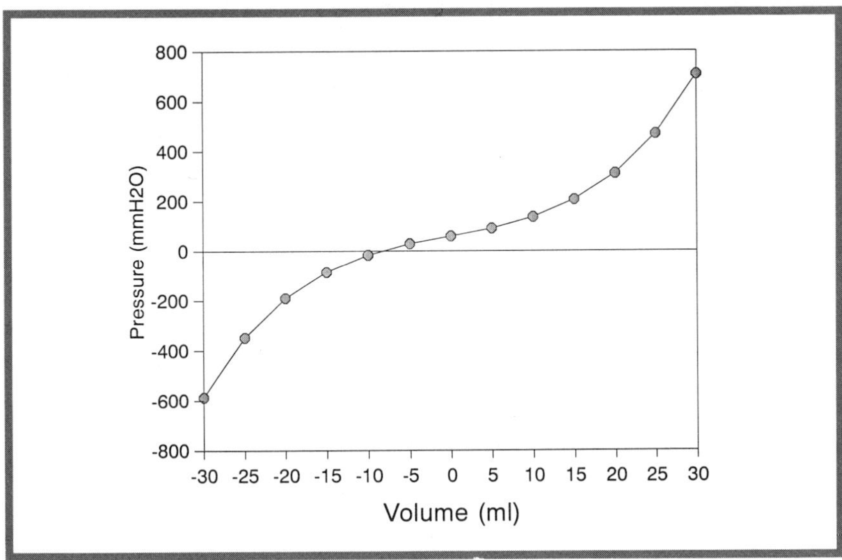

FIGURE 3-14
Graph of mathematical model of pressure-volume relationship for the positive-negative exponential function.

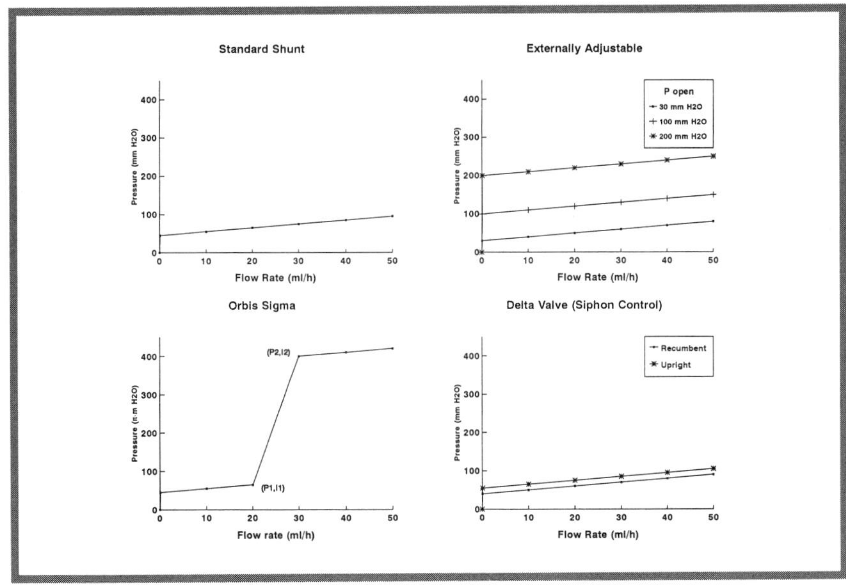

FIGURE 3-15
Graphs of mathematical models for four types of shunts—a standard differential pressure shunt, an adjustable differential pressure shunt, a flow-control Sigma shunt, and an antisiphon device.

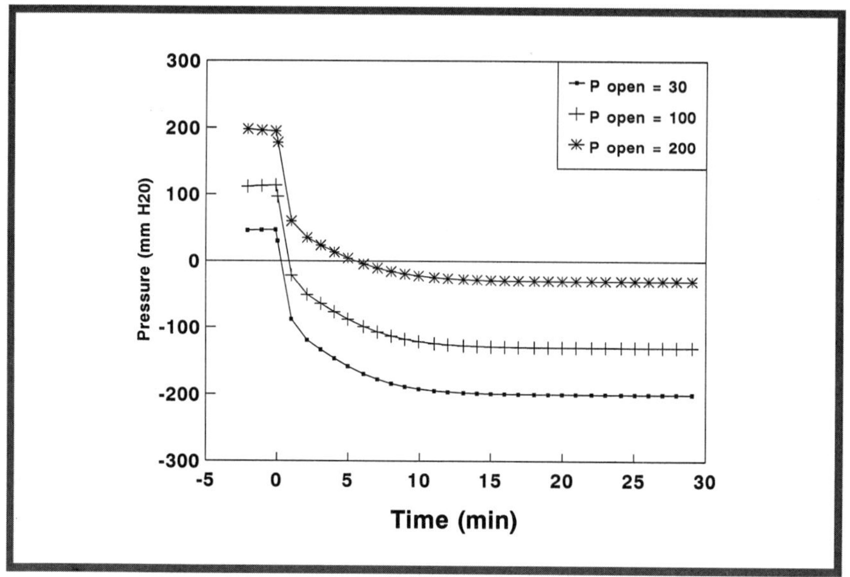

FIGURE 3-16
Computer pressure simulation in a hydrocephalic patient before and after assuming the upright posture with an adjustable differential pressure shunt in place. As the opening pressure in the shunt is increased, the negative pressure in the upright position is less, but with an exact corresponding increase in the equilibrium pressure in the supine position.

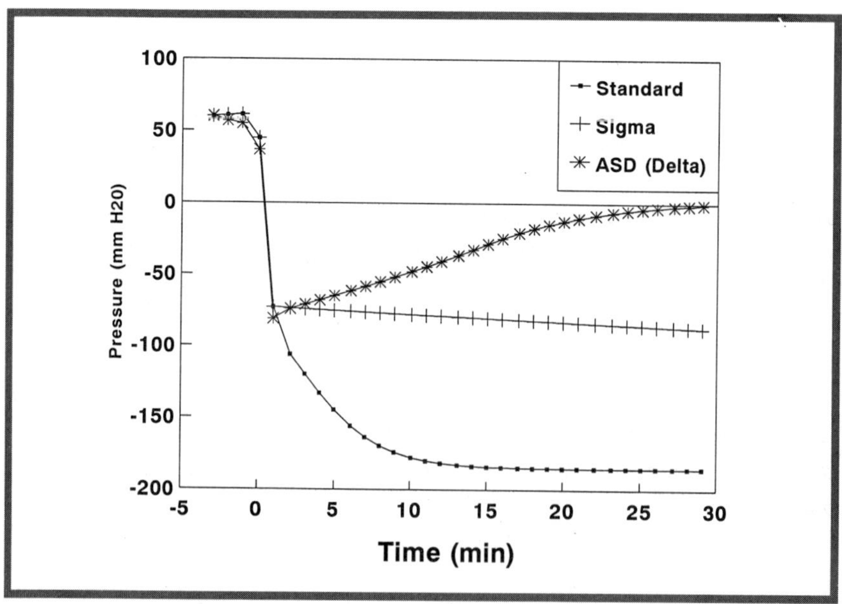

FIGURE 3-17
Computer pressure simulation comparing three types of valves in the horizontal and upright position--a standard differential pressure valve, a flow control sigma valve, and an antisiphon device.

TABLE 3-7 MODEL PARAMETERS FOR HUMAN HYDROCEPHALIC PATIENT SIMULATION

I_f	.33 cc/min
k	(PVI=28)
P_h	250 mm H_2O
P_o	168 mm H_2O
P_{ss}	140 mm H_2O
R_o	98 mm H_2O/ml/min
Standard Shunt	
P_{open}	45 mm H_2O
R_1	60 mm H_2O/ml/min
Externally Adjustable	
P_{open}	40,110,200 mm H_2O
R_1	60 mm H_2O/ml/min
Orbis Sigma	
P_{open}	45 mm H_2O
P_1	70 mm H_2O
P_2	400 mm H_2O
R_1	60 mm H_2O/ml/min
R_2	2,000 mm H_2O/ml/min
R_3	60 mm H_2O/ml/min
Delta Valve	
P_{open}	40,55 mm H_2O (horizontal, vertical)
R_1	20 mm H_2O/ml/min
ℓ	0

standard one-way valve, a Cordis Orbis Sigma, and a siphon prevention device (the PS Medical Delta Valve) were simulated in both the horizontal and vertical position (Figure 3-17). Again, the correspondence with the mechanical model and the two patients shunted with a standard valve and the Sigma is reasonable. One can see that as the opening pressure of the externally adjustable device is increased, the magnitude of the negative pressure decreases, but with an exactly corresponding increase in resting pressure in the horizontal position. The Delta valve placed at the level of the foramen of Monro raises the pressure above a normal negative value. The Sigma delays the onset of excessive negative pressures, at least during the course of the simulation.

The results of both the mechanical and computer models illustrates the efficacy of this approach. The correspondence between the results of the model simulation and as much data as can be obtained from actual patients is quite good. This indicated that simulation of new or modified shunt designs can be performed with some confidence. There is a problem, however, with this approach in that actual structural deformation and alteration in the brain parenchyma that occurs with the hydrocephalic process and its treatment have not been simulated. Nagashima has made an initial attempt at this by using finite element analysis (51). However, as little information exists on the physical characteristics of the brain and the nature of the boundary conditions at both the ventricular wall and skull surface, much of this modeling really amounts to trying to fit the model output to experimental data (CT scans) rather than being able to predict ventricular size sometime in the distant future. Further efforts should be directed to developing simplified structural models that can be tested systematically.

REFERENCES

The following "F" references are standards from the references labeled 1,2,4,38,40. (Storer RA, ed. Annual book of AST standards, Vol. 13. Philadelphia : American Society for Testing and Materials, 1987.)

1. F 748-82 Practice for selecting generic biological test methods for materials and devices.
2. F 981-86 Practice for assessment of compatibility of biomaterials (non-porous) for surgical implants with respect to effect of materials on muscle and bone.
3. International Standards Organization. ISO/DIS 10993-1.
4. F 361-80 Practice for assessment of compatibility of Metallic materials for surgical implants with respect to effect of materials on tissue (Discontinued 1987 – Replaced by F 981).
5. F 469-78 Practice for assessment of compatibility of nonporous polymeric materials for surgical implants with regard to effect of materials on tissue (Intent to withdraw).
6. F 602-87 Criteria for implantable thermoset epoxy plastics.
7. F 604-87 Classification for silicone elastomers used in medical applications.
8. F 619-79 Practice for extraction of medical plastics (1986).
9. F 647-85 Practice for evaluating and specifying implantable shunt assemblies for neurosurgical applications.
10. F 702-81 Specification for polysulfone resin for medical applications (1985).
11. F 719-81 Practice for testing biomaterials in rabbits for primary skin irritation (1986).
12. F 749-82 Practice for evaluating material extracts by intracutaneous injection in the rabbit.
13. F 750-82 Practice for evaluating material extracts by systemic injection in the mouse.
14. F 755-82 Specification for selection of porous polyethylene for Use in surgical implants
15. F 756-82 Practice for assessment of the hemolytic properties of materials.
16. F 763-82 Practice for short-term screening of implant materials.
17. F 813-83 Practice for direct contact cell culture evaluation of materials for medical Devices.

18. F 881-84 Specification for silicone gel and silicone solid (nonporous) Facial Implants.

19. F 895-84 Test method for agar diffusion cell culture screening for cytotoxicity.

20. F 720-81 Standard practice for testing guinea pigs for contact allergens : guinea pig maximization test (1986).

21. F 55-82 Specification for stainless steel bar and wire for surgical implants.

22. F 56-82 Specification for stainless steel sheet and strip for surgical implants.

23. F 67-83 Specification for unalloyed titanium for surgical implant applications.

24. F 136-84 Specification for wrought titanium 6A1-4V ELI alloy for surgical implant applications.

25. F 138-86 Specification for wrought steel bar and wire for surgical implants (special quality).

26. F 139-86 Specification for stainless steel sheet and strip for surgical implants (special quality).

27. F 560-86 Specification for unalloyed tantalum for surgical implant applications.

28. F 601-86 Practice for fluorescent penetrant inspection of metallic surgical implants.

29. F 603-83 Specification for high-purity dense aluminum oxide for surgical implant spplication.

30. F 746-87 Test method for pitting or crevice corrosion of metallic surgical implant materials.

31. Agranoff J, ed. Modern plastics encyclopedia. Volume 57. New York: McGraw-Hill, 1980:10A.

32. Baumeister T. Mark's standard handbook for mechanical engineers, 8th edition. New York: McGraw-Hill, 1978.

33. F 86-84 Practice for surface preparation and marking of metallic surgical implants.

34. F 640-79 Tests methods for radiopacity of plastics for medical use (1987).

35. Office of the Federal Regulations National Archives and Records Administration. Code of Federal Regulations 21 Part 820, Good manufacturing practices for medical devices: general. Revised as of April 1, 199, Washington: U.S. Government Printing Office.

36. Omega Engineering. Omega compleste pressure, strain, and force measurement handbook and encyclopedia, Volume 26. Stamford: Omega Engineering Inc., 1988.

37. Spiegel MR. Schaum's outline of theory and problems of statistics. New York: McGraw-Hill, 1961.

38. Chilton RH. Chemical engineer's handbook, 5th ed. New York: McGraw-Hill, 1973.

39. ASTM standard F 647-85. In: Storer RA, ed. Annual book of ASTM Standards, Vol. 13. Philadelphia: American Society for Testing and Materials, 1987.

40. ISO standard 7197: 1988 (E).

41. ASTM standard F 647, draft 4/13/92 (revised 6/9/92). In: Storer RA, ed. Annual book of ASTM Standards, Vol. 13. Philadelphia: American Society for Testing and Materials, 1987.

42. Ahearn E, Randall K, Cipoletti G, Johnson R. Computer simulation of shunt performance in hydrocephalus. In: Proceedings of the North East Bioengineering Conference 14th. New York: IEEE, 1988:194–197.

43. Brophy J, Ahearn E, Randall K, Cipoletti G, Johnson R. Comparative computer simulation of shunt performance in hydrocephalus. In: Proceedings of the Annual Conference on Engineering in Medicine and Biology 12th. New York: IEEE, 1990, Volume 3:1192–1193.

44. Davson H: Formation and drainage of the cerebrospinal fluid. In: Shapiro K, Marmaou A, Portnoy H, eds. Hydrocephalus. New York: Raven Press, 1984:3-40.

45. Friden H, Ekstedt J. The human cerebrospinal fluid space volume/pressure relationship: a five parameter model with general applicability. In: Ishii S, Hagai H, Brock M, eds. Intracranial pressure V. Berlin: Springer Verlag, 1983:261–268.

46. Gaab MR, Haubitz I, Brawanski A, Faulstich J, Heisler HE. Pressure-volume diagram, pulse amplitude, and intracranial pressure volume: analysis and significance. In: Ishii S, Hagai H, Brock M, eds. Intracranial pressure V. Berlin: Springer Verlag, 1983:261–268.

47. Guinane JE. An equivalent circuit analysis of cerebrospinal fluid hydrodynamics. Am J Physiol 1972;223(2):425–430.

48. Hakim CA. The physician and physicopathology of the hydraulic complex of the central nervous system. PhD thesis, Massachusetts Institute of Technology, 1985.

49. Kimura M, Tamaki N, Kose S, Takamori T, Matsumoto S. Computer simulation of intracranial pressure using electrical R-C circuit. In: Hoff JT, Betz AL, eds. Intracranial Pressure VII. Berlin: Springer Verlag, 1989:295–298.

50. Marmarou A, Shulman K, Rosende R. A nonlinear analysis of the cerebrospinal fluid system and intracranial pressure dynamics. J Neurosurg 1978;48:332–344.

51. Nagashima T, Tamaki N, Matsumoto S, Horwitz B, Seguchi Y. Biomechanics of hydrocephalus: a new theoretical model. Neurosurg 1987;21(6):898–904.

52. Rekate HL, Williams F, Chizeck HJ, Elsakka W, Ko W. The application of mathematical modeling to hydrocephalus research. Concepts Pediatr Neurosurg 1988;8:1–14.

53. Sainte-Rose C, Hooven MD, Hirsch JF. A new approach to the treatment of hydrocephalus. J Neurosurg 1987;66:213–226.

54. Drake JM, Tenti G, Sivalsganathan S. Computer modeling of siphoning for CSF shunt design evaluation. Pediatr Neurosurg 1994;21:6–15.

55. Olivero WC, Rekate HL, Chizeck HJ, Ko W, McCormick JM. Relationship between intracranial and sagittal sinus pressure in normal and hydrocephalic dogs. Pediatr Neurosurg 1988;14:196–201.

56. Horton D, Pollay M. Fluid flow performance of a new siphon-control device for ventricular shunts. J Neurosurg 1990;72:926–932.

57. Portnoy HD, Schulte RR, Fox JL, Croissant PD, Tripp L. Anti-siphon and reversible occlusion valves for shunting in hydrocephalus and preventing post-shunt subdural hematomas. J Neurosurg 1973;38:729–738.

58. Lofgren J, von Essen C, Zwetnow NN. The pressure-volume curve of the cerebrospinal fluid space in dogs. Acta Neurol Scandinav 1973;49:557–574.

59. Yamada S, Ducker TB, Perot PL. Dynamic changes of cerebrospinal fluid in upright and recumbent shunted experimental animals. Child's Brain 1975;1:187–192.

60. Shapiro K, Fried A, Marmarou A. Biomedical and hydrodynamic characterization of the hydrocephalic infant. J Neurosurg 1985;63:69–75.

Chapter 4

CEREBROSPINAL FLUID SHUNT COMPONENTS

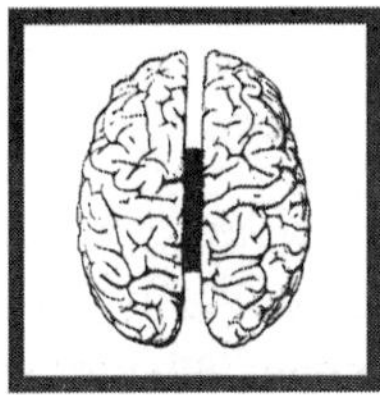

4 Cerebrospinal Fluid Shunt Components

In this chapter, we will outline the available shunt systems and components. There is a bewildering array of shunt components and configurations offered by the various manufacturers. These change rapidly and many custom products are available so that describing every possible combination is impossible. We will, however, try to outline the main shunt components available.

Every shunt is basically composed of three components: a proximal catheter for access to the CSF, a valve system, and a distal catheter, which diverts CSF toward a drainage cavity. Several miscellaneous accessories can be added to the basic system and the whole system put together as a unitized, or "unishunt," system or separately in pieces. Most manufacturers offer a variety of proximal catheters, distal catheters, and valves. The proximal catheters, of which there are many variations (probably related to the fact that proximal obstruction is the most common cause of shunt failure), and distal catheters, of which there are fewer variations, will be described as groups with no attempt to identify the manufacturer unless there is really something different about the design. The valves, however, will be described by manufacturer because, while it is usually quite obvious what particular design or feature is contained in proximal and distal catheters from inspection of the device or even the catalogue, inspection of the valve and the enclosed information often fails to reveal the type of valve mechanism, how many valves are contained, or, in some cases, even where the valve is situated.

We have included a table of pressures for the different categories of valve as supplied by the manufacturer when available. We have also plotted flow versus pressure curves wherever the information was available. The graphs have all been plotted on the same scale and on the same axes to allow for easier comparison. Some manufacturers supply a range of values on the graph. As these are variable and not always quantifiable, we have simply plotted a line through the middle of the range.

PROXIMAL VENTRICULAR CATHETERS CONNECTORS

VENTRICULAR CATHETERS

All ventricular catheters are made of silicone rubber. They vary in terms of their length, internal and external diameter, stiffness, shape, tip configuration, and radiopaque markings (Figure 4-1). Free ventricular catheters normally come either straight, and usually 15 cm to 23 cm, or preshaped. The catheter is then cut to appropriate length. In preshaped catheters, the curve for the burr hole is already fashioned as either a right angle or greater than 90° ("angular" catheter). The intracranial length of the preshaped catheters varies from 3 to 10 cm. In unitized systems, the length of the ventricular catheters is fixed and varies between 5 to 13 cm, although custom lengths are also available.

The internal and external diameters of these catheters range from 1.3/2.5, 1.6/3.2, 1.5/3.1, 1.4/2.7, to 1.0/2.7 for the regular diameters. Besides these regular-sized catheters, several manufacturers offer small-diameter catheters for neonatal patients–1.0/2.1, 1.2/2.5–in order to "minimize injury to the brain." It is easy to understand that catheters of different wall thickness and made of silicone of various grades will display variable stiffness. However, there does not appear to be any particular rationale for the different catheter wall thickness or internal diameter.

There are basically three types of tip configuration. First is standard tubing with distal holes. The number, position, shape, and diameter of the holes are variable between manufacturers. The holes are normally distributed over at least the distal 1 cm of the ventricular catheter. The second is standard tubing to which flanges or fins of various size, configuration, stiffness, etc. are added.

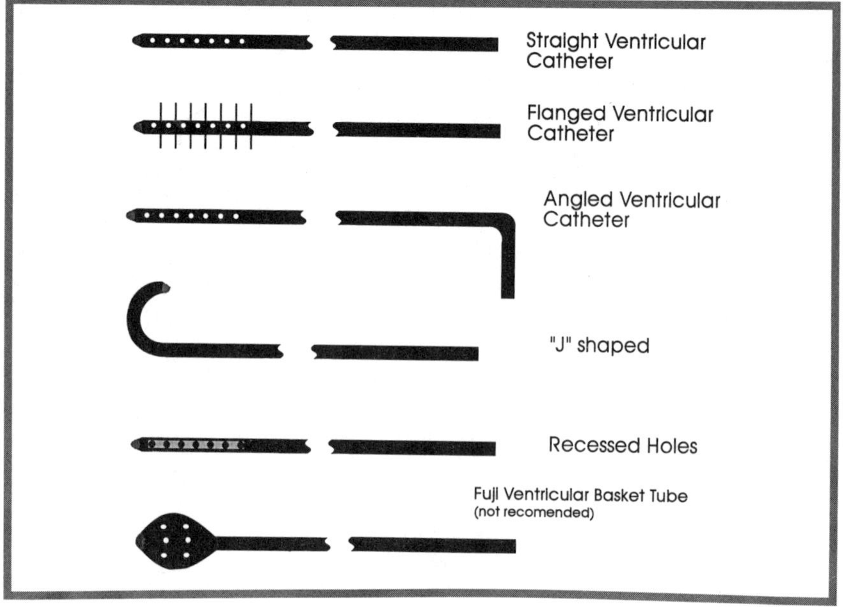

FIGURE 4-1

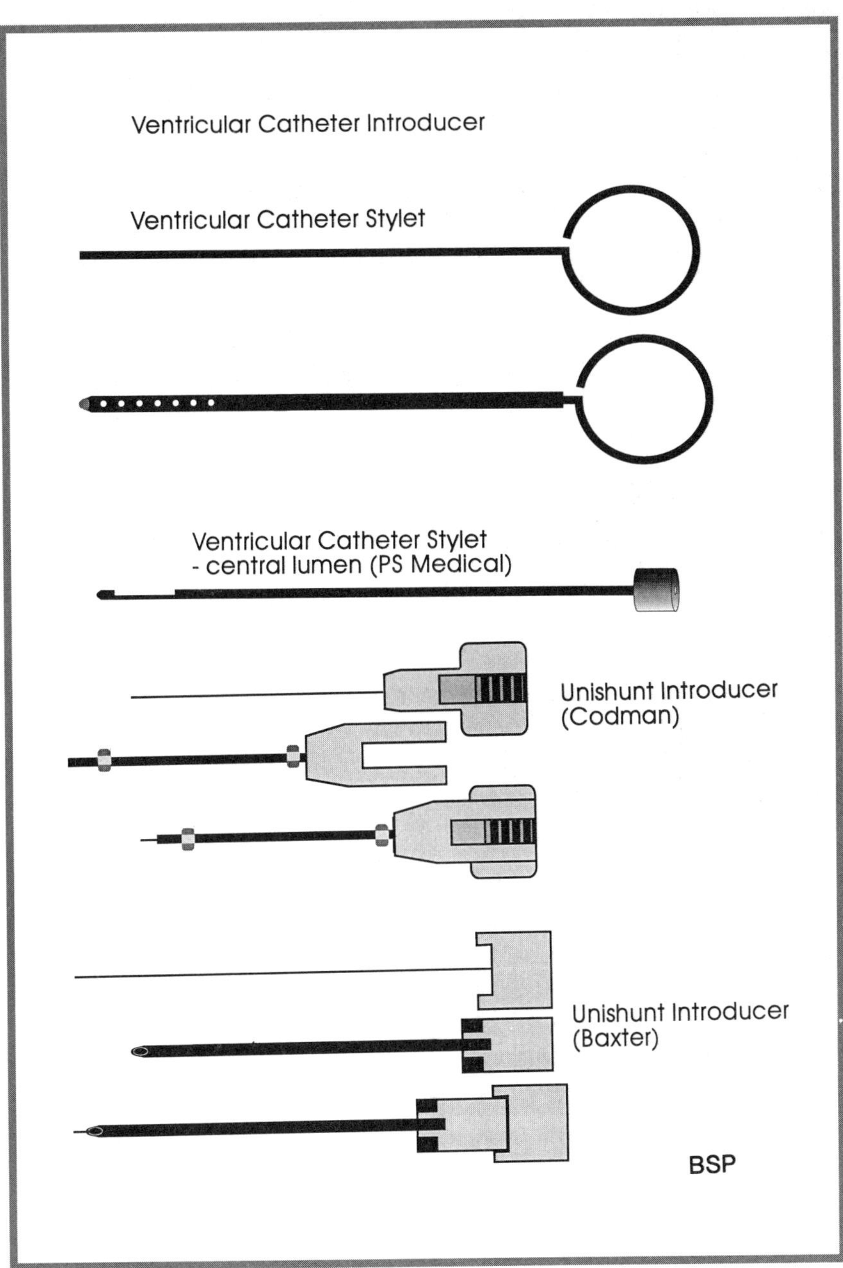
Ventricular Catheter Introducer
Ventricular Catheter Stylet
Ventricular Catheter Stylet
- central lumen (PS Medical)
Unishunt Introducer
(Codman)
Unishunt Introducer
(Baxter)
BSP

FIGURE 4-2A AND, 4-2B

These are designed to keep the brain from entering the catheter during passage through the brain. The third type is a "grooved" distal tip where the holes are recessed. The proximal end of the shunt is normally tapered and occluded with a radiopaque marker. Several other tip modifications have been or are now again available. The Hakim catheter is "J" shaped with the holes on the inside curve of the "J." This is supposed to protect the holes from ingrowth of choroid plexus or brain. At one time a ventricular catheter with an inflatable tip was available. This tip was, again, meant to keep the surrounding brain structure away from the catheter holes. However, what if, on occasion, the balloon failed to deflate and the catheter was removed with the balloon inflated? Fuji now offers a ventricular basket catheter with a ballooned tip with contained holes. As far as we are aware, there is no evidence that the type of holes, flanges, curves, etc., makes any difference to the incidence of proximal obstruction. Some of the more elaborate tips carve a larger swath through the brain, although this also may be of no consequence.

The catheter itself may be barium impregnated over its entirety or may have radiopaque markers (tantalum) added to nonradiopaque tubing or to barium-impregnated tubing. The markers are usually at 2- or 5-cm intervals along the catheter and allow the surgeon to calculate the amount of tubing inside the brain.

VENTRICULAR CATHETER INTRODUCERS

Free ventricular catheters are introduced using a metallic central stylet that is withdrawn to verify free flow of CSF once the ventricle is entered (Figure 4-2A-C). New designs of the stylet contain a central lumen, which provides immediate evidence of ventricular cannulation. In unishunts, an external stylet is (to date) necessary. These consist of a central stylet made usually of plastic and an outer rigid metal sheath. The stylet is introduced into the tip of the catheter through one of the distal openings and holds the catheter more proximally. It is necessary to keep the ventricular catheter under some tension to keep the stylet in place. When the stylet is removed, the ventricular catheter tip is freed and CSF flows along the introducer sheath and the shunt. These introducers are slightly more difficult to use, and verifying the ventricle has been entered is also more difficult, but avoids the connectors, ties, etc., of nonunitized systems.

CONNECTORS

Getting the catheter out of the brain and onto the surface of the skull involves making a 90° turn at the burr hole. There are several ways of doing this. The simplest is to simply bend the catheter and allow the dura and overlying skin to maintain the shape. While most catheters will not kink, the inherent stiffness of some is such that the tip of the catheter will tend to lie along the wall of the ventricle in the direction of the bend as the catheter attempts to straighten. Rigid right angle connectors (Figure 4-3) with lumen avoid this problem but involve ties and the possibility of losing the ventricular catheter at revision. External right angle guides accomplish the same thing without connectors but may be awkward to put in place. Finally, burr hole reservoirs and valves redirect the flow

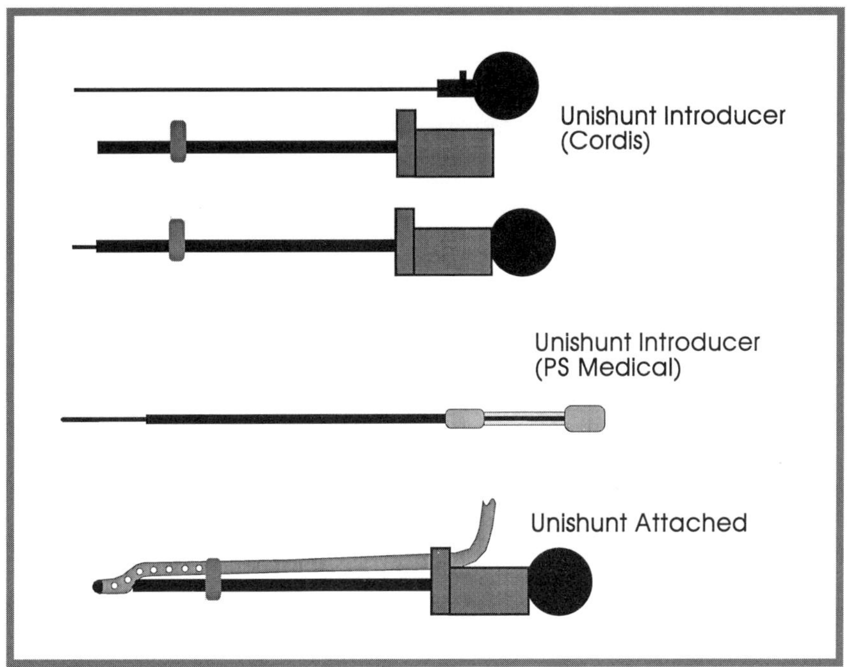

FIGURE 4-2C

of CSF at 90° but involve connectors and the possibility of losing the ventricular catheter. New snap-on systems avoid any ties but require a special holding instrument.

CSF SHUNT VALVES

STANDARD DIFFERENTIAL PRESSURE VALVES

In this section, we will only discuss "standard valves." These are valves that simply open or close to a pressure differential. Valves or additional devices that function from quite a different mechanism will be discussed in subsequent sections. It is not often obvious when looking at a shunt just what valve or valves are present although they all are grouped into one pressure category or another. While some would argue that this is all that is really necessary, we think it is of considerable interest to know just what kind of valve is present and where it is situated. Most companies tend to manufacture one or two types of valves so we have grouped the valves according to mechanism.

A valve unit often contains several additional components, including the valve, reservoir or pumping chamber, occluders, etc., so that the valve may be tested, CSF sampled, etc. Most valves are placed either proximally or distally although, theoretically, a valve can be placed anywhere along the course of the shunt line.

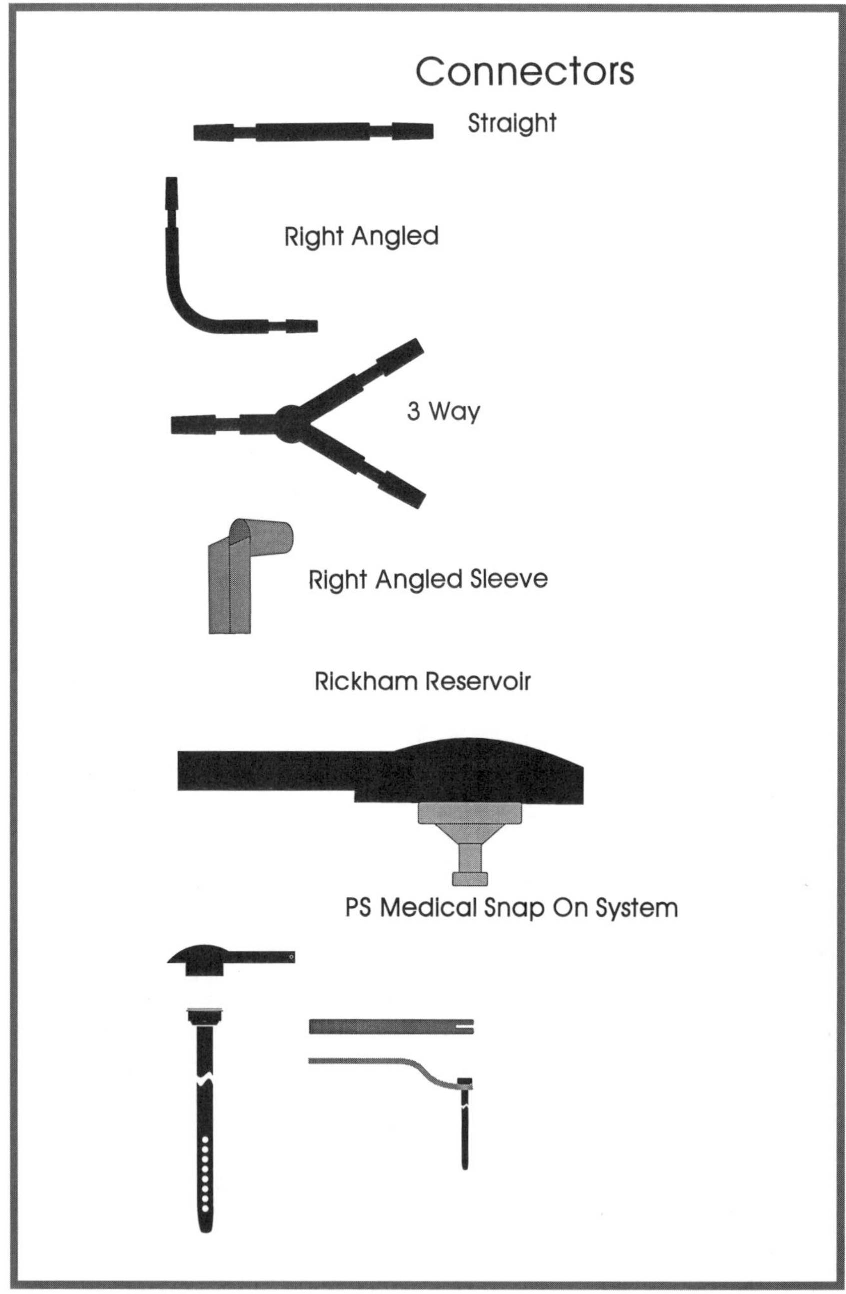
Connectors
Straight
Right Angled
3 Way
Right Angled Sleeve
Rickham Reservoir
PS Medical Snap On System

Figure 4-3

Proximal Slit Valves

Codman Holter Valve

The Codman Holter valve consists of two silicone slit valves with internal springs to prevent invagination of slits (Figure 4-4A,B). Valves are housed in stainless steel adapter assemblies separated by a silicone-housed pumping chamber. This valve comes in three sizes and shapes. The Holter straight valves are cylindrical in shape; the Holter elliptical valve has a larger pumping chamber; and the Holter minielliptical valves, advised for pediatric use or where extensive skin tension should be avoided, are 20% smaller than the standard elliptical valves.

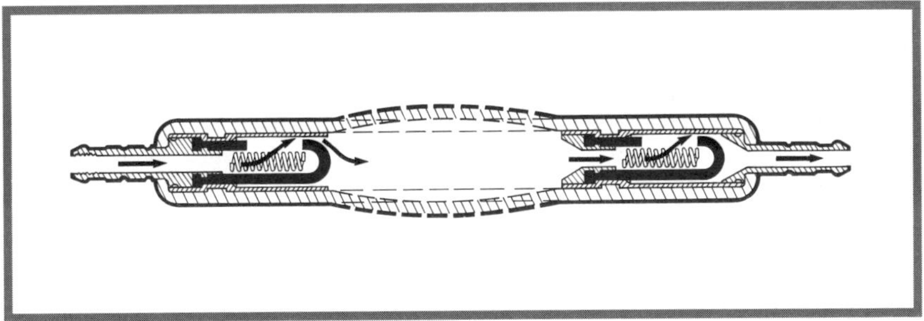

Figure 4-4A

Category	Pressure (mm H_2O) (Flow = 8.6 cc/hr)	Code
High Pressure	76–110	H
Medium Pressure	41–75	M
Low Pressure	11–40	L
Extra Low Pressure	0–10	EL

Phoenix Holter-Hausner Valve

The Phoenix Holter-Hausner valve is a cruciform slit valve that consists of two silicone slit valves housed in a stainless steel valve assembly bonded into a silicone body, the center of which is a flat-based pumping chamber with a flange for attachment to the periosteum (Figure 4-5). The extension of the silicone body over the adapters overlaps the ends of the proximal and distal catheters for added connection security. A simplified version using the same valve mechanism consists of a thimble-shaped silicone elastomer slit valve housed in a stainless steel adapter assembly. The valve housing is encased in a .25 cm thick elastomer sheet.

Codman Denver Shunt

The Codman Denver shunt is a single cruciform slit valve. The very large pumping chamber is designed to allow both proximal and distal flushing by rolling a finger along the chamber in the direction of flushing (Figure 4-6A,B).

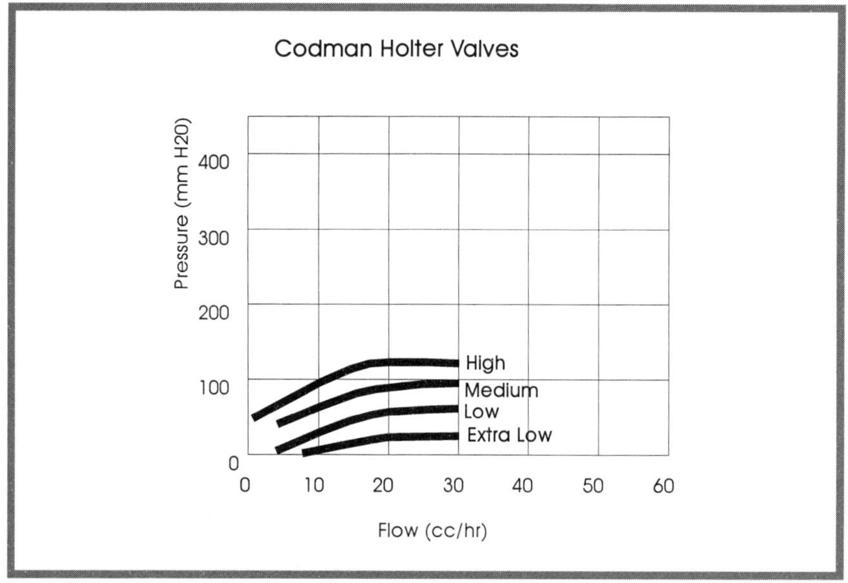

Figure 4-4b

When rolling the finger proximally, the cruciform slits invert, temporarily allowing proximal flow and flushing.

Category	Flow Rate (cc/hr) (Pressure = 100 mm H_2O)
Low Flow Rate (High Pressure)	6-17
Standard Flow Rate (Medium Pressure)	18-59
High Flow Rate (Low Pressure)	60-120

Radionics Standard Shunt Valve System

The Radionics standard shunt valve system has a single silicone membrane in apposition to a Teflon base, acting to create a slit valve in stainless steel housing (Figure 4-7A,B). The Teflon-silicone interface is designed to prevent sticking. It has a distal integral pumping chamber and is usually configured with an additional proximal reservoir. It is also available in a mini system for infants.

Category	Pressure (mm H_2O) (Flow = 5 cc/hr)	Pressure (mm H_2O) (Flow = 40 cc/hr)	Code
High Pressure	175	175	•••
Medium Pressure	75	100	••
Low Pressure	35	35	•

Chhabra Slit in Spring

This cylindrical side-walled slit valve girdled in stainless steel is spring-designed to protect and support the slit valve while maintaining the opening pressure. The distal silicone reservoir is categorized in Figure 4-8.

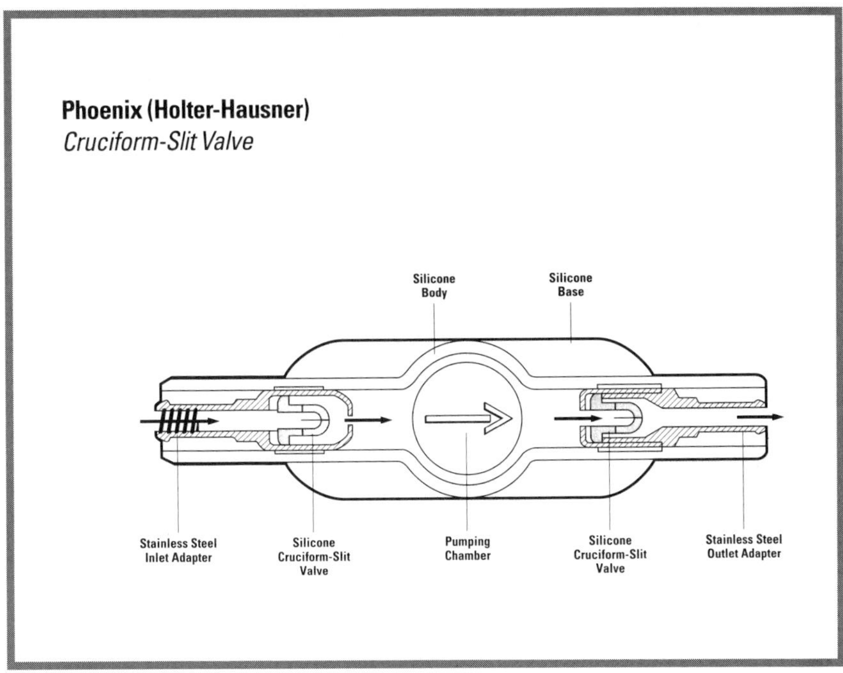
Phoenix (Holter-Hausner)
Cruciform-Slit Valve
Silicone Body
Silicone Base
Stainless Steel Inlet Adapter
Silicone Cruciform-Slit Valve
Pumping Chamber
Silicone Cruciform-Slit Valve
Stainless Steel Outlet Adapter

FIGURE 4-5

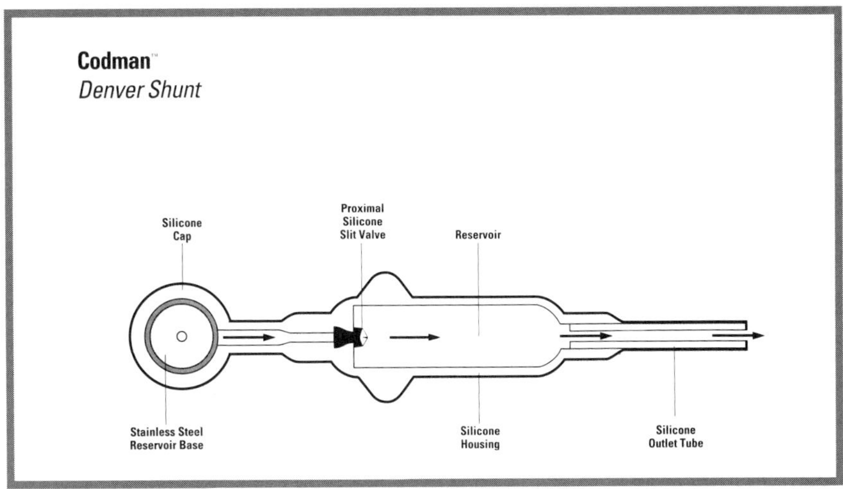
Codman™
Denver Shunt
Silicone Cap
Proximal Silicone Slit Valve
Reservoir
Stainless Steel Reservoir Base
Silicone Housing
Silicone Outlet Tube

FIGURE 4-6A

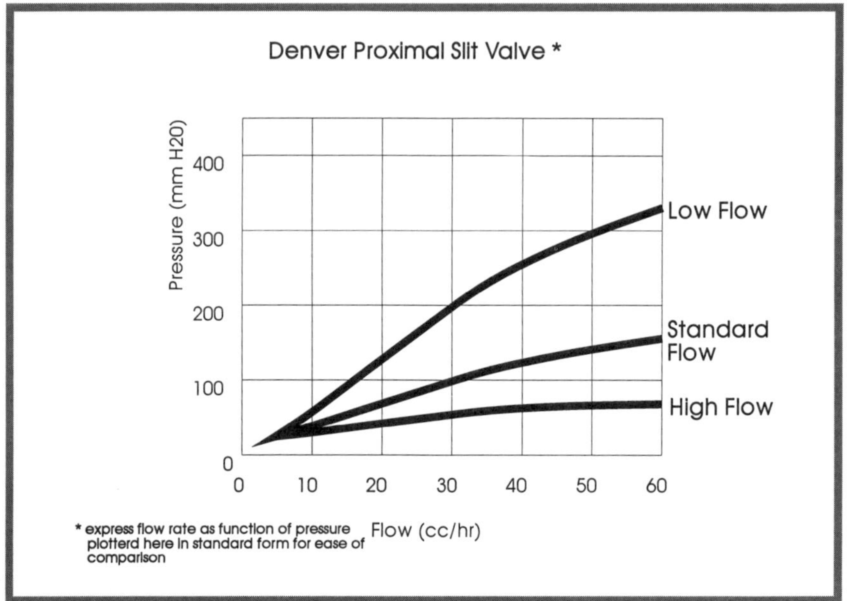

FIGURE 4-6B

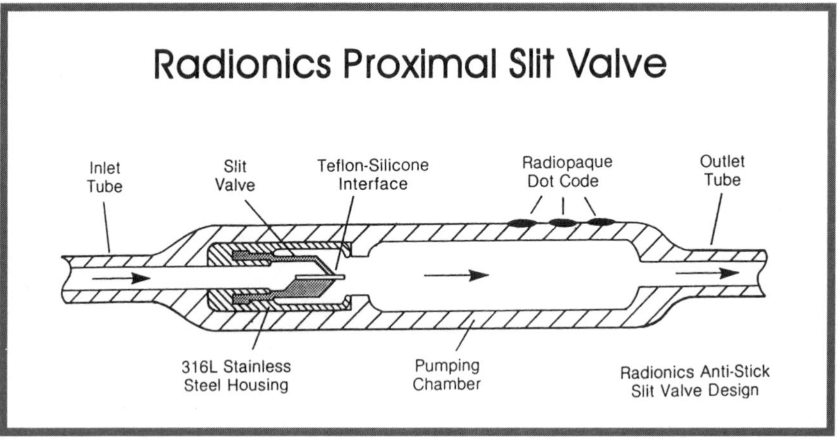

FIGURE 4-7A

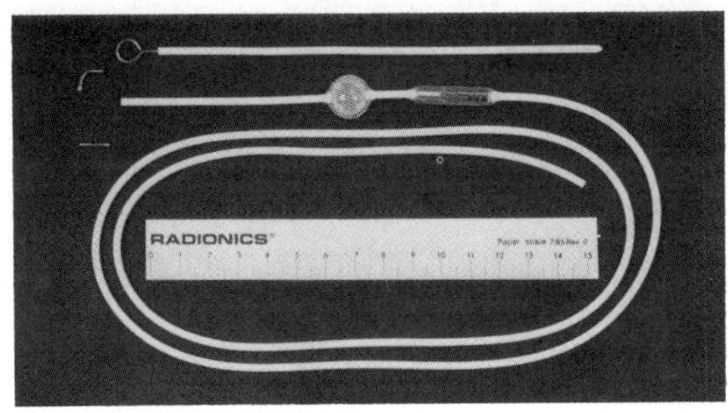

FIGURE 4-7B

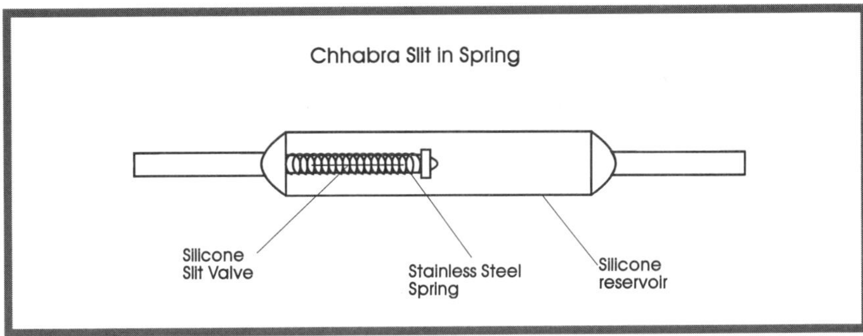

FIGURE 4-8

CATEGORY	PRESSURE (MM H_2O) (FLOW = 5 CC/HR)	PRESSURE (MM H_2O) (FLOW = 40 CC/HR)	CODE
High Pressure	175	175	•••
Medium Pressure	75	100	••
Low Pressure	35	35	•

DIAPHRAGM VALVES
CODMAN ACCU-FLO (BURR HOLE)

This is a flexible ribbed silicone membrane housed in a silicone base and covered with a silicone dome (Figure 4-9).

CATEGORY	PRESSURE (MM H_2O) (FLOW = 5 CC/HR)	PRESSURE (MM H_2O) (FLOW = 50 CC/HR)	CODE
High Pressure	100	220	•••
Medium Pressure	45	140	••
Low Pressure	2	75	•

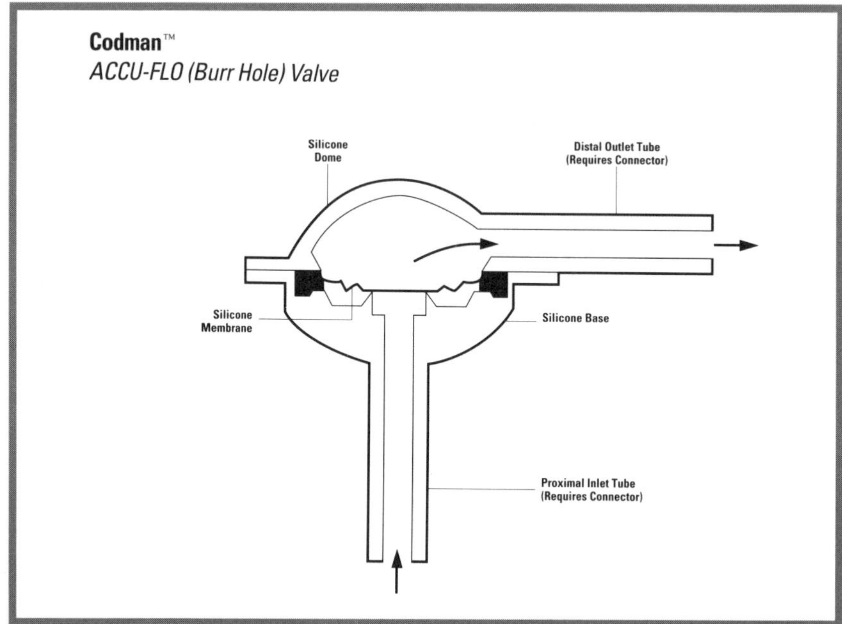

FIGURE 4-9

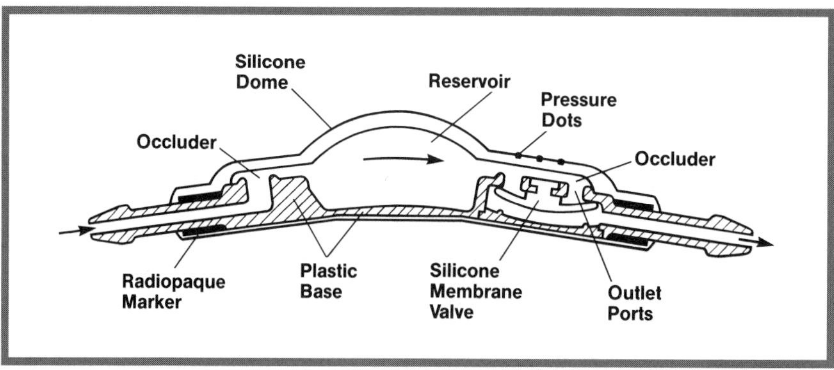

FIGURE 4-10

PS Medical Flow-Control Valve (Contoured)

This valve has a similar silicone membrane diaphragm. By compressing the silicone dome against a plastic base, proximal and distal occlusion sites allow flushing and testing both proximally and distally (Figure 4-10). There are integral plastic connectors. The contoured valve is available in three sizes—regular, small, and ultra-small. The small sizes are proposed for use in premature and full-term infants. The diaphragm valve is available without flushing chamber or occlusion sites as a "button valve," also for use in preterm infants (Figure 4-11A,B).

PS Medical Flow-Control Valve (Cylindrical)

These dual silicone membrane diaphragm valves are mounted horizontally in a plastic base (Figure 4-12). A silicone reservoir is between the valves, which are available with a proximal antechamber with a plastic needle guard (same pressure designation as contoured valves).

PS Medical Flow-Control Valve (Burr Hole)

This silicone membrane diaphragm is housed in a polypropylene base (Figure 4-13A,B). An overlying needle shield is in a silicone dome. It is available in two sizes, one for 12- and one for 16-mm burr holes. It has integral polypropylene plastic connectors (same pressure designation as contoured valves).

Category	Pressure (mm H_2O) (Flow = 5 cc/hr)	Pressure (mm H_2O) (Flow = 50 cc/hr)	Code
High Pressure	120	200	•••
Medium Pressure	60	130	••
Low Pressure	10	70	•
Low-Low Pressure	5	40	

V. Mueller Heyer Schulte Pudenz Flushing Valve (Burr Hole)

This is a single silicone membrane diaphragm valve on a silicone base with a silicone dome (Figure 4-14).

V. Mueller Heyer Schulte Low Profile Valve

This single silicone membrane diaphragm valve is in a silicone housing, has proximal and distal occluder sites, and a silicone dome with a plastic needle guard. It is available with integral plastic connectors, an integral antisiphon device, and/or an on-off device (Figure 4-15A,B).

Category	Closing Pressure (mm H_2O)	Code
High Pressure	111–180	•••
Medium Pressure	55–94	••
Low Pressure	15–44	•

MITER VALVES

V. Mueller Heyer Schulte In-Line Valve

This single silicone miter valve is housed in silicone and has a distal silicone flushing chamber (Figure 4-16A,B).

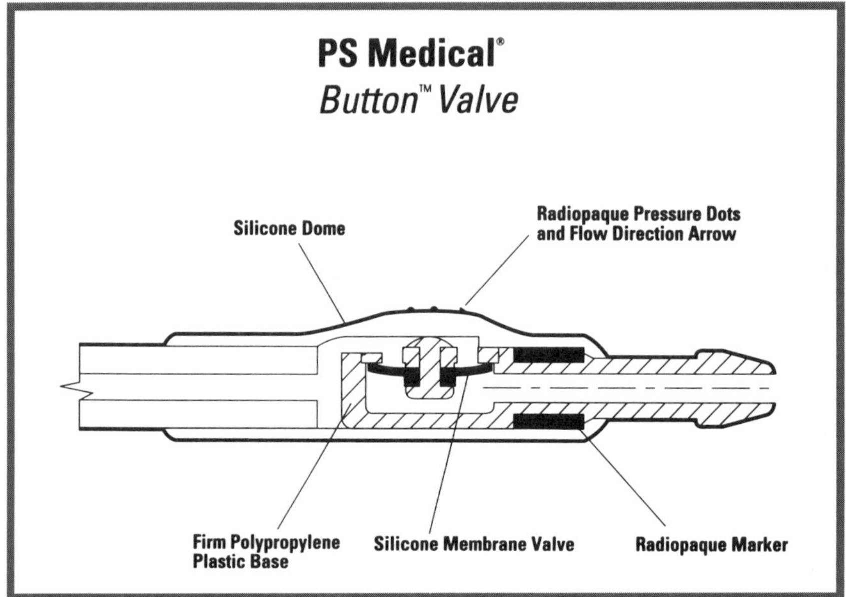

FIGURE 4-11A

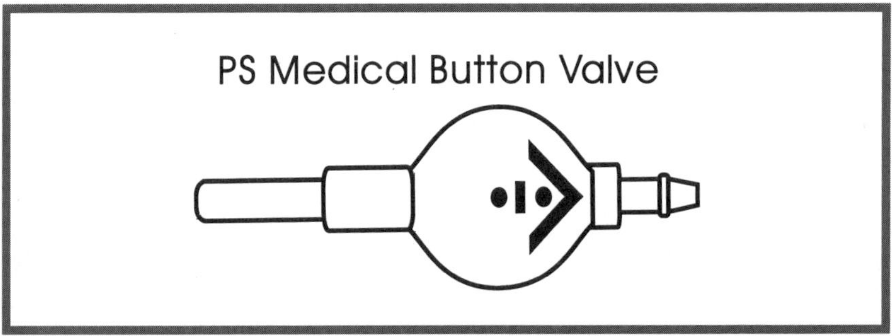

FIGURE 4-11B

V. Mueller Heyer Schulte Mishler Flushing Device

This device is a single silastic miter valve located in a silastic septum which separates chambers of silastic dome and silastic base. It is available with an integral antisiphon device and/or an on-off device (Figure 4-17).

CATEGORY	CLOSING PRESSURE (MM H_2O)	CODE
High Pressure	95–150	•••
Medium Pressure	55–94	••
Low Pressure	15–54	•

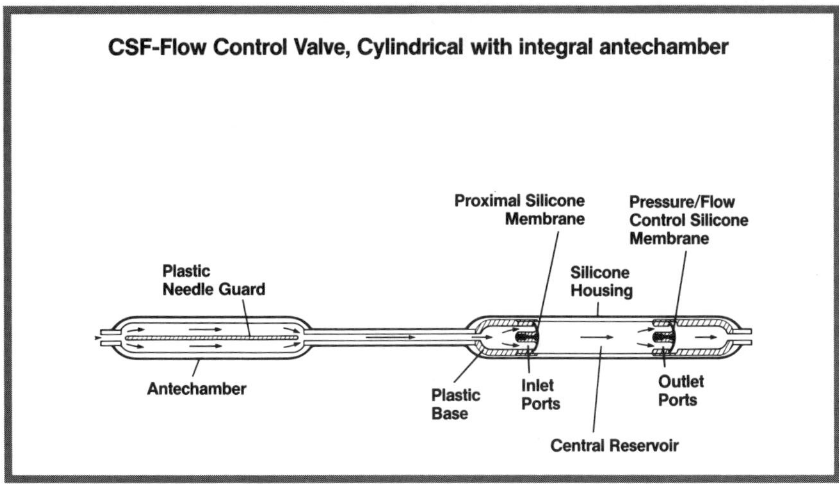

FIGURE 4-12

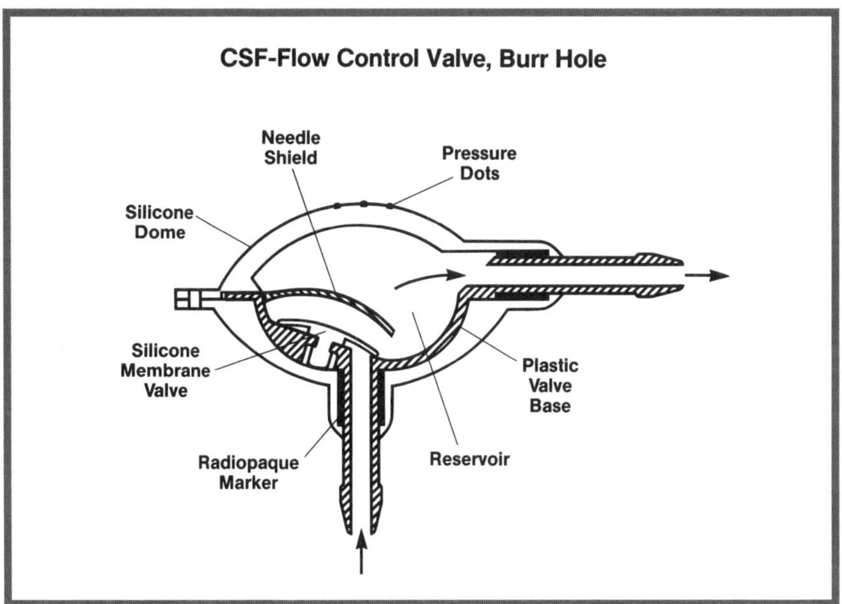

FIGURE 4-13A

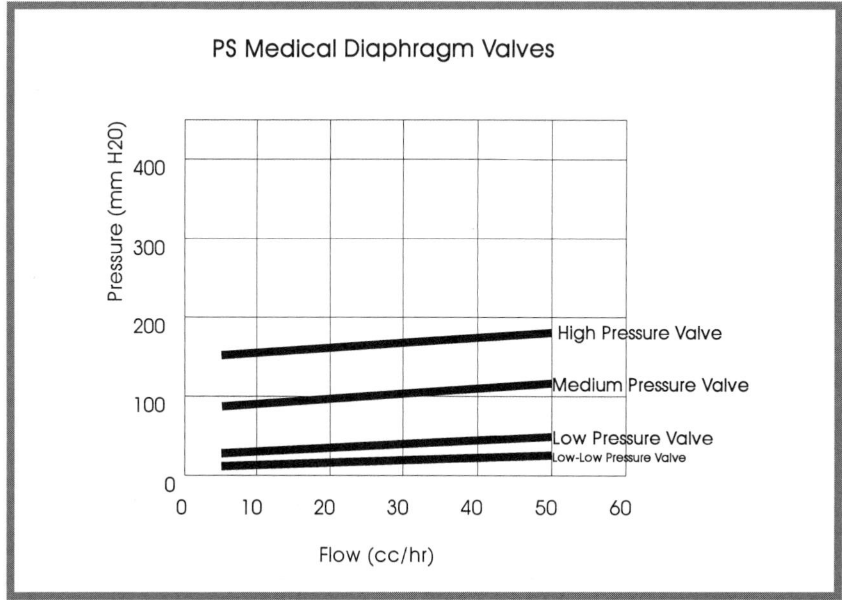

FIGURE 4-13B

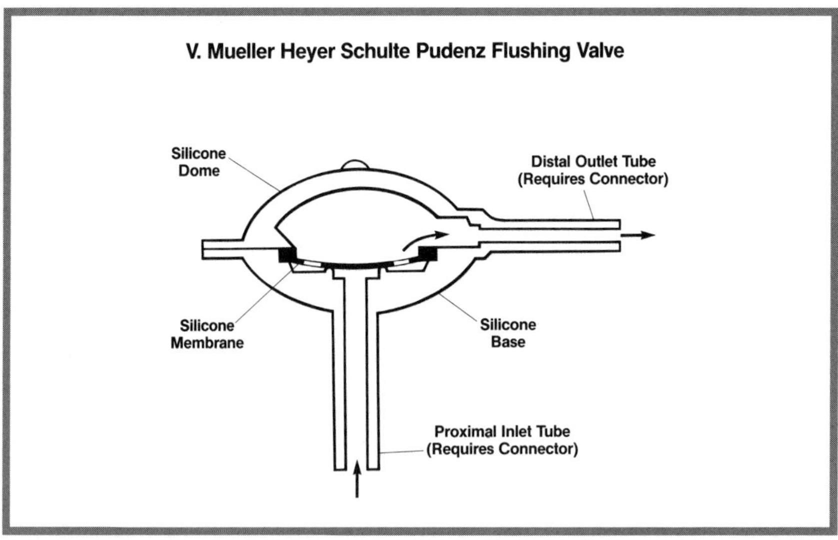

FIGURE 4-14

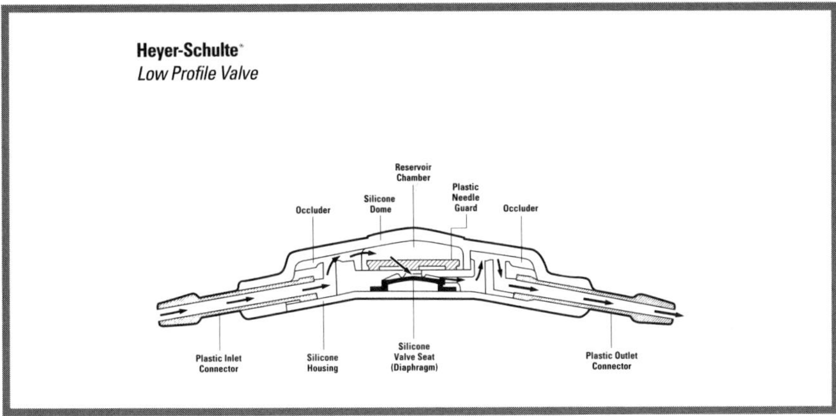

FIGURE 4-15A

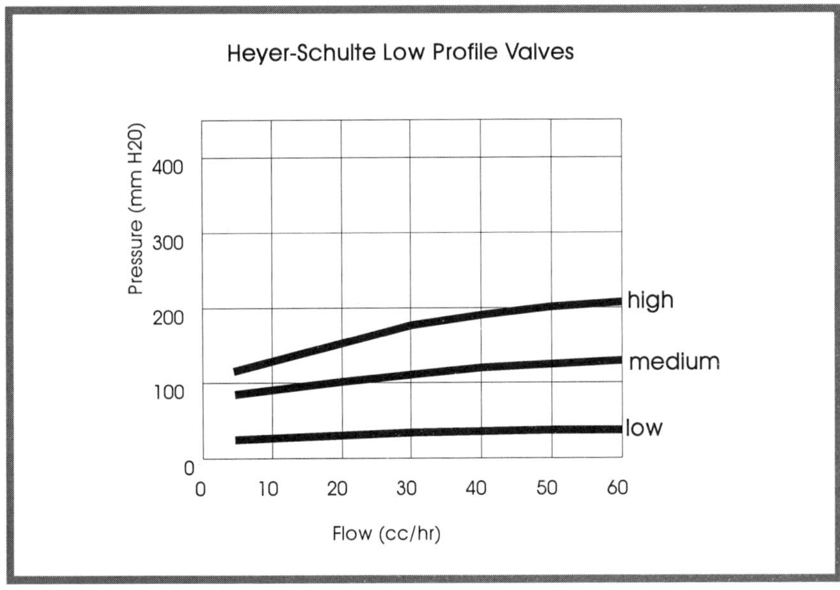

FIGURE 4-15B

RADIONICS CONTOUR FLEX VALVE

Remarkably similar in appearance to the PS Medical diaphragm valve, this Radionics valve has a polypropylene base that is segmented, ostensibly to allow for flexion. Integral connectors, silastic dome and reservoir, and proximal and distal occluders are basically the same as in the PS Medical valve (Figure 4-18A,B).

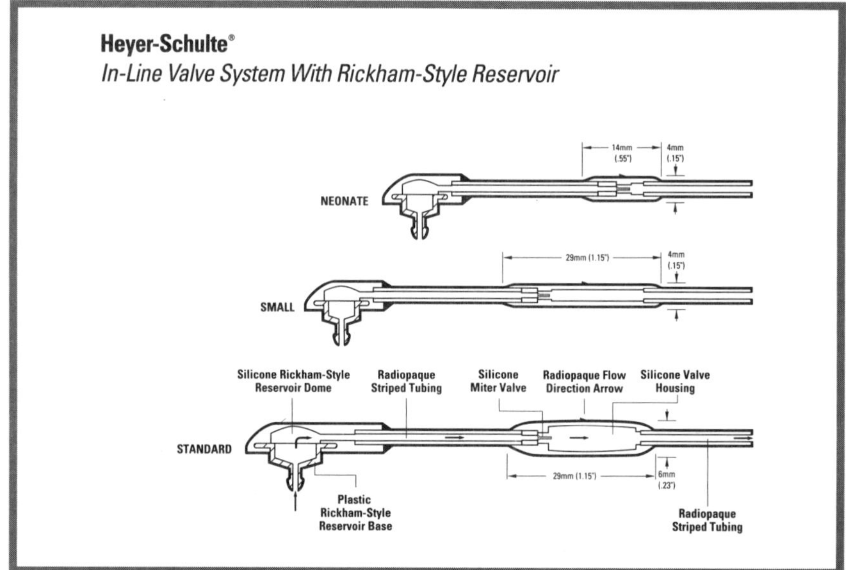

FIGURE 4-16A

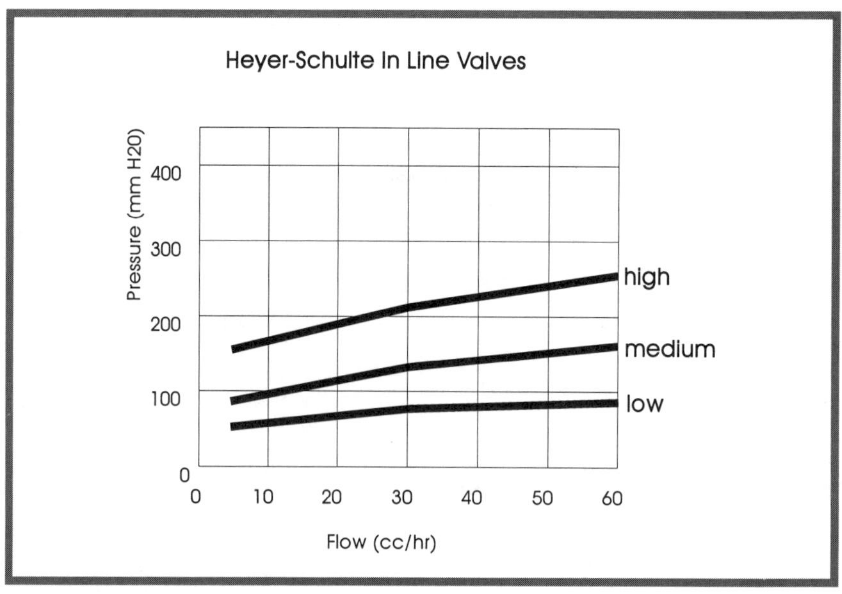

FIGURE 4-16B

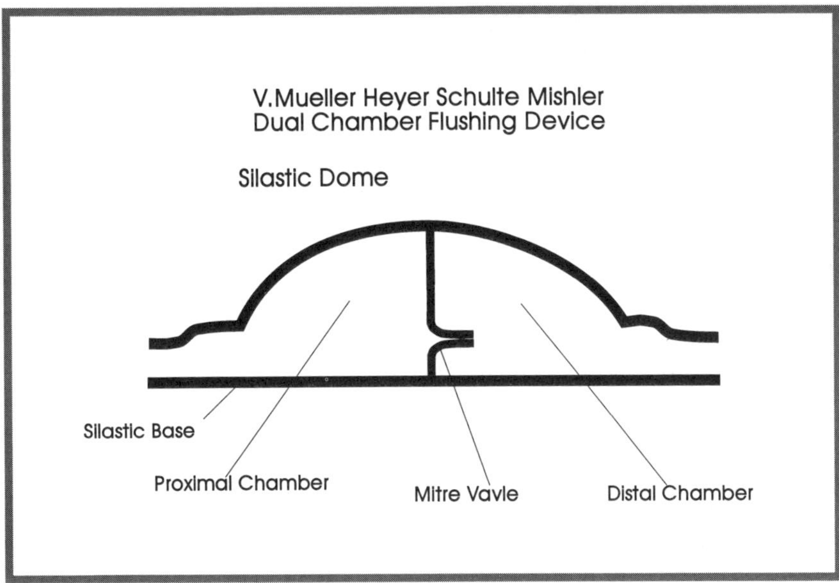

FIGURE 4-17

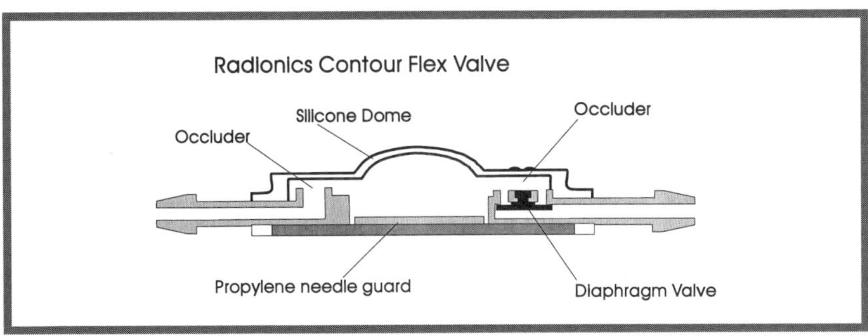

FIGURE 4-18A

CATEGORY	PRESSURE (MM H_2O) (FLOW = 5 CC/HR)	PRESSURE (MM H_2O) (FLOW = 40 CC/HR)	CODE
High Pressure	120	200	•••
Medium Pressure	60	130	••
Low Pressure	10	70	•

Fuji Flushing Device (Flat Bottom)

The Fuji flushing device is a single silastic miter valve located in a silastic inlet with a silastic dome reservoir (Figure 4-19). It also comes as a dual-domed chamber with a miter valve between chambers. This allows proximal and distal flushing.

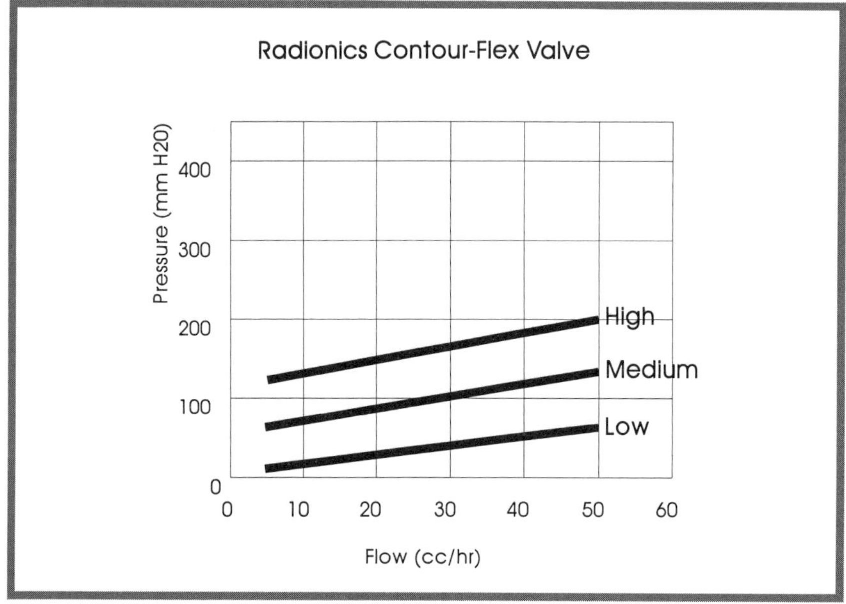

FIGURE 4-18B

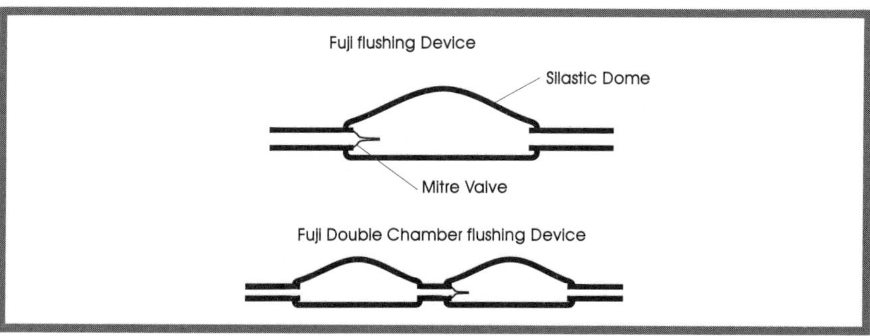

FIGURE 4-19

BALL AND SPRING VALVES

Cordis Hakim Valve

The Cordis Hakim is a dual-spring ball valve. The inlet valve is a synthetic ruby ball seated in a stainless steel valve seat (Figure 4-20A,B). The stainless steel spring is calibrated by a micro-adjustable telescopic fulcrum. The chassis is titanium. The total pressure of the valve unit is controlled by the inlet valve; the outlet valve functions as a check valve only. There is an interposed translucent flushing chamber. It is available with a proximal silastic antechamber with a stainless steel needle guard and integral connectors, or as a unitized system. A pediatric valve is smaller and has helical springs.

CATEGORY	CLOSING PRESSURE (MM H_2O) (FLOW < 1.5 CC/HR)	OPERATING PRESSURE (MM H_2O) (FLOW = 5 CC/HR)	CODE
Very High Pressure	136-165	170-230	Green
High Pressure	91-135	120-170	Brown
Medium Pressure	56-90	80-120	Yellow
Low Pressure	21-55	40-80	White
Very Low Pressure	5-20	15-40	Blue

Codman Medos Hakim Valve System

In this system, a synthetic ruby ball sits in a synthetic valve seat (Figure 4-21). The base is titanium. A clear silastic reservoir leads to a second valve that is a helical spring type. It has a proximal antechamber with a titanium needle stop for CSF access.

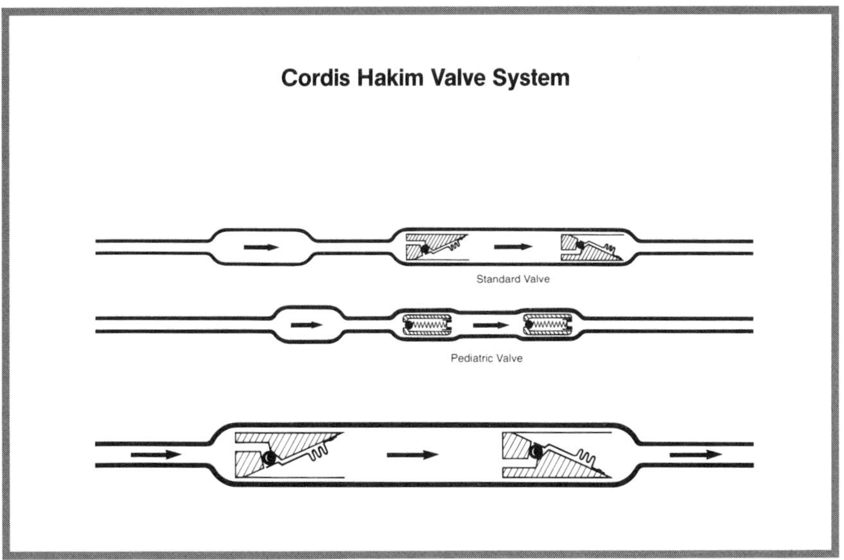

FIGURE 4-20A

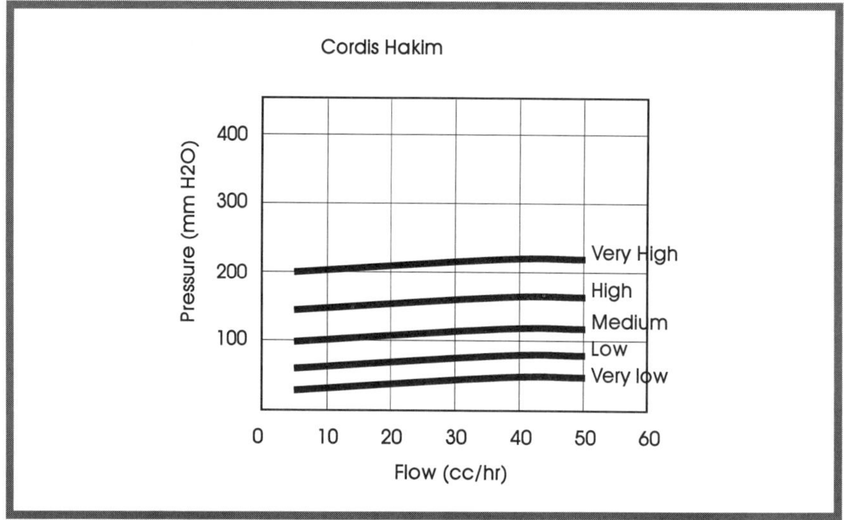

FIGURE 4-20B

EXTERNALLY ADJUSTABLE DIFFERENTIAL PRESSURE VALVES

ADJUSTABLE SPRING BALL VALVES

Codman Medos Programmable Hakim Valve System

This proximal spring valve is adjustable (Figure 4-22A-C). Its stainless steel spring fulcrum is incrementally raised on a polyethersulfone cam and stepper motor. The motor contains a magnet that is turned by an external magnetic field. Radiopaque markers provide the opening pressure setting. The base is titanium. Operating pressure is adjustable from 30 to 200 mm H_2O in eighteen 10-mm increments.

Sophysa Adjustable Valve

The spring in this valve is semicircular (Figure 4-23A-C). The spring is attached to one end of a pivoting bar or rotor, which contains two micro-magnets. Rotation of the bar changes the force on the ball by altering the fulcrum of the spring. A second spring adjacent to the first stops the rotor in three positions (model SU3), ranging in pressure from 50 to 170 mm H_2O (at 50 cc/hr). The rotor is moved using an external magnet. Position of the rotor is checked with a compass. Note--the bar will also move in the strong magnetic field of MRI. The model SU8 has eight positions over the same pressure range.

CATEGORY	PRESSURE (MM H_2O) (FLOW = 5 CC/HR)	PRESSURE (MM H_2O) (FLOW = 50 CC/HR)
High Pressure	110*	170
Medium Pressure	75*	110
Low Pressure	20*	50

* Values estimated from graph.

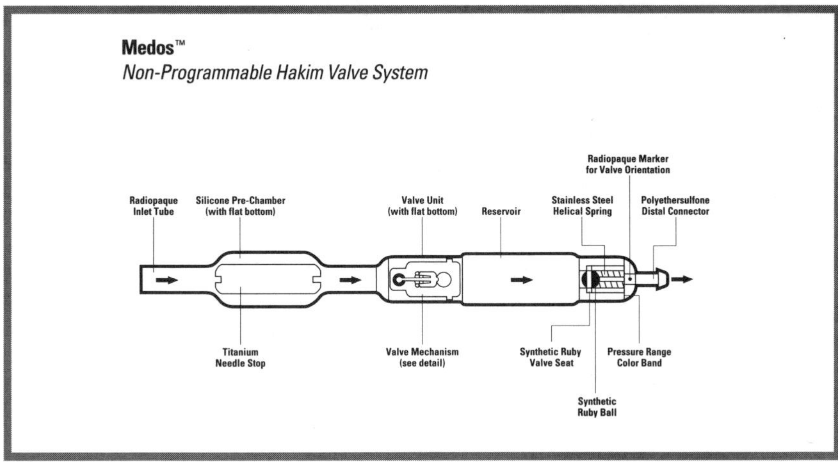

FIGURE 4-21A

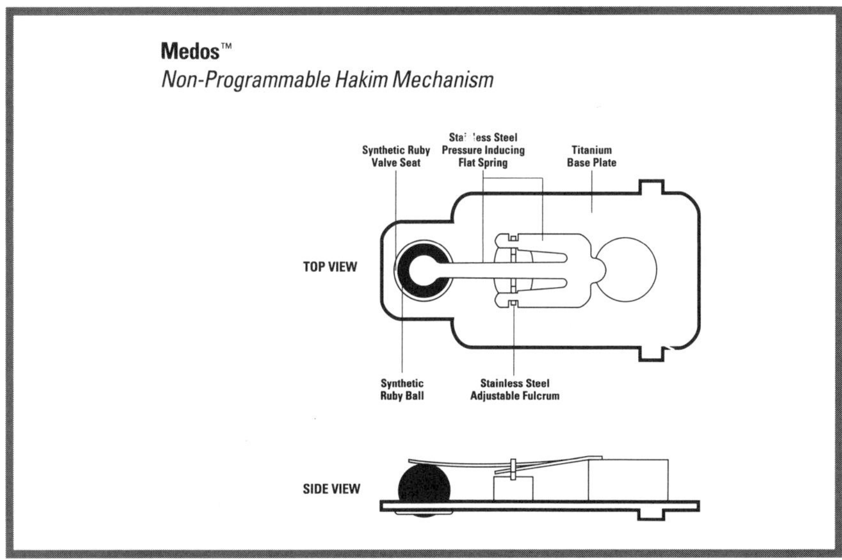

FIGURE 4-21B

OTHER ADJUSTABLE VALVES

MDM Multipurpose Adjustable Valve

This is basically a valve with two parallel proximal slit valves, one medium pressure (medium flow) and one high pressure (low flow) (Figure 4-24A,B). The channel to each valve can be occluded by moving the metallic ball along a silastic

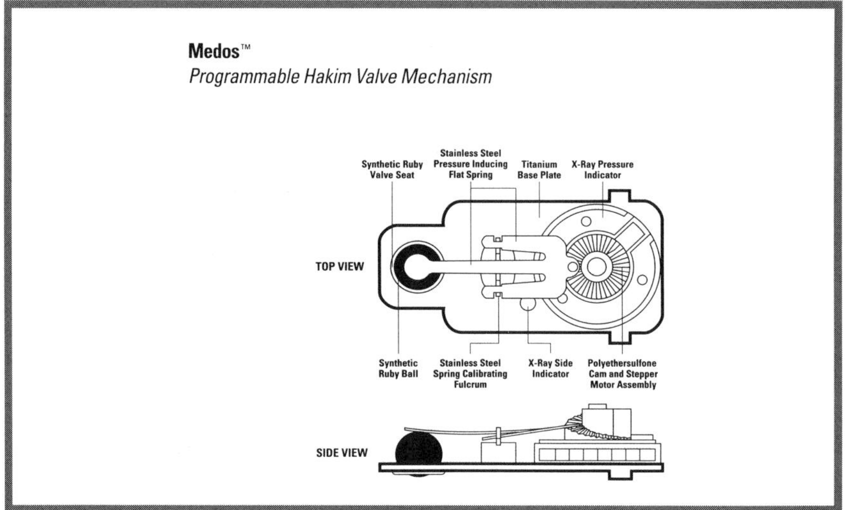

FIGURE 4-22A

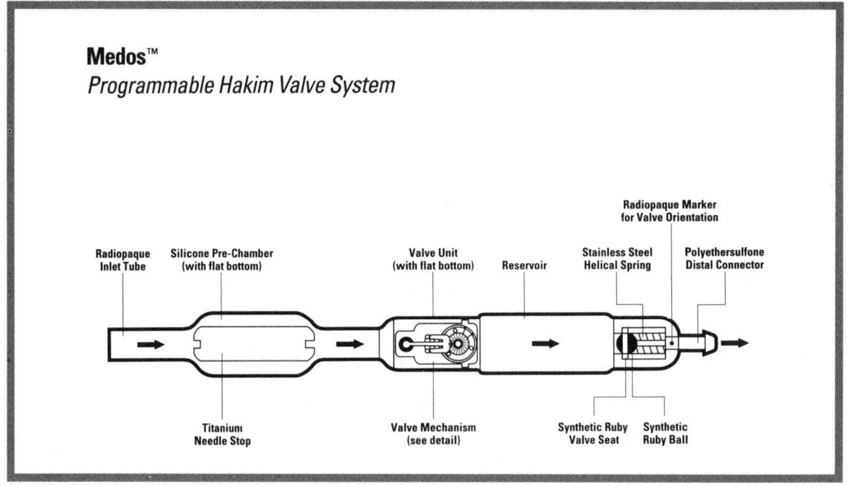

FIGURE 4-22B

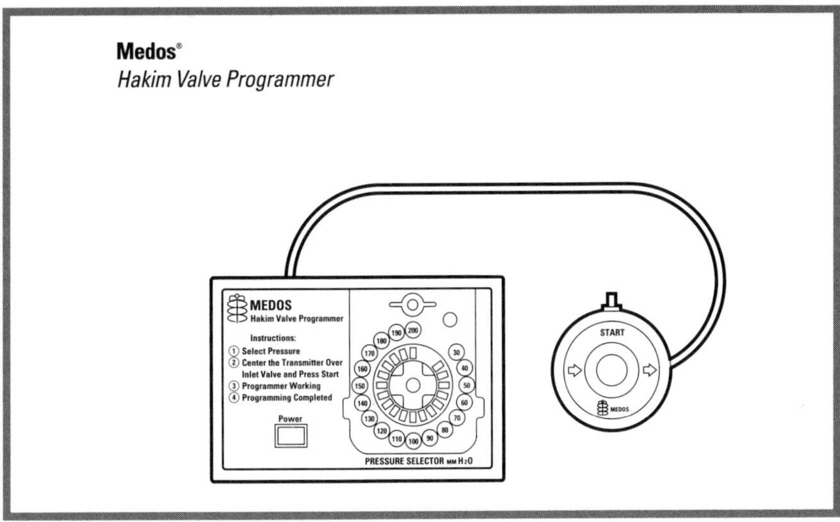

FIGURE 4-22C

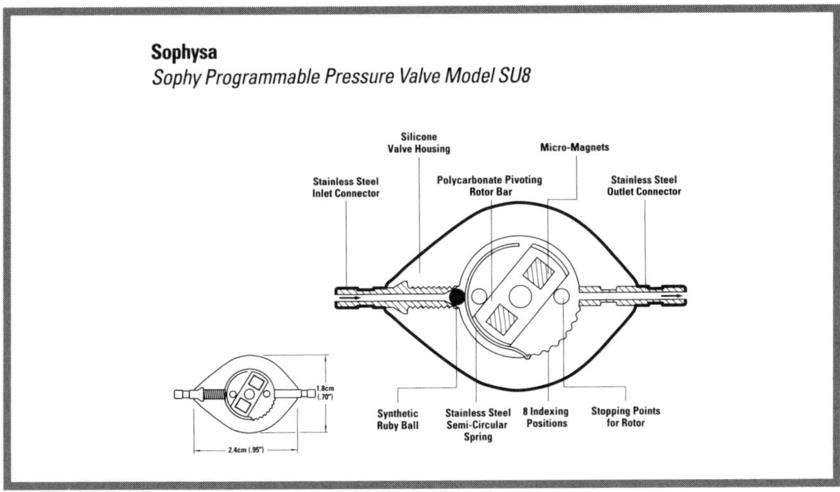

FIGURE 4-23A

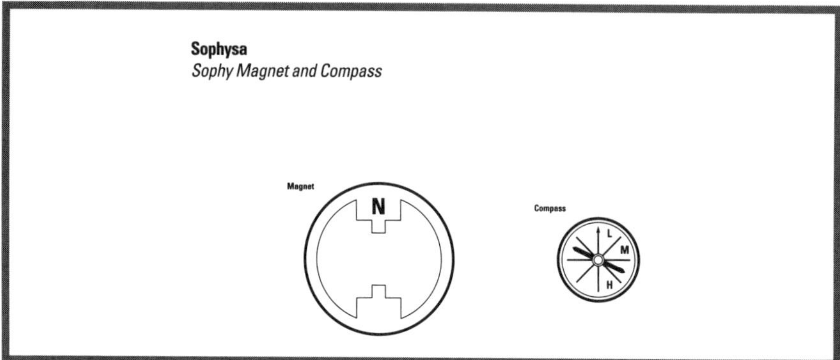

FIGURE 4-23B

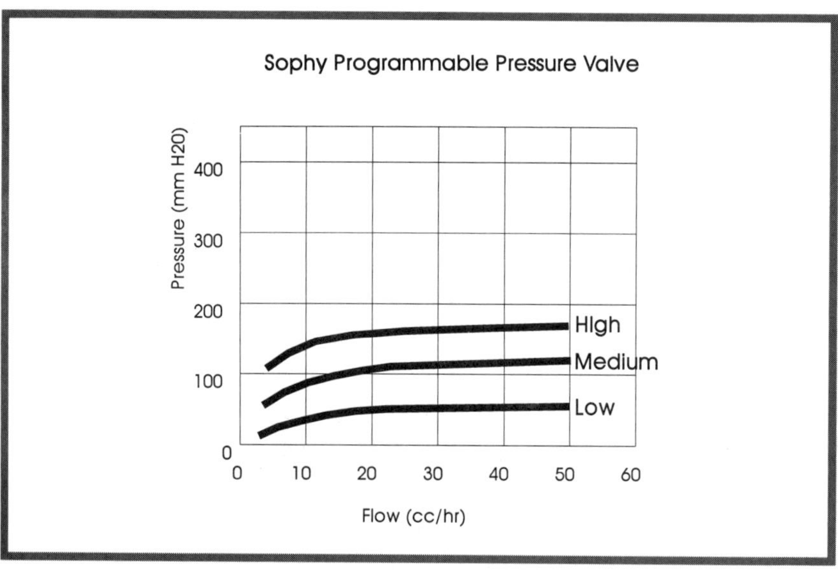

FIGURE 4-23C

sleeve. This leads to four possible settings. The valve is a high pressure valve with the low flow channel open, a medium pressure valve with the medium flow channel open, and a low pressure valve with both channels open (high flow) (see Chapter 2 for information about adding valves together). Finally, with both channels occluded, the valve is completely blocked off, and, in this sense, the valve also functions as an on-off device (see below).

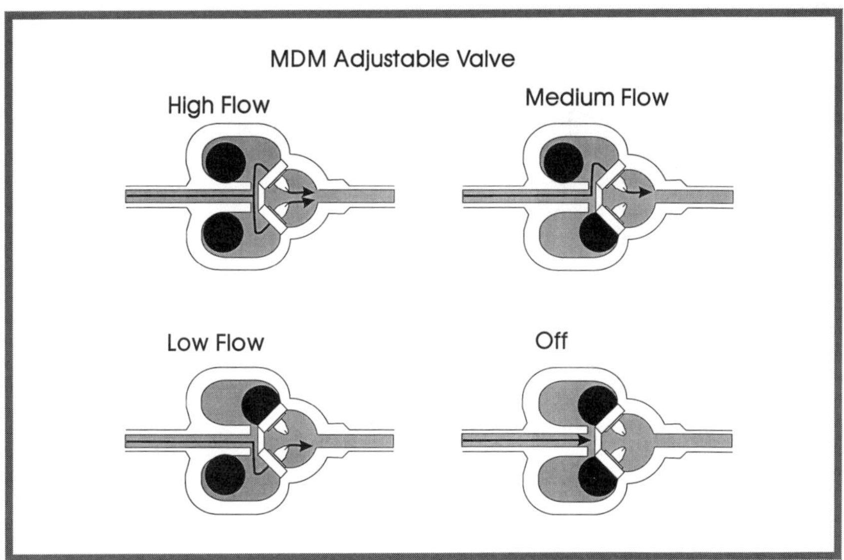

FIGURE 4-24A

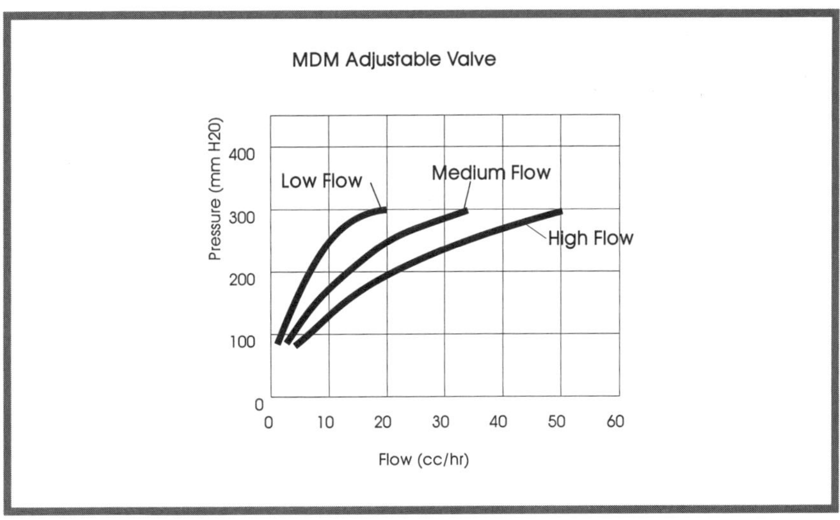

FIGURE 4-24B

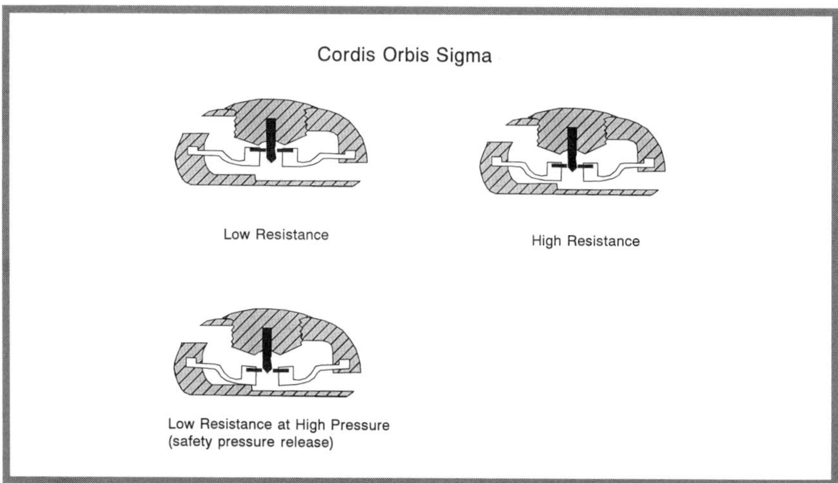

FIGURE 4-25A

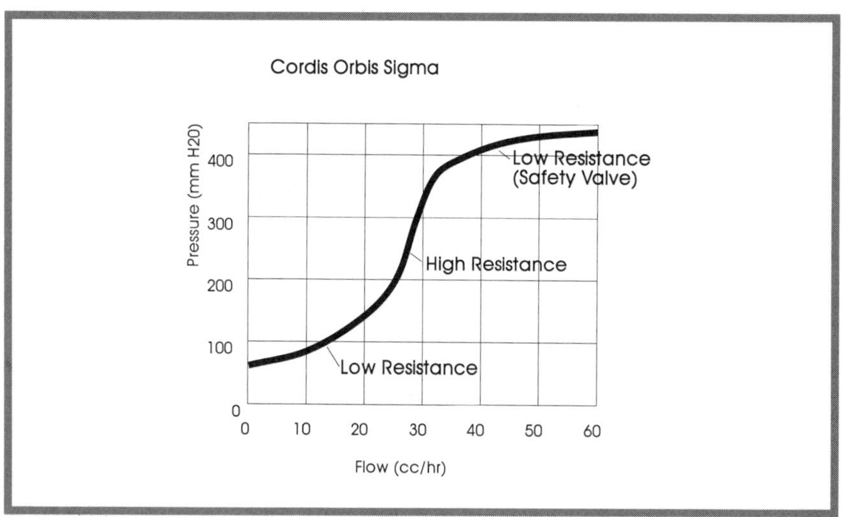

FIGURE 4-25B

FLOW-CONTROL VALVE

CORDIS ORBIS SIGMA

A flexible silicone diaphragm houses a synthetic ruby ring seat that moves along a synthetic ruby flow-control pin according to differential pressure (Figure 4-25A,B). The synthetic ruby pin is contoured so that the opening around the pin decreases as the diaphragm descends with increased pressure. This increases the resistance and limits the flow. The valve housing is polysulphone encased in silastic. It is available as a unishunt or separately, with integral connectors.

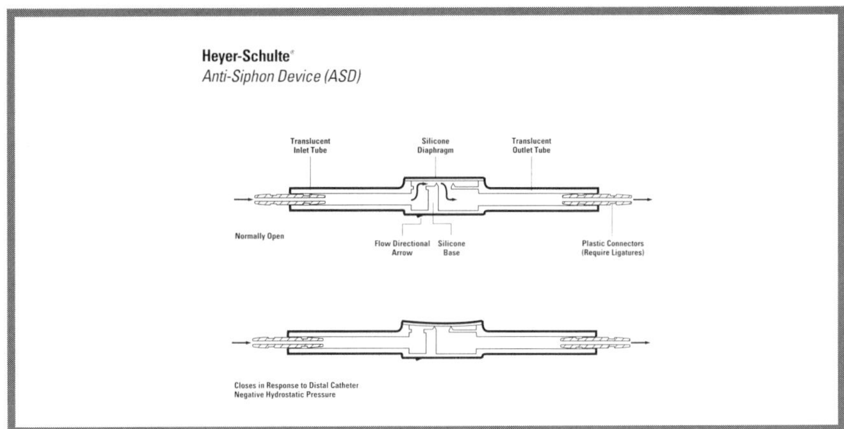

FIGURE 4-26

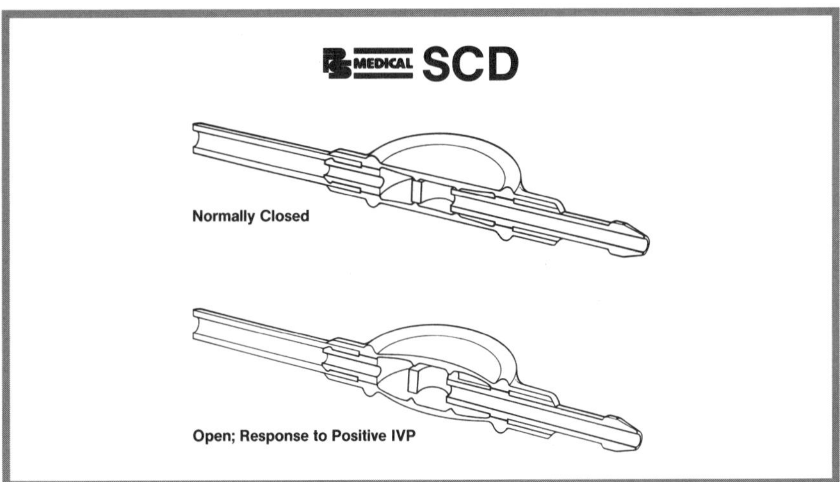

FIGURE 4-27

STAGE	VALVE MODE	PRESSURE (MM H_2O)	(FLOW CC/HR)	FUNCTION
I	Low Differential Pressure (DP) — Low Resistance	40–80 to 40–120	5–18	drains at DPs close to opening pressure
II	Flow Regulation — Variable Resistance	120–130	18–30	reduces or prevents over - drainage
III	Safety Valve/ High DP — Low Resistance	320–450 to 320–540	30–50	prevents intracranial hypertension

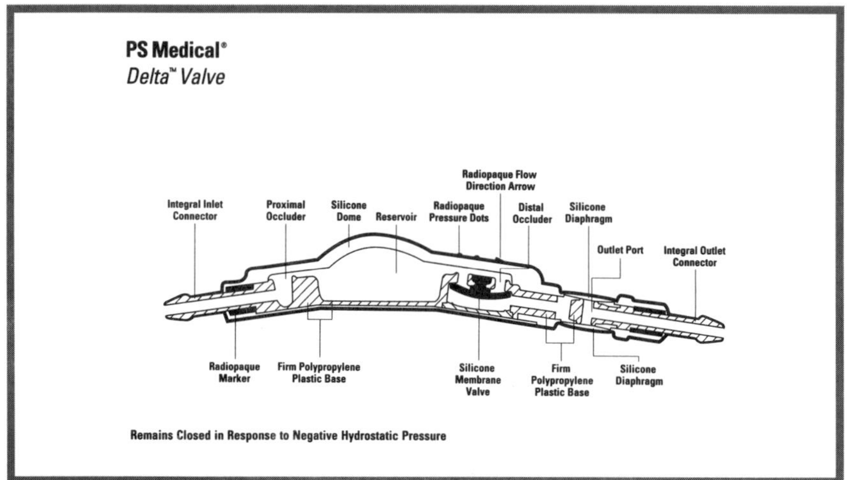

FIGURE 4-28A

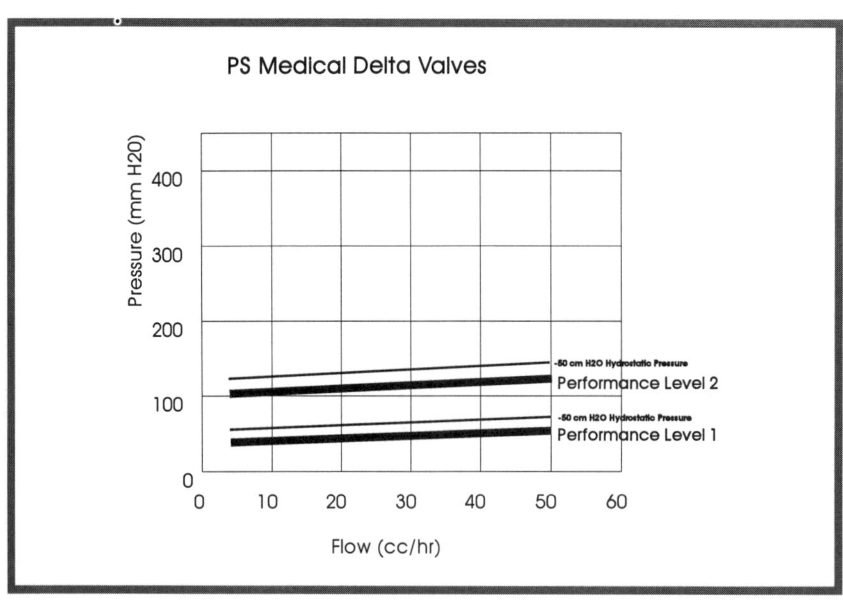

FIGURE 4-28B

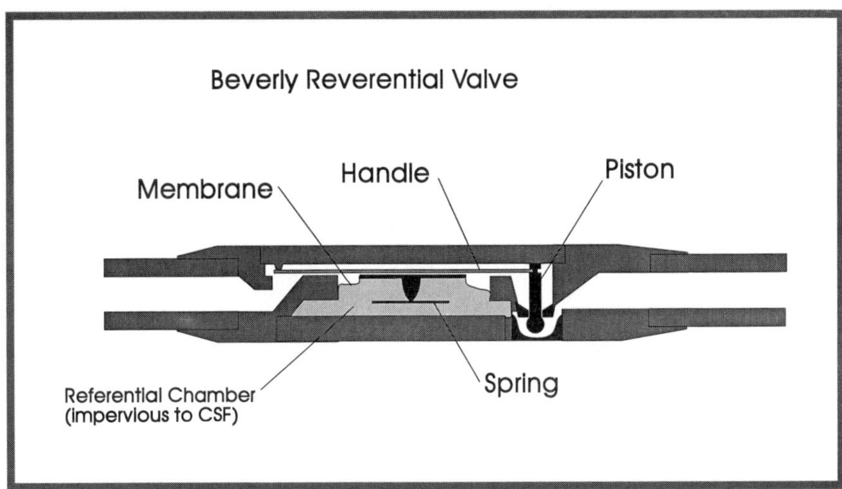

FIGURE 4-29A

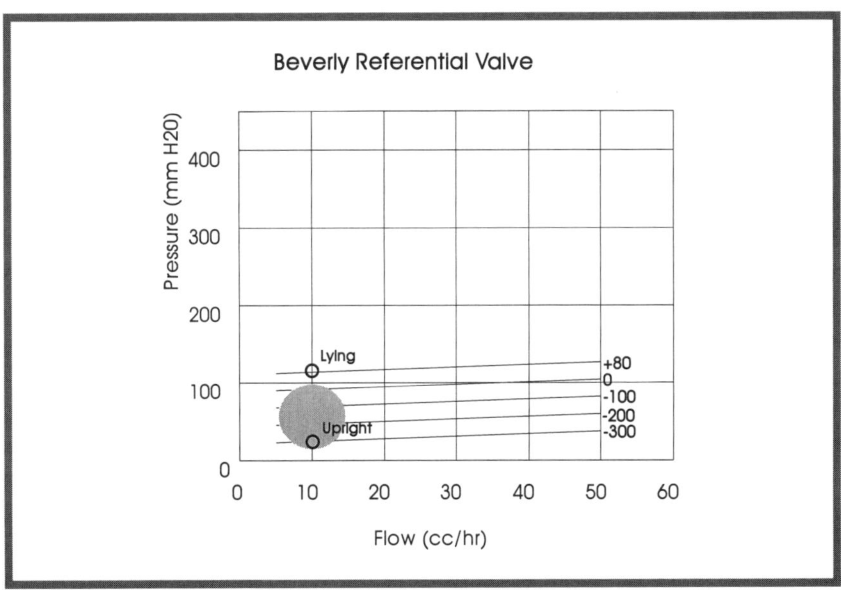

FIGURE 4-29B

DIFFERENTIAL PRESSURE SIPHON-REDUCING DEVICES

V. Meuller Heyer-Schulte Antisiphon Device

This flexible silicone diaphragm moves in response to the difference in pressure across the diaphragm (Figure 4-26). With internal negative pressure, the diaphragm moves against its silicone base to increase resistance. It is available separately or integrated with valves and/or an on-off device.

PS Medical Siphon-Control Device

This device has dual flexible silicone diaphragms that move in response to differences in pressure across them (Figure 4-27). Internal negative pressure causes both diaphragms to move against the polypropylene plastic base. The device is available separately or integrated into several valves.

PS Medical Delta Valve

This valve has a siphon-control device integrated into a contoured flow-control diaphragm valve (Figure 4-28A,B). The design of this siphon control device is slightly different in that there is minimal increase in resistance with negative distal pressures. It is available in three varieties of opening pressure: levels 1, 1.5, and 2. Level 1.5 has a pressure/flow profile midway between level 1 and 2 on the graph.

Beverly Referential Valve

With the Beverly referential valve, a piston acts essentially as a diaphragm valve. The referential chamber, presumably set at atmospheric pressure, acts as much like the siphon-reducing devices (Figure 4-29A,B). When pressure in the chamber falls below zero, the chamber moves against a handle, closing the piston and increasing resistance. Unlike the other siphon-reducing devices, this one appears impervious to the effects of overlying tissue capsule pressure.

GRAVITY-ACTUATED SIPHON-REDUCING DEVICES

Cordis Horizontal-Vertical Lumboperitoneal Valve

This inlet spring ball valve contains a synthetic ruby ball in a stainless steel seat held by a helical spring (Figure 4-30A,B). The outlet valve consists of a synthetic ruby ball in a stainless steel seat held in place by variable weights of stainless steel balls. In the vertical position, the weight of the balls acts to increase the opening pressure of the valve. In the horizontal position, the steel and ruby balls fall away from the valve seat, reducing opening pressure to that of the inlet valve only. Increasing the tension in the helical spring and/or the number of steel balls provides a range of opening pressures for children to large adults.

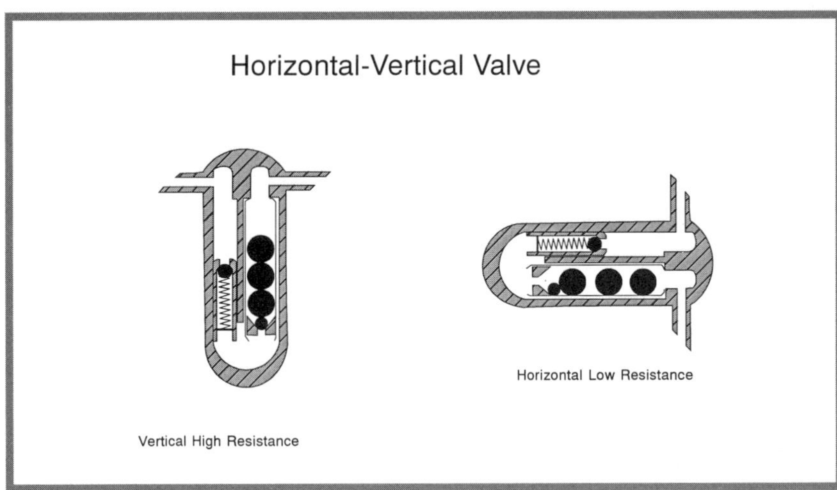

FIGURE 4-30A

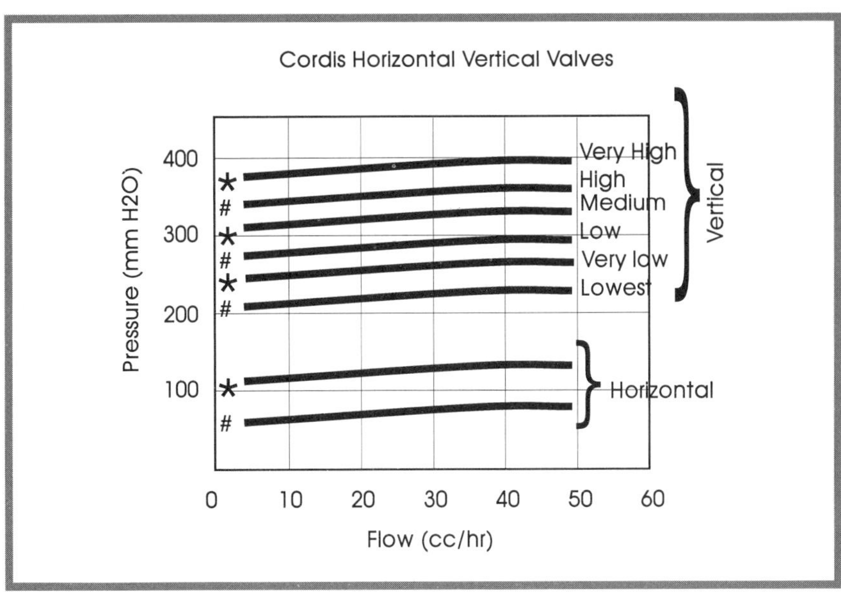

FIGURE 4-30B

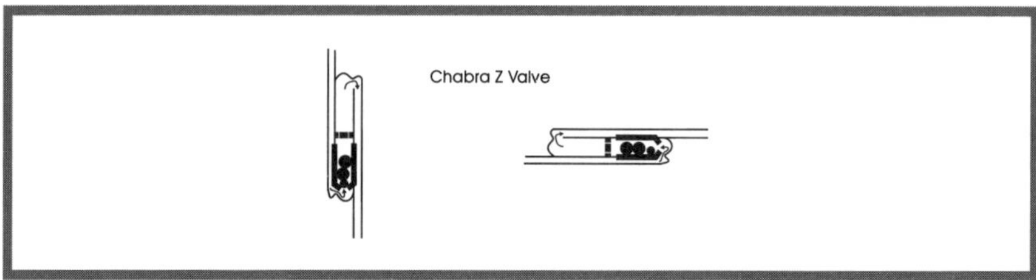

FIGURE 4-31A

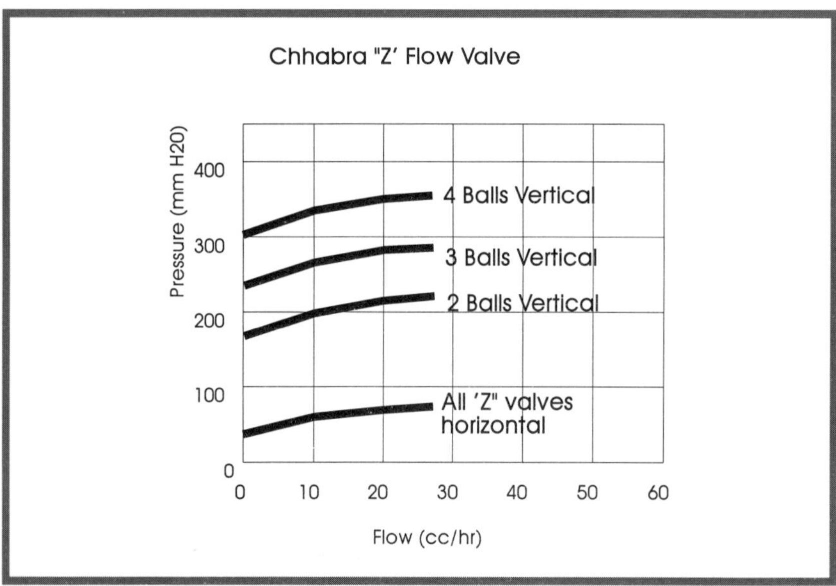

FIGURE 4-31B

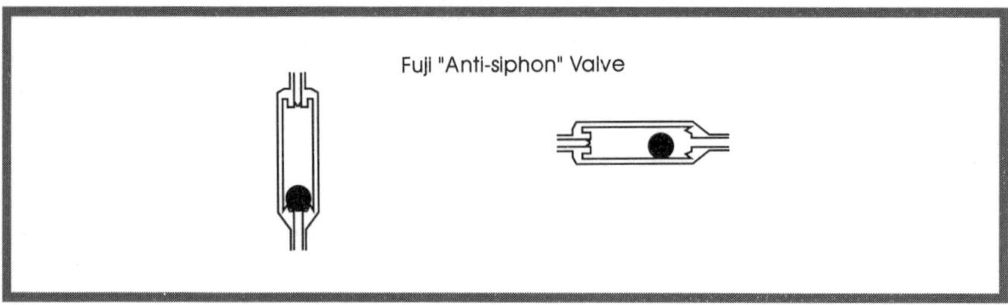

FIGURE 4-32

Category	Closing Pressure ($mm\ H_2O$) — Horizontal (Flow < 1.5 cc/hr)	Closing Pressure ($mm\ H_2O$) — Vertical (Flow < 1.5 cc/hr)	Code
Large Adults	85–125	325–445	Green
Large Adults — extreme ventricular enlargement	50–80	290–400	Brown
Large Children and Normal-Sized Adults	85–125	265–365	Yellow
Large Children and Small Adults — extreme ventricular enlargement	50–80	230–320	White
Small Children	85–125	250–285	Blue
Small Children — extreme ventricular enlargement	50–80	170–240	Red

Chhabra "Z" Flow Valve

In the Chhabra "Z," a synthetic sapphire ball rests in a stainless steel housing. An additional two to four stainless steel balls increase the opening pressure in the upright position (Figure 4-31A,B). These fall away in the horizontal position. The reservoir is silastic.

Category Distance between vertex and second or sixth intercostal space	Pressure ($mm\ H_2O$) — Horizontal (Flow=5 cc/hr)	Pressure ($mm\ H_2O$) — Vertical (Flow=25 cc/hr)	Code
to 38 cm	40-60	160-200	2 balls
39-47 cm	40-60	220-260	3 balls
48 cm or more	40-60	290-330	4 balls

Fuji Anti-Siphon Ball Valve

A single ball rests in a valve seat in upright position, increasing the resistance. The valve seat must be slightly differently shaped from the ball or the ball will become plugged (Figure 4-32). The reservoir is silastic.

Sophysa Hydrostatic Pressure Valve

This Sophysa valve has a synthetic ruby ball in a stainless steel valve seat with a stainless steel semicircular spring, as with an adjustable configuration (Figure 4-33A,B). The stainless steel wheel balance rotates under the influence of

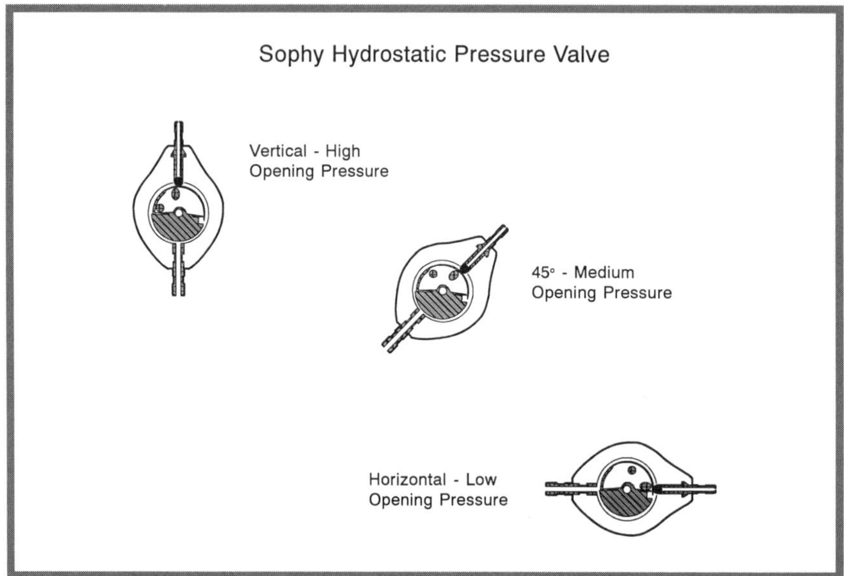

FIGURE 4-33A

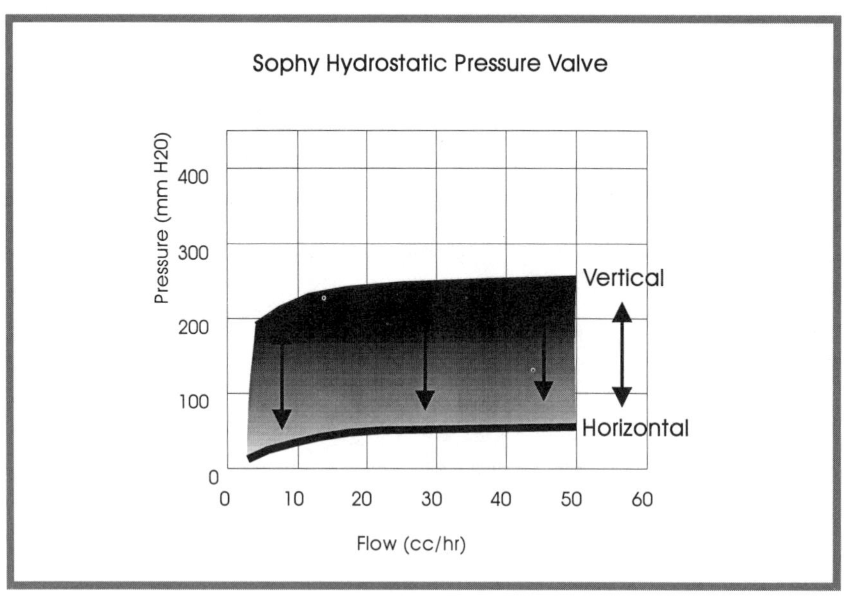

FIGURE 4-33B

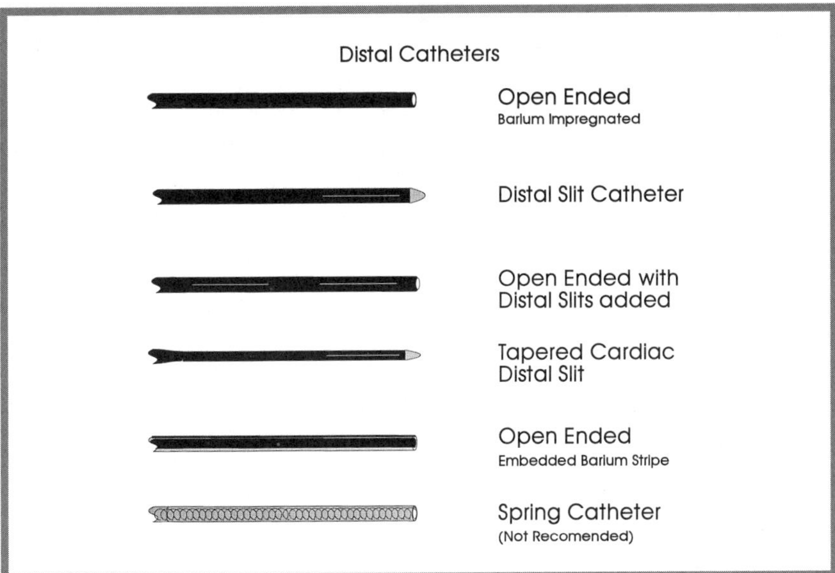

FIGURE 4-34

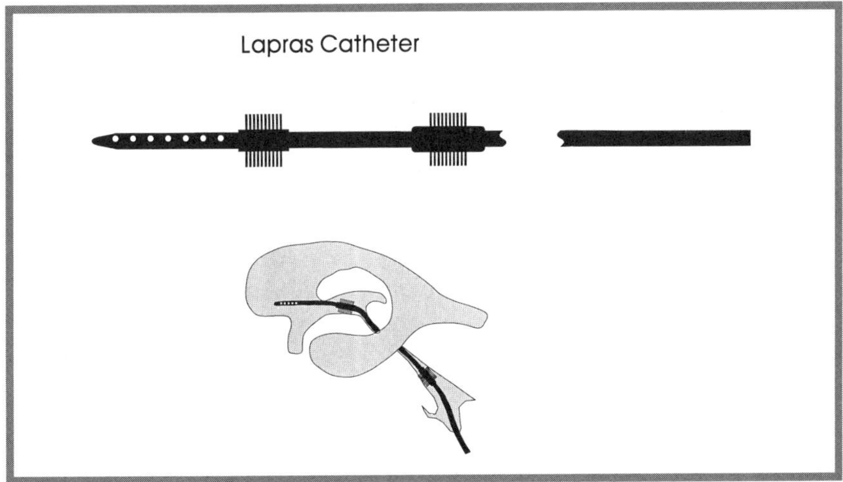

FIGURE 4-35

gravity, increasing the opening pressure in the upright position. The wheel rotates only in one direction, however. Therefore, it may not operate correctly according to position and direction of rotation of the head, i.e., if the patient lies face down, as opposed to back down, the wheel may not be able to rotate.

Category	Pressure (mm H_2O) (Flow = 50 cc/hr)
Vertical position	250
Horizontal position	50

DISTAL CATHETERS AND VALVES

PERITONEAL CATHETERS

There is not much to choose from for peritoneal catheters. They are simply shunt tubing of various lengths. They may be open-ended or closed with distal slit valves (Figure 4-34). Some manufacturers include more than one set of slits, more proximally, to avoid the problem of debris collecting in the blind tip and occluding the slit valves. Presumably, these would also eventually be occluded too, should the shunt remain in place long enough. Other manufacturers include slits with open-ended peritoneal catheters. The slits are supposed to act as safety valves should the open end be obstructed by an abdominal viscus. (Does this really happen?) The only other modification to peritoneal catheters has been the addition of an internal spring. This spring is supposed to prevent the catheters from kinking. Most catheters today are kink-resistant, and the spring has a nasty habit of eroding through the wall of the tubing, through the wall of the bowel, etc. One company offers what can only be described as a "snake-like" distal catheter, which is supposed to uncoil with growth. We all know that this catheter will be encased in a fibrous tract long before it has a chance to unwind, and, besides, there does not appear to be any strict limit on how much tubing can be put into the peritoneal cavity. In the Codman unishunt series, which have distal slit valves, this is the only valve; there is no valve in the proximal reservoir.

Codman Distal Slit Valves

Category	Closing Pressure (mm H_2O)	Code
High Pressure	90–140	•••
Medium Pressure	50–90	••
Low Pressure	20–50	•

Baxter V. Mueller Pudenz and Raimondi Peritoneal Catheters

Category	Closing Pressure (mm H_2O)	Code
High Pressure	95–144	•••
Medium Pressure	55–94	••
Low Pressure	15–54	•

Cardiac and Vascular Distal Catheters

Cardiac catheters, which actually preceded peritoneal catheters historically, are essentially the same, except that they are not open-ended but have distal slit valves (Figure 4-34). Some varieties of pediatric cardiac catheters are tapered. These catheters can, of course, be put into other venous channels, including the jugular vein, the jugular vein against the flow, the superior saggital sinus, etc. Some of the ancient varieties are not barium-impregnated but clear tubing with a radiopaque tip. Being visible on fluoroscopy helps to position these catheters. If the clear tubing were to fracture and embolize, it would be difficult to know how much had broken, if any were left behind following transvascular removal, etc.

Internal Shunts

The Lapras catheter is a single piece of tubing with holes and flanges at both ends (Figure 4-35). It is meant to connect the third with the fourth ventricle in cases where the aqueduct is likely to become occluded with tumor or even apparently in cases of congenital or acquired aqueduct stenosis, the catheter being utilized like a trochar. The flanges prevent migration of the catheter out of the aqueduct.

Lumboperitoneal (LP) Shunts

Proximal End

There are just two varieties of lumboperitoneal shunt proximal catheters (Figure 4-36A-C). The "percutaneous" type is narrow silicone tubing, .7mm inside and 1.5 mm outside diameter, which is passed through a Tuohy needle into the lumbar thecal sac. The tip is open and angled and there are several side holes. The "T" tube type has a distal "T," which must be introduced through a laminectomy and dural opening. It is, however, much less likely to migrate. The one-piece percutaneous LP shunts have a much narrower internal diameter and a higher resistance to flow, as mentioned in Chapter 2. As one-piece systems, they usually have distal slit valves. However, the proximal catheter can be cut and connected to any variety of valves and miscellaneous devices. A special connector is required to go from the narrow tubing to standard diameter devices. If you add an antisiphon device here, it will not work (see Chapter 2).

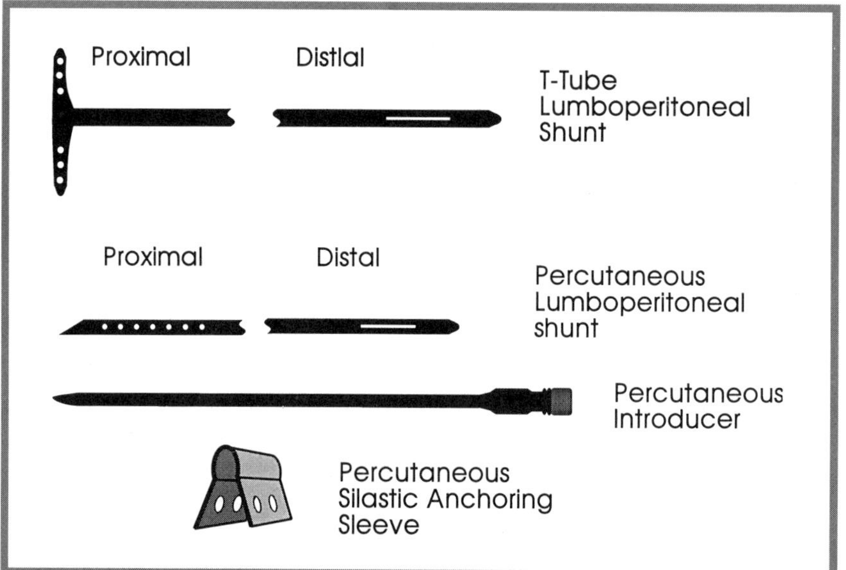

FIGURE 4-36A

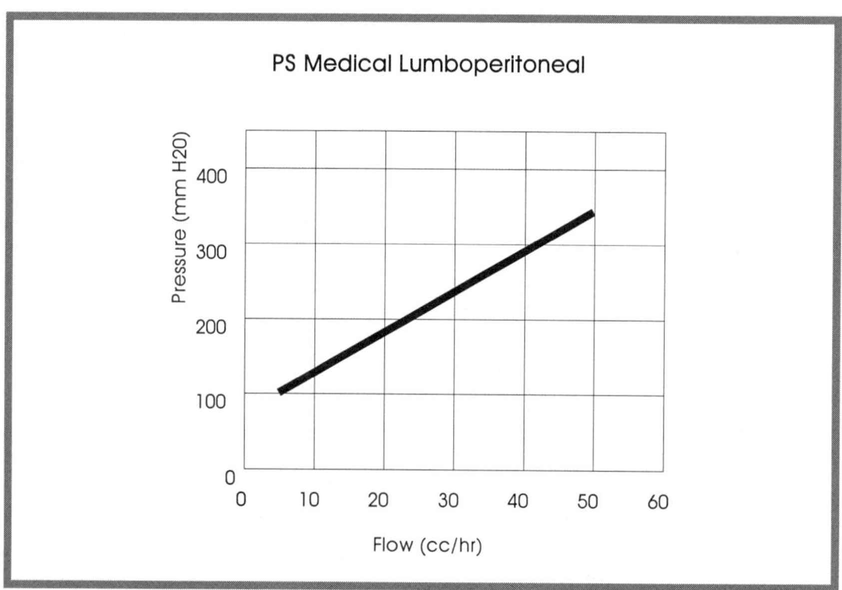

FIGURE 4-36B

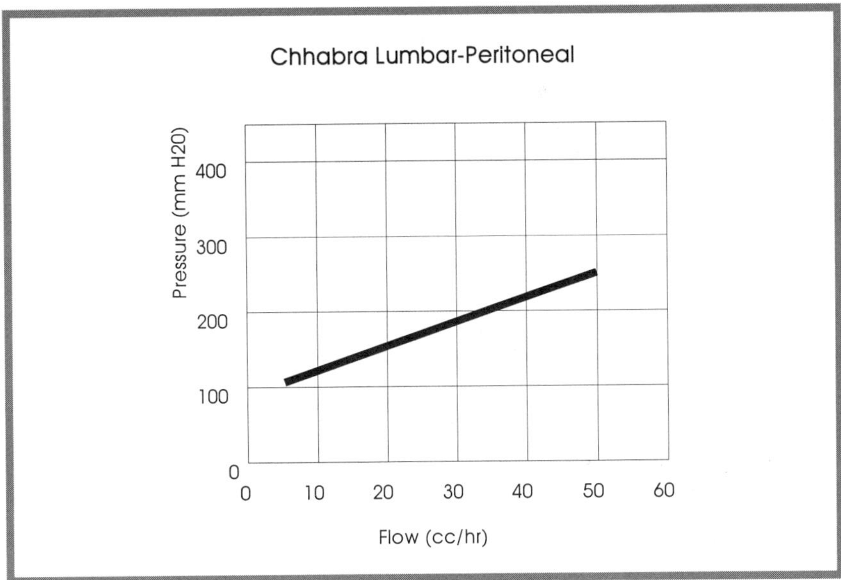

FIGURE 4-36C

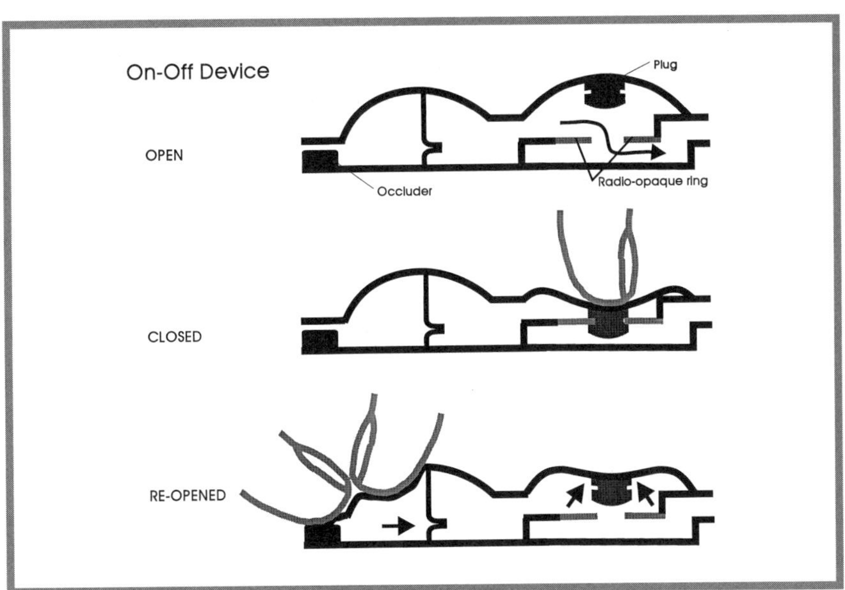

FIGURE 4-37

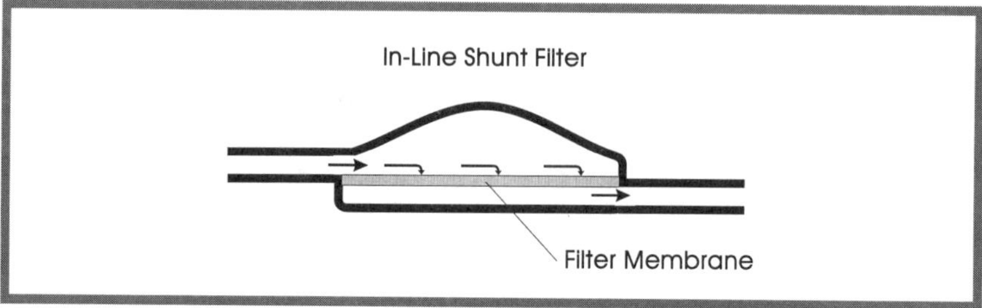

FIGURE 4-38

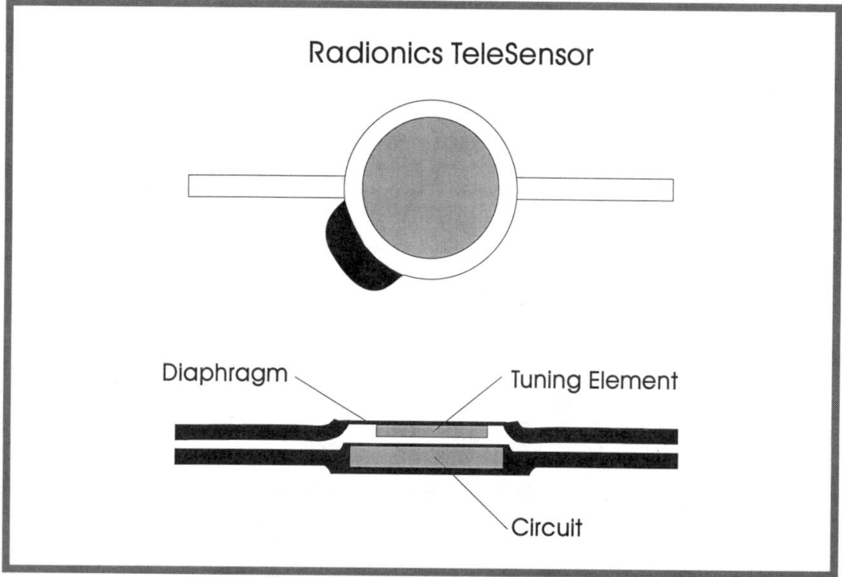

FIGURE 4-39A

MISCELLANEOUS ACCESSORIES

ON-OFF DEVICE

A radiopaque plug is attached to the silastic dome and is pressed into the radiopaque ring to occlude flow (Figure 4-37). The plug is dislodged by increasing the pressure in the lower chamber. This is accomplished by occluding flow above the valve reservoir and flushing the reservoir into the on-off valve. Tangential x-rays will show the relative position of the plug and ring to confirm the status of the device. These x-rays may be difficult to obtain and interpret. It is possible to inadvertently occlude or open the device by direct pressure. Patients (particularly children), family members, etc., may also manipulate the device themselves.

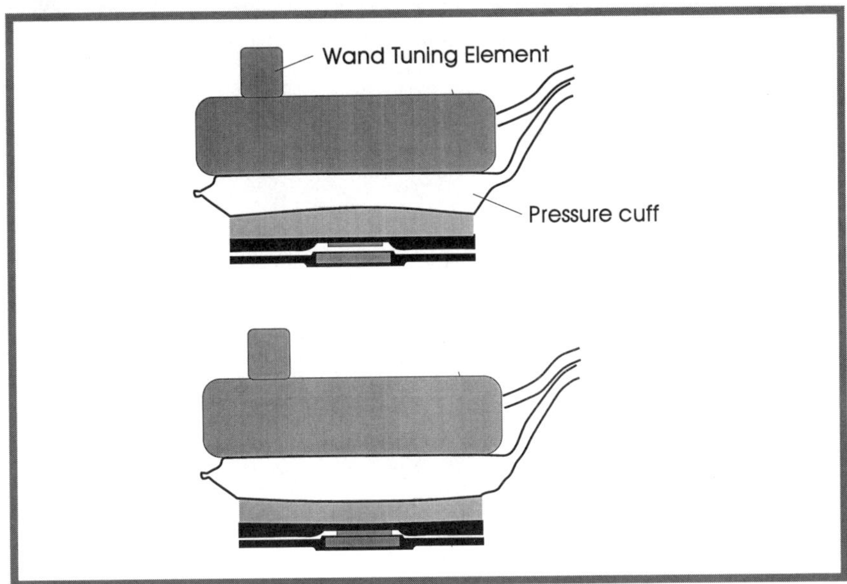

FIGURE 4-39B

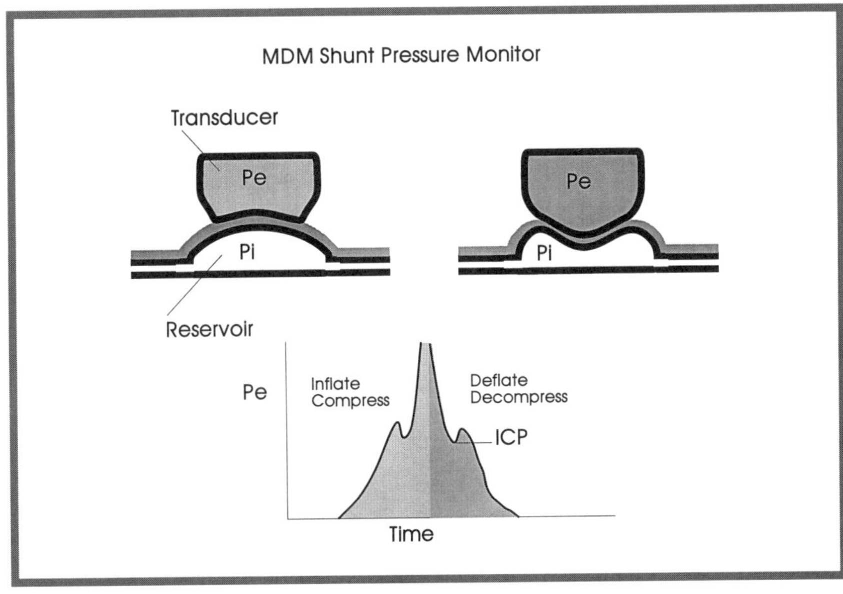

FIGURE 4-40

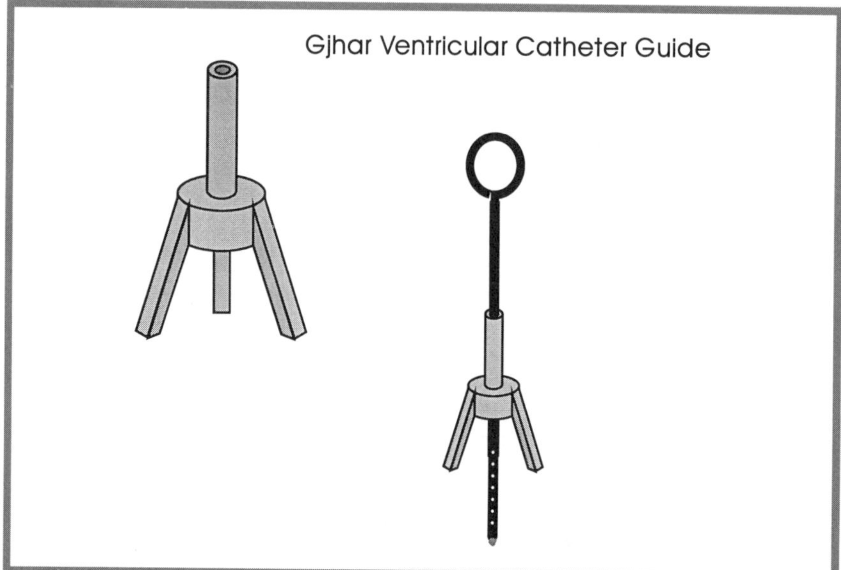

FIGURE 4-41

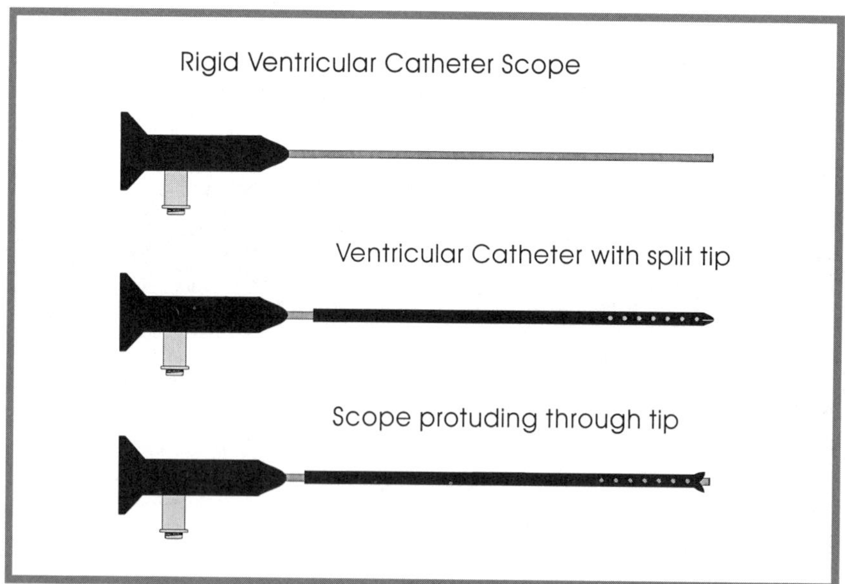

FIGURE 4-42A

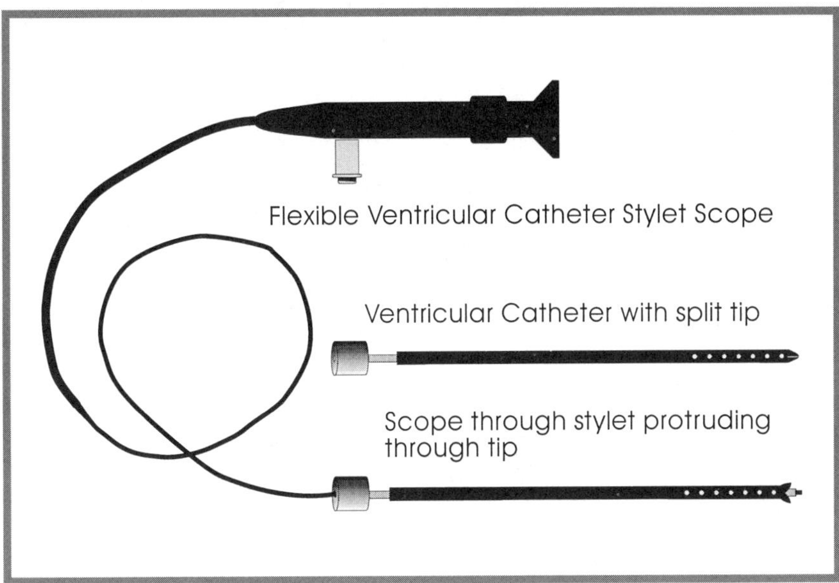

FIGURE 4-42B

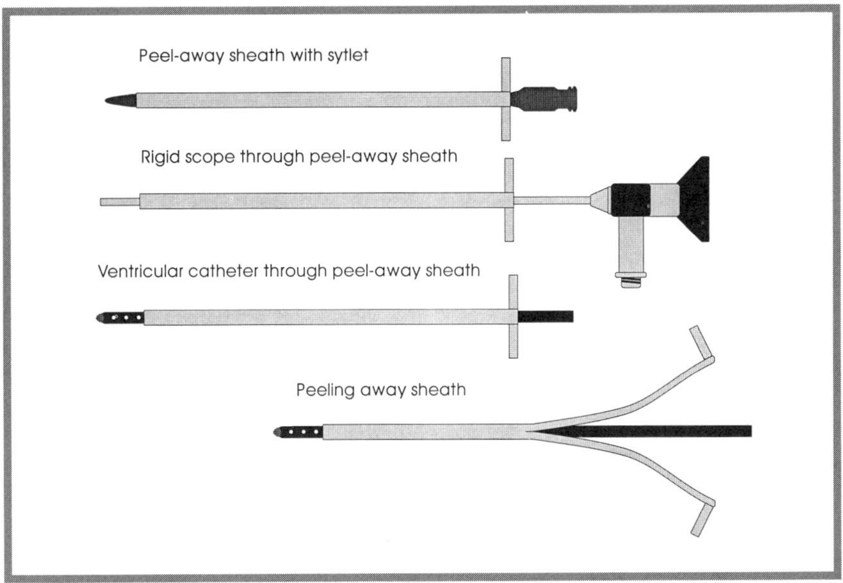

FIGURE 4-43A

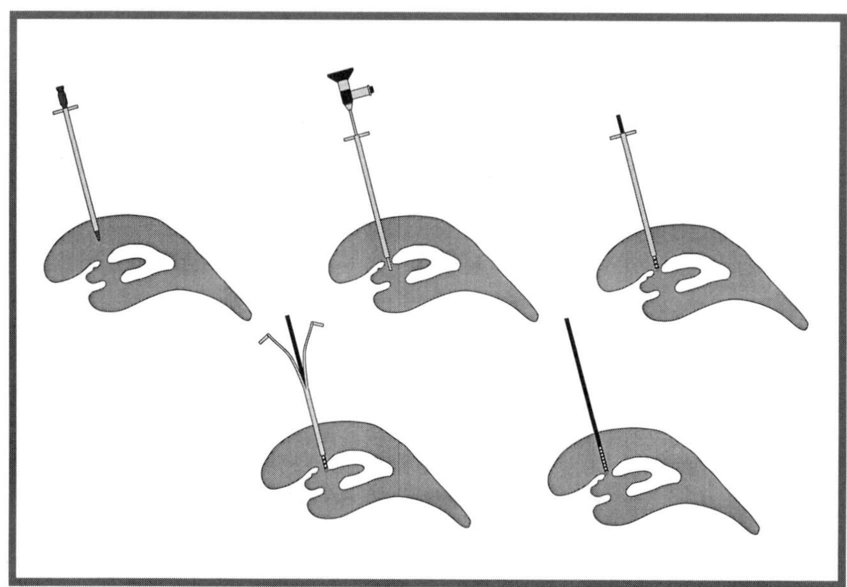

FIGURE 4-43B

HOLTER IN-LINE SHUNT FILTER

This is a 3.9-micron cellulose filter with an area of 68 mm^2 supported in a stainless steel mesh and encased in silicone. It is designed to filter malignant cells (Figure 4-38). Proof of clinical efficacy is lacking and the filter easily clogs with protein, any cells, and debris.

RADIONICS TELE-SENSOR PRESSURE TRANSDUCER

The quest for information on how the shunt is performing has led to a number of ingenious measuring devices. The first was the implantable pressure transducer manufactured by Radionics (Figure 4-39A,B). This device contains a radio frequency receiver mounted on a moveable diaphragm. When an inflatable pressure cuff is placed over the dome, the pressure that moves the dome into a closed position is the pressure in the shunt.

MDM ICP MONITOR

This system uses the force required by a transducer to deform a silastic dome to calculate intracranial pressure (Figure 4-40). The "dicrotic notch" on the down slope of the force measurement corresponds to the intraluminal pressure.

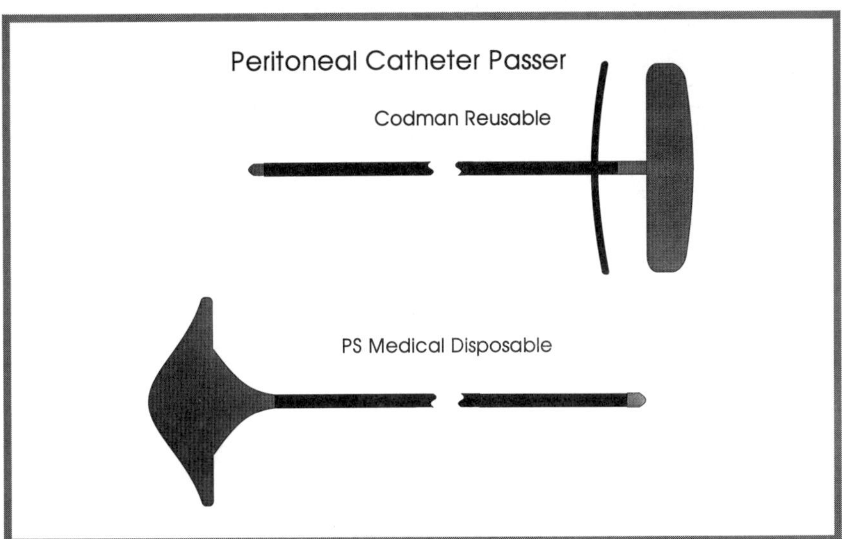

FIGURE 4-44

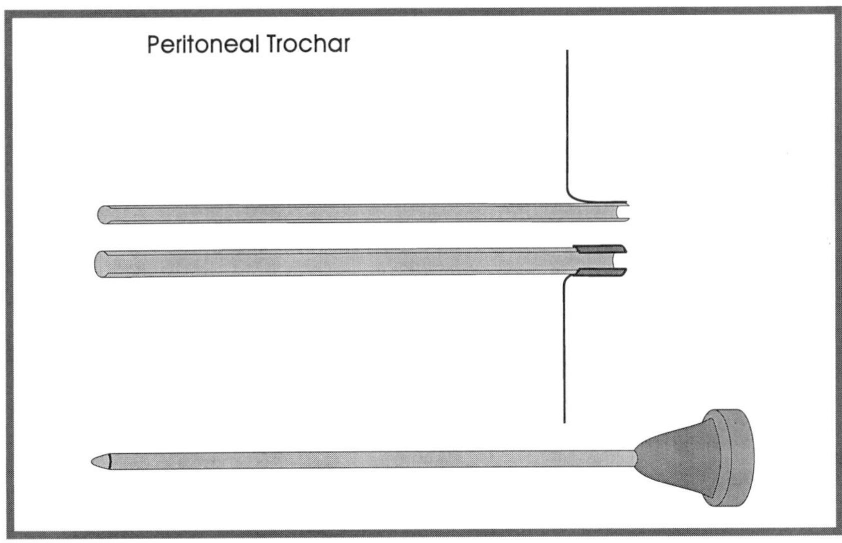

FIGURE 4-45

AIDS TO SHUNT INSERTION

GJHAR GUIDE

This tripod is designed to aid hitting the ventricles from the coronal approach (Figure 4-41), based on the principle that the skull is basically a sphere in which the ventricles are in the center. As any trajectory perpendicular to the surface of a sphere takes one to the center, this tripod ensures that the trajectory is perpendicular. A side slit ensures that either unishunts or separate ventricular catheters can be inserted into the frontal horn.

VENTRICULOSCOPES

Ventriculoscopes are increasingly coming into use in neurosurgery, and, naturally, are being applied to shunt insertion (Figure 4-42A,B). The rationale is that one can accurately position the tip of the catheter under direct vision. All the different designs--rigid, flexible, and steerable--can be adapted for shunt insertion (Figure 4-42A,B). Using a peel-away sheath, any type of scope can be used to position the sheath in the ventricle (Figure 4-43A,B). The length of ventricular catheter necessary to reach the end of the sheath is advanced down the sheath, and then the sheath is peeled away. Newer scopes are specifically designed for shunt insertion. One design consists of a small diameter rigid scope that acts as the ventricular catheter stylet and protrudes from a slit in the tip of the catheter once inside the ventricle. Smaller flexible scopes go down a hollow ventricular stylet in an analogous manner. Several questions arise about the use of scopes--do they really reduce the incidence of shunt malfunction, does the shunt move after the scope is withdrawn, and does the increased handling and surgery time increase the risk of infection?

TUNNELING DEVICES

An essential device for placing a shunt without interval incisions, a tunneling device is basically a metal tube with a central trochar that can be bent to various contours to assist with shunt subcutaneous passage (Figure 4-44). Those with detachable handles can be passed from either the upper or lower incision. Those with fixed handles can only be passed from below when implanting a unishunt. Just try to pass the valve through the tube in this situation!

PERITONEAL TROCHARS

Peritoneal trochars are not universally used or loved. For those who do use them, they are a simple means of quickly entering the peritoneal cavity, although there is always that "moment of truth" when you plunge into the peritoneal cavity and wait to see if something untoward will occur (Figure 4-45). Much like the tunneling devices, they have an outer sheath and an inner trochar. Other peel-away systems, much like the ventricular catheter placement with scopes and often employed in placing peritoneal dialysis catheters, can also be used. Of course, one can also pass a scope down the sheath and, after inflating the abdominal cavity with CO_2 gas, and place the catheter under direct vision.

Chapter 5

SHUNT COMPLICATIONS

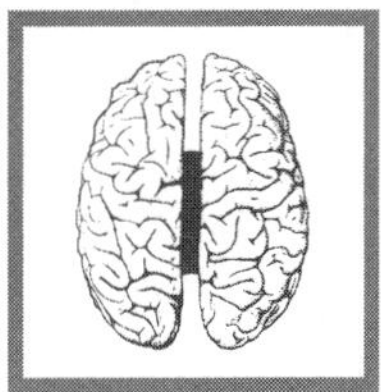

5 Shunt Complications

MECHANICAL FAILURE

Shunt complications are numerous (1-8). To quote R. McLaurin (9), it can be said that "the history of the evolution of ventricular shunting for hydrocephalus is largely a history to prevent the complications of shunting." These complications can be categorized into three groups: (1) "mechanical" failure related to improper function of the device, (2) infection related to implanted foreign material, and (3) functional failure resulting from an inadequate flow rate of a functioning shunt.

Efforts to reduce shunt complications are of considerable interest because these complications have significant adverse consequences. Clinically, there is a low but real percentage of death or neurological impairment related to shunt mechanical complications (10). It is also a painful and psycologically disturbing additional operation for the patient and his or her family. Finally, from an economical point of view, each malfunction doubles the cost of the treatment.

In trying to reduce the rate of shunt malfunction, it is necessary to define and understand the causes of these complications. Factors related to shunt failure have three potential origins: the surgeon, the patient, and the shunt. Shunt complications are in fact more often related to some combination of factors.

The importance of these factors, which may seem to be self-evident and is often taken for granted, should not be underestimated. These factors are often critical in determining the outcome of a shunt operation.

THE SURGEON

Even if the ideal shunt existed, it would be quickly rendered useless by improper surgical technique during implantation. Shunt failure rate is known to be higher in inexperienced hands, and shunt surgery must be seen as technically demanding. The efforts toward the reduction in shunt infection focus on the surgical environment and technique. The same type of focus is required on the problem of shunt mechanical failure.

While analogies of CSF shunts to plumbing are perhaps inevitable and somewhat regrettable, there is at least one advantage to this type of comparison. While common sense and skill are usually employed in typical home repairs, it is often lacking in the application to shunting situations. For anyone who has faced a plumbing problem at home, it is easy to understand that, sooner or later, drainage problems are unavoidable. However, the best material properly installed and correctly utilized has the greatest chance for problem-free longevity. The situation is the same for shunts; complications are perhaps inevitable, but, for a large part, they are quite preventable.

However, perhaps because of the analogy to plumbing, shunt surgery is not usually considered very difficult or prestigious. Very often, the surgery is delegated to people not very well trained in this particular surgical field. Most neurosurgical services, particularly pediatric, perform as many shunt revisions as insertions. Faced with this horrendous failure to adequately treat hydrocephalus with a single procedure and inundated with shunt complications, many accept these complications as inevitable. Believing that their own individual efforts and equipment are the best possible, surgeons usually cling to what they were "brought up on" with almost religious fervor. Alternatively, the problem of hydrocephalus treatment is seen from a single viewpoint, and the accorded solution is a modification of some facet of the shunt procedure or equipment with no data to support this effort. This has led to a bewildering array of shunt equipment (11), fueled in part by the shunt companies' willingness to please individual surgeons and by competition for market share, with innovative technology seen as providing a competitive edge.

A procedure that improves the condition of more than 100,000 patients per year worldwide is also worthy of our best talent, experience, and attention.

THE PATIENT

Hydrocephalus is a condition, not a disease, and no two hydrocephalic patients are exactly alike. Each case must be considered carefully. One must not forget that, for the patient, the best shunt is no shunt. This is, of course, in the presence of a valid alternative. In many cases, it is possible to avoid a shunt. This is particularly true in the treatment of "obstructive" hydrocephalus due to a blockage of the CSF pathways localized between the aqueduct of Sylvius and the outlets of the fourth ventricles; endoscopic fenestration of the floor of the third ventricles is successful in up to 90% of correctly selected patients (12). In tumors associated with hydrocephalus, normal CSF circulation can be reestablished after removal of the tumor in a significant number of cases (13).

However, despite this progress, a large number of patients still need to be shunted. In those patients, several factors need to be taken into consideration because of their potential effect on the occurrence of shunt complications:

- Patients Age (14–17): The younger the patient, the thinner the skin, the physiologically lower the intracranial pressure, and the greater the potential for growth; the older the patient, the higher the differential pressure applied to the shunt. From a theoretical point of view, it is quite impossible to get a shunt to match the needs of both a newborn or premature infant, as well as that of an adolescent or an adult. The requirements are not the same from one age to another: small valve contour, low CSF pressures in the youngest patients, resistance to overdrainage phenomenon in the oldest.

• Ventricular Configuration (18–21) (e.g. multilocution, Dandy-Walker cyst, etc.): Several anatomical conditions are predisposed to shunt problems and require special care. For instance, a multiloculated and enlarged ventricle can be treated by several shunts resulting in a complex drainage system and increased risk of malfunctions. Fenestration of the loculations prior to a single shunt insertion can simplify the situation and reduce the risk of malfunction. Dandy-Walker malformation is another example. On one hand, one can choose to insert the shunt in the lateral ventricles, which is easier, but increases the risk of a trapped fourth ventricle; on the other hand, one can shunt the cyst, which is more difficult, but carries less risk of secondary aqueduct stenosis.

• CSF Composition (e.g., debris, blood) (22): Ideally, in order to minimize the probability of obstruction, the CSF should be normal at shunt insertion. Often, this is not the case. Debris can be present in the CSF after treatment of ventriculitis or after surgery involving the ventricles. Blood clots form in the ventricles from a variety of sources. Clearly, debris or blood clots in the CSF can promote obstruction of the drainage system at various levels (the most vulnerable part of a shunt varies according to the design of that shunt). In these circumstances, inserting a temporary external ventricular drain pending CSF normalization, prior to inserting a shunt may reduce the risk of malfunction.

These examples illustrate just how complicated patients with hydrocephalus may be and how many possible treatment strategies are available. One must spend considerable time analyzing each particular clinical case in terms of the patient, the status of the ventricular system, and the state of the CSF, and try to determine an optimal strategy. Finally, one should never forget that a commitment to a shunt is usually life-long, and, like marriage, not to be entered into lightly.

THE SHUNT

A shunt is a mechanical device in which two different characteristics have to be considered: the design of the shunt and the hydrodynamic properties of the system.

From the hydrodynamic standpoint, it seems that an ideal shunt is possible to define while actually quite impossible to manufacture. To quote H. Pornoy (1), it can be said that "an ideal valve should be flow controlled. Such a valve would have to continuously determine the formation rate and the rate of outflow through natural channels and regulate the flow through the valve so as to remove only the excess fluid." Excess fluid is defined as the percentage of the CSF secretion rate not able to be reabsorbed through natural channels under physiological intracranial pressure conditions. At present, there is no mechanism that can accomplish these requirements. The wide number of available systems, differing in terms of their hydrodynamic properties, shape, configuration, and material, as well as the accessories that can be added, attest to the attempts to achieve the ideal shunt, but none of them succeeding completely.

As the perfect shunt does not exist and as there are many unknowns regarding the treatment requirements in hydrocephalus, one can take the attitude that all shunt systems are essentially the same, and it really makes no difference which one is used. However, we think, particularly with the newer shunt designs (23), that there are significant differences between the shunt designs and their hydrodynamic properties, and despite the uncertainties, one is obliged to logically consider all the available information, including clinical trials.

"BEST COMPROMISE"

One must never lose sight of the fact that any choice among the numerous possibilities that exist in the treatment of hydrocephalus is usually the result of a compromise between two or more risk factors. The shunt characteristics, including configuration, hydrodynamic properties, and material, are a compromise between ease of insertion, risk of disconnection, risk of early or late obstruction, expense, and ease of manufacture. As far as the patient is concerned, one often compromises between the pressure-flow requirements at the time of surgery and those later on in life. As far as the surgeon is concerned, compromises occur as well at many stages during the course of patient management.

DEFINITION OF SHUNT MECHANICAL FAILURE

Definition of shunt mechanical failure is not easy, and the literature is often quite confusing. Many of the reported series of shunt failure are difficult to interpret or compare for two main reasons: (1) the debate that surrounds what constitutes a shunt failure and (2) the types of statistical analysis applied to these series.

While problems directly related to the shunt (e.g., proximal obstruction of the ventricular catheter) are universally acknowledged as shunt complications, problems related to imperfect shunt function (e.g., subdural collection, postural headache) are sometimes more difficult to interpret (24,25). Finally, some shunts are inserted with deliberate plans to revise, i.e., lengthen the peritoneal catheter or upgrade the valve, at some time in the future. While carried out in an elective and planned fashion, we would still maintain that as far as the patient is concerned, this represents a complication. In terms of imperfect shunt function, any problem that requires a subsequent operation seems a reasonable definition of shunt complication. In fact, we would broaden this concept to hold that any subsequent surgical procedure related to the treatment of hydrocephalus represents a shunt complication. We would also include any death directly related to a shunt failure where no operation took place.

In effect, causes of shunt failure are clearly time-related events with different onsets. Whereas an improperly tied connector or improper placement will manifest itself very quickly, problems such as degeneration and fracture of the tubing may take many years. For this reason, it is necessary to have a sufficient follow-up to detect those shunt failures that occur late after surgery. Because of the time-related nature of these events, and because patients are followed for various periods of time, or lost to follow-up, survival analysis (life-table analysis) is required to adequately assess the probability of each type of shunt failure at different times after surgery. The multiplication of variables and the interaction between them that arises in the analysis of subsequent shunt failure in the same patient makes the statistical interpretation of the results questionable.

CLASSIFICATION

Classification of shunt mechanical complications can be assessed in several different ways:

- They can be related to the function of the shunt and then divided into two groups: underdrainage and overdrainage.
- They can be related to the different components of the device: complications at the level of the ventricular catheter, complications of the valve system, complications related to connectors, etc.
- They can also be classified according to their mechanisms: improper placement of the ventricular catheter, improper placement of the distal tubing in the drainage cavity, overdissection of the subcutaneous tissue, migration of the shunt system, clots, choroid plexus, etc.

Actually, it seems logical to use these three different classifications together, the first one giving the net effect for the patient, the second the site of the complication along the shunt system, and the third the mechanism of that complication. Finally, it is possible to relate these complications to the surgical technique, the patient, or the device itself. This is of the greatest interest because it allows us to better identify and understand the interactions between these three factors (all together or separately) and shunt malfunction. This basic knowledge is mandatory to optimize, at present, the treatment of hydrocephalus and define areas for future progress

INCIDENCE OF FAILURE

We previously referred to shunt mechanical complications as being time-related. This is better understood when looking at the survival functions of different series of shunted patients (5,6,26) (Figure 5-1). These series from the literature show that month after month, year after year, shunt complications continue to occur. All these pediatric patients were treated with "conventional" pressure-regulating systems. It is interesting to note that, from East to West, from North to South, in the past and at present, the results are very similar. The risk for a patient to experience a shunt failure is maximum in the first few months after surgery, ranging from 25% to 40% at one-year follow-up. Later on, after this critical period, the risk remains around 4% to 5% per year. The mean survival time for a shunt in these series was about five years.

An analysis of the time of occurrence of each type of complication and distribution over the follow-up in a large pediatric series (6) (Figure 5-2) shows significant differences; some types of shunt failure tends to occur soon after surgery and some later; for some failures, the period "at risk" is quite short while others

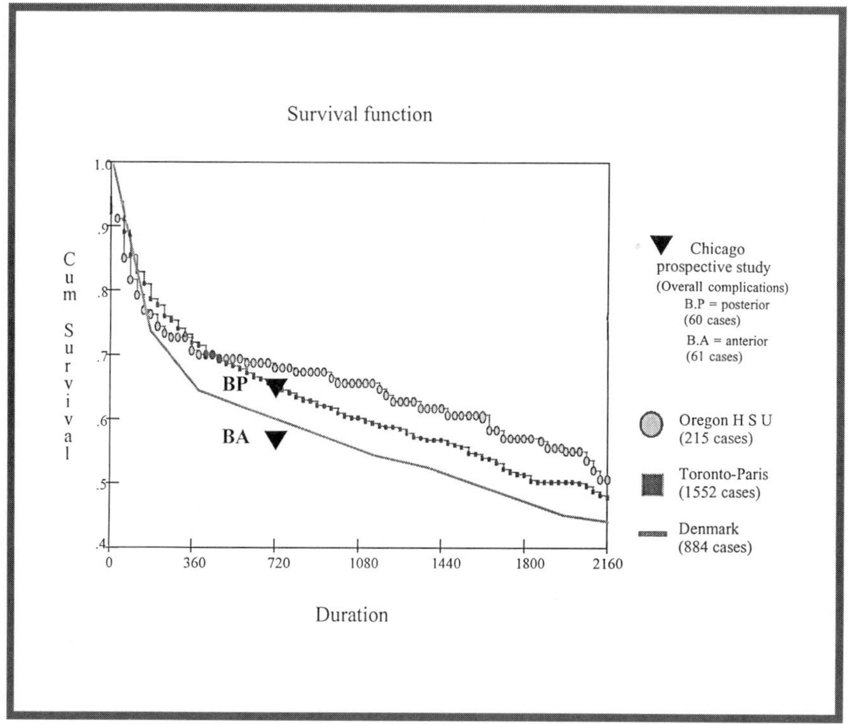

FIGURE 5-1
Survival function of four pediatric series of patients treated with "conventional" shunts. The time interval for analysis was one month over a period of six years. The cumulative proportion of shunts not revised (that "survived") is represented by the Y axis. The X axis is the length of follow-up (in days) after the first shunt insertion.

are spread all along the follow-up period. For a particular type of shunt failure, the causative factors are frequently not the same over time. For example, the ventricular catheter can be occluded soon after surgery by a ventricular clot or later by the choroid plexus. It is also probable that these factors are not the same in children as in adults.

As mentioned previously, there are several possible classifications for shunt failure. As it is virtually impossible to determine retrospectively the actual causes of many complications, most of the reported data give only an approximation of what really happened. However, based on these data, it can be assumed that the largest group of shunt complications is shunt obstruction. A breakdown of shunt failure in a large pediatric series (6) showed that shunt obstruction was responsible for 56% of shunt mechanical complications and fracture for 15% (Figure 5-3). Altogether, obstruction and fracture were responsible for more than two-thirds of shunt failure in this particular series.

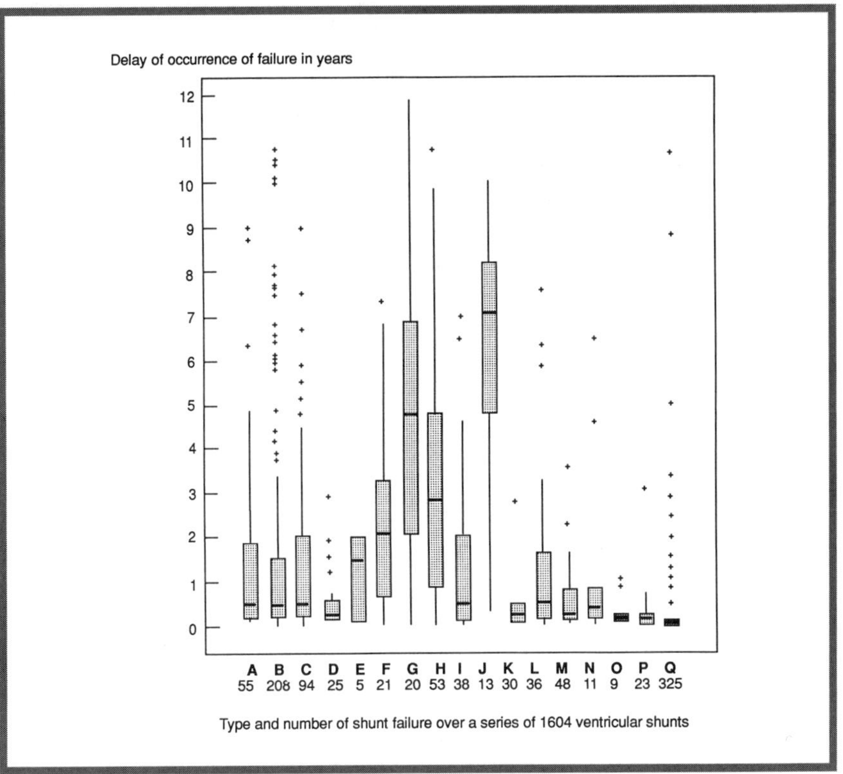

FIGURE 5-2
Multiple box and wisker plot of delay of occurrence of shunt complications (years) versus type of complications. The central box covers the middle 50% of the data values, between the lower and the upper quartile; the "wiskers" extend out to the extremes, while the central line is at the median. The shunt complications are codified as follows: A = shunt obstruction without precision of the site of obstruction in the patientís file; B = ventricular catheter obstruction; C = valve obstruction; D = obstruction of an accessory (millipor filter, antisiphon device); E = peritoneal pseudocyst; F = fracture or disconnection of the ventricular catheter; G = fracture or disconnection of the distal catheter; H = disconnection at the level of the reservoir; I = migration of the shunt; J = lengthening procedure because of a distal catheter becoming too short; K = improper placement of the ventricular or distal catheter; L = post-shunt isolated ventricles (lateral or fourth); M = "classical" manifestations of overdrainage (subdural collection, slit-ventricles syndrome, orthostatic hypotension, craniosynostosis); N = no evidence of shunt malfunction found at the time of surgery; O = miscellaneous; P = skin problems; Q = shunt infection. The number under each code letter represents the total number of this particular complication observed over the 12-year follow-up period.

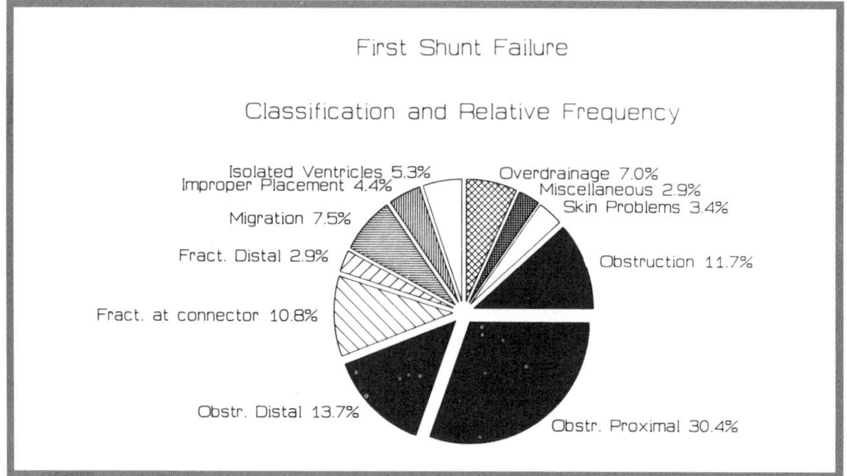

FIGURE 5-3
Relative frequency of first shunt complications in a pediatric series.

ANALYSIS OF SPECIFIC SHUNT COMPLICATIONS

In this section, an analysis of each type of shunt mechanical complication will be made. However, while several observations and, occasionally, recommendations for procedures to avoid these complications can be made, what frequently emerges is the enormous complexity of interrelated factors. Attempts to avoid one set of predisposing causes often leads to increased exposure to others. The management of these complications when they occur requires careful analysis so that other unexpected problems do not ensue.

OCCLUSIONS

As shown in the previous section, shunt occlusion represent about one-half of shunt complications in pediatric series. This percentage is smaller in adult series but still significant.

It is interesting to note that risk for shunt obstruction varies during the follow-up period. The risk is highest in the immediate postoperative period. In the series reported in the previous section (6), the probability of occurrence of a shunt obstruction was about 7% in the first postoperative month then dropped to 2% to 4% for the four following months. After month five, the probability of such a complication was less than 0.5% per month for the next ten years (Figure 5-4). This variation's risk results from certain causes of shunt obstruction occurring more commonly during particular time periods. Debris or clot in the CSF or misplacement of the proximal catheter is probably a cause in these early occlusions, whereas choroid plexus ingrowth, ependymal reaction, or immune reaction predominate in delayed occlusion (22,27,28).

A shunt can be occluded at three different levels: (1) at the entry point (proximal occlusion), (2) at the level of the valve system (valve obstruction), and

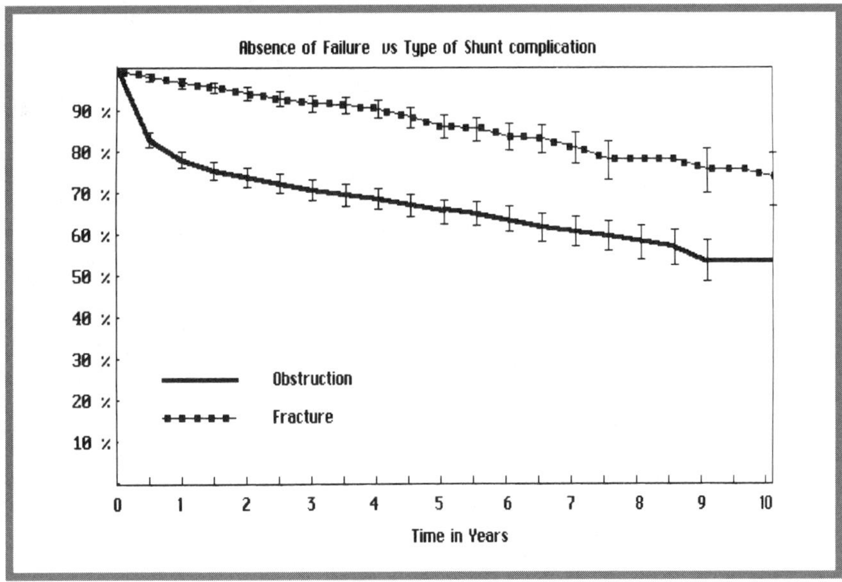

FIGURE 5-4

Probability of nonoccurrence of two different types of shunt complications: obstruction and fracture. The obstruction curve demonstrates a two-step slope, with a risk maximum in the immediate postoperative period, while the risk of fractures or disconnection appears more constant over the follow-up period.

(3) at the level of the distal end (distal catheter occlusion). Factors influencing these occlusions are still being investigated, but nevertheless, an analysis of the potential causes of these types of shunt failure can still be made.

PROXIMAL OCCLUSIONS

An inert catheter floating in a pristine cavity filled with pure water has no reason to become obstructed. However, silicone catheters are not entirely inert (29), the CSF may contain various debris or tissue, and the cavity can become contracted to the point of putting in apposition the shunt catheter and wall (30), or the choroid plexus floating in the CSF may naturally be swept along by the CSF current in the direction of the proximal catheter (Figure 5-5).

CSF Contents

Blood or cellular debris have a propensity to block the lumen and distal holes on ventricular catheters. A period of temporary external drainage would appear to be a solution to this problem.

Catheter Tip Location

Catheter location is probably one of the most ancient controversies in the treatment of hydrocephalus. This debate is centered on standard teaching,

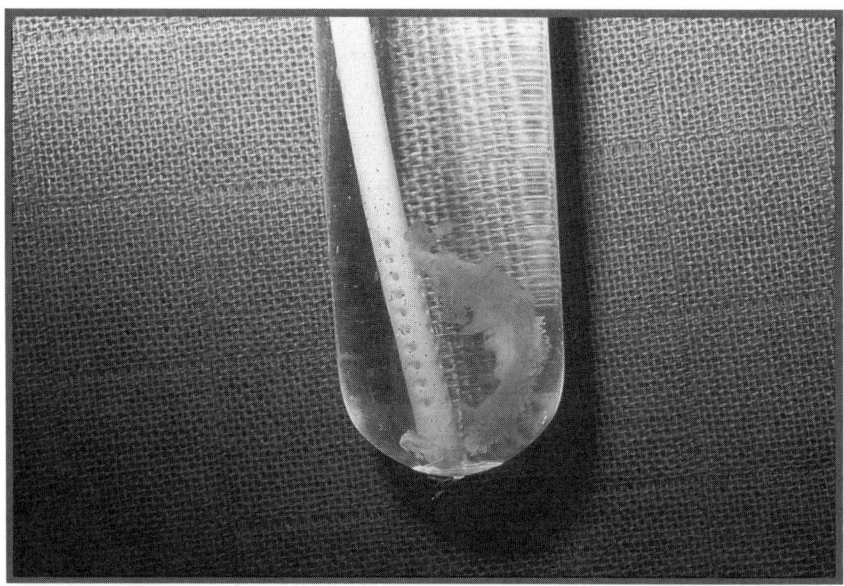

FIGURE 5-5
Ingrowth of the choroid plexus into the ventricular catheter. This type of complication is promoted in small ventricles where the holes of the catheter are close to the choroid plexus. At shunt revision time, there is a risk of avulsion of the plexus and intraventricular bleeding when the attached ventricular catheter is pulled out without intraluminal cauterization, as in this case.

which dictates that the choroid plexus is the agent responsible for proximal catheter obstruction. Conventional wisdom states that the ventricular catheter has to be placed in front of the foramen of Monro to avoid the choroid plexus. However, a ventricular catheter inserted in the frontal horn via an occipital route can be pulled back onto the choroid plexus due to head growth, or alternately, collapse of the ventricles may cause the catheter to migrate into the surrounding brain. Moreover, there are several other tissues besides the choroid plexus that may obstruct the catheter. These include ependymal cells, glial tissue, connective tissue, and leptomeninges (22,28,29,31). Two clinical studies have examined the issue of ventricular catheter placement. One retrospective study (32) found lateral ventricular catheters placed via the frontal route had a lower obstruction rate than catheters placed occipitally. A recent prospective randomized study (26) found the opposite, when all the shunt complications were taken into account! In another pediatric study, already mentioned (6), an analysis of proximal obstruction versus catheter tip location showed fewer proximal obstructions when the catheter was intended to be placed in the posterior part of the ventricles via an occipital route than when it was pushed in the direction of the frontal horn (Figure 5-6). Actually, it is probable that there is no one ideal place to locate the tip of the ventricular catheter; probably, the lowest risk location is the place that remains larger after ventricular decompression drainage, this place varying from one patient to another (33-35).

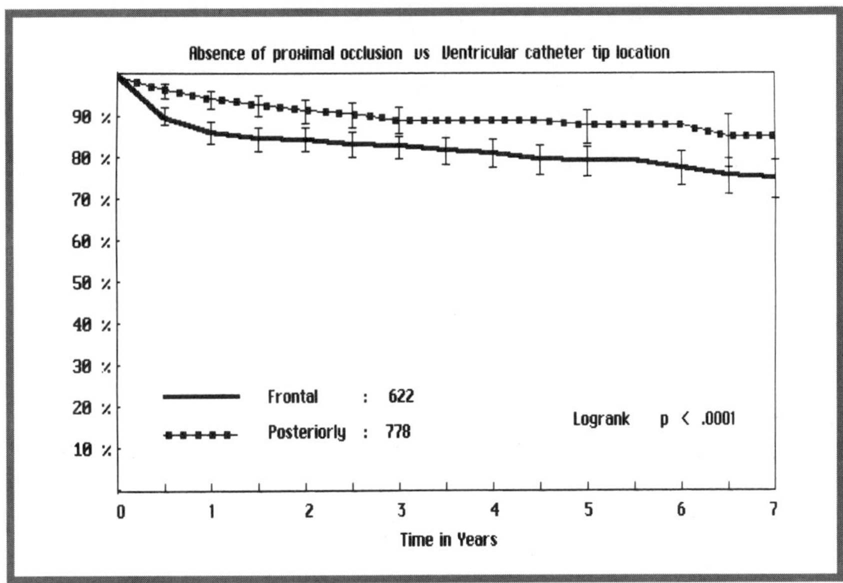

FIGURE 5-6
Correlation between tip location of ventricular catheters (inserted via an occipital route) and occurrence of proximal obstruction.

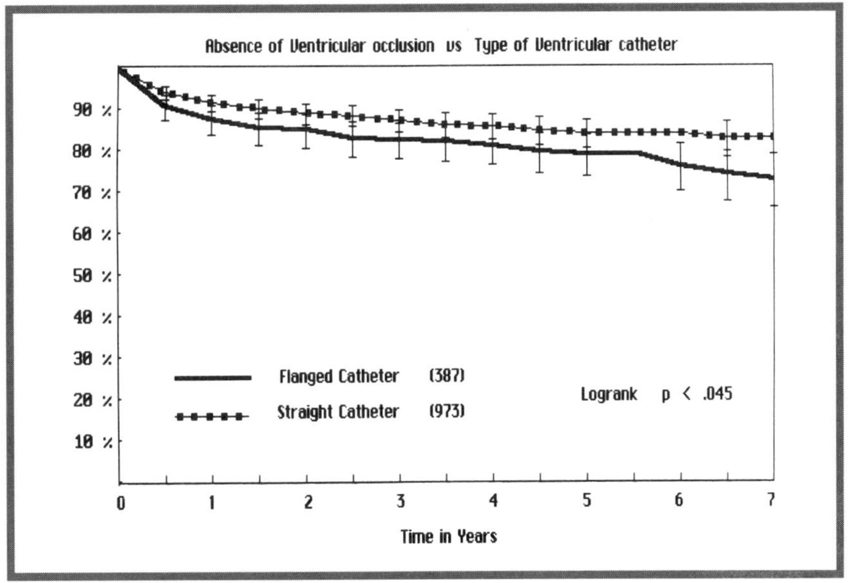

FIGURE 5-7
Probability of occurrence of a proximal obstruction in two groups of patients shunted with different types of ventricular catheter, flanged and "regular."

Other confounding factors include catheter stiffness and the method of contouring the ventricular catheter around the burr hole. Because of the elasticity of silicone rubber, catheters not held rigidly at right angles will tend to lie against the ventricular wall no matter where they are placed. It has also been suggested that ventricular catheters be placed with assistance (e.g. endoscope, x-rays, ultrasound, etc.) to ensure ideal placement (36,37). While this avoids insertion into the temporal horn or brain parenchyma , these methods carry their own risk of morbidity, and catheters may still obsturct from causes unrelated to placement.

When faced with an occluded and stuck ventricular catheter, one is at risk of major hemorrhage if the attached catheter is simply avulsed. In some cases, it is possible to overcome this problem by coagulating on the metal stylet inserted to the tip of the ventricular catheter or by using the coagulation wire of an endoscope; frequently, this allows a sufficient retraction of the invading choroid plexus to withdraw the catheter easily and safely.

Type of Ventricular Catheter

Several ventricular catheter tip designs (flanged, recessed holes) have been proposed to keep the holes of the ventricular catheter away from the walls of the ventricles and the choroid plexus (38). However, there is no evidence that these devices are able to prevent proximal occlusion from occurring. Moreover, they may promote firm attachment of the choroid plexus to the tubing (Figure 5-7).

TABLE 5-1

	Ventricular Size		
Mechanical Complication	Slit	Normal	Enlarged
None	55.7	78.3	69.3
Failure	44.3	21.7	36.1

Cross-tabulation of ventricular size by shunt mechanical complications showing the percentage of complications significantly higher ($p = 3.7E^{-3}$) in patients developing slit ventricles on the CT during in the postoperative period.

TABLE 5-2

	Ventricular Size		
Typed Shunt Occlusion	Slit	Normal	Enlarged
Proximal obstruction	81.3	8.1	21.4
Other obstruction	18.7	91.9	78.6

Cross-tabulation of ventricular size by types of shunt occlusion, showing that almost all the shunt malfunctions in patients having slit ventricles are proximal obstruction. ($p = 5E^{-7}$).

Ventricular Size

The size of the ventricle is an important factor in delayed proximal catheter occlusion (6,39,40). Wherever the tip of the proximal catheter may be located, collapsed ventricles secondary to overdrainage phenomenon put into contact the holes of the ventricular catheter with the walls of the ventricles (or, even worse, with the choroid plexus). Slit-like ventricles after shunting are common in patients treated with conventional pressure-regulating devices; this condition can be as frequent as 40% in the reported pediatric series (6). The risk of proximal occlusion in this situation is almost inevitable (Tables 5-1, 5-2). Not all parts of the ventricular system are distended to the same degree (33). In children, particularly those with congenital anomalies, the occipital horns remain large, and catheter tips thus located may have a lower risk of obstruction, as previously suggested.

Occurrence of slit-like ventricles is related to the patient's age at shunt insertion time (potential of brain growth), existence of brain atrophy, prior shunting, brain compliance (which is related to the acuteness of hydrocephalus), and the hydrodynamic properties of the shunt. All available shunts overdrain more or less. However, it appears that a reduction of overdrainage, as obtained with newly developed shunts (23), and the subsequent decrease of the number of slit-like ventricles after shunting may reduce the incidence of proximal obsruction. In a series of patients treated with a flow-regulating device (41), the correlation between slit-ventricles and proximal obstruction disappeared. As shown in Figure 5-8, decreased "delayed" ventricular obstruction dramatically improved the shunt survival curve. The probability of shunt malfunction at Five-years follow-up was 25% as compared with the "classical" value of 50%.

VALVE OBSTRUCTIONS

The second component at risk for obstruction is the valve system itself. Some occlusions are rarely due to an improper manufacturing of the device, which mandates a patency check test at shunt insertion time. This also raises the issue of manufacturing standards and recommendations for shunt testing during manufacture. Besides this manufacturing problem, shunt valves create areas of flow restriction, more or less marked depending on the type of valve, and dead space, which predisposes to accumulation of debris and tissue colonization, which can lead to occlusion. Limitation of overdrainage, achieved by severe flow restriction in the valve system, can increase the risk of valve obstruction (41).

Valve obstruction occurs under three different cirucmstances: (1) at shunt insertion time, there is always a risk of contamination of the valve with clot or parenchymal tissue or other debris from the ventricular catheter; (2) bacterial proliferation in a shunt system can first appear as a valve occlusion (31); and (3) cellular immune reaction, as suggested in well-documented cases of sterile shunt malfunctions, may lead to late valve obstruction (29). In other words, valve obstruction may result from active phenomena (bacterial proliferation, development of an immune reaction) or a passive phenomena (accumulation of debris).

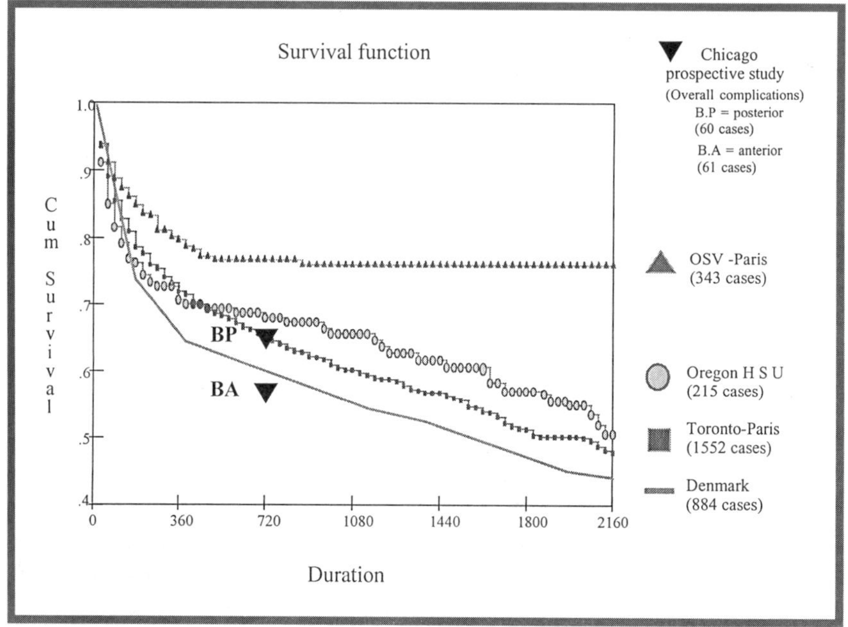

FIGURE 5-8

Effect of overdrainage limitation on shunt survival function: patients treated with "conventional" shunts (the same as Figure 5-1) are compared with a pediatric series shunted with a flow-regulating system (Orbis-Sigma valve—OSV). It is interesting to note that the risk of complications were similar in the first few months after surgery, while it is reduced by half at five years in the OSV series; these results are explained by the absence of shunt fracture and fewer "delayed" proximal obstructions (only one was observed after two years postoperatively) in that group.

Valve obstruction can be at least partly prevented by improving the valve design in order to avoid dead space and avoiding introduction of debris or clots in the valve at shunt insertion time.

DISTAL OBSTRUCTIONS

The risk of distal occlusion varies according to the site of drainage and the design of the distal catheter.

Distal slit catheters (the slits may or may not function as valves) of closed-ended distal tubing carry a higher risk of occlusion (Figure 5-9). There is dead space beneath the slits, which promotes progressive debris accumulation leading to plugging of the catheter. This tissue is composed of granulomatous nodules of relatively acellular fibrin clumps surrounded by a large number of macrophages, a few mesothelial cells, lymphocytes, and fibroblasts. Some of the macrophages form multinucleated giant cells. The risk of this type of obstruction does not exist with open-ended distal tubing.

In ventriculoatrial shunts, there is a risk of occlusion when the tip of the

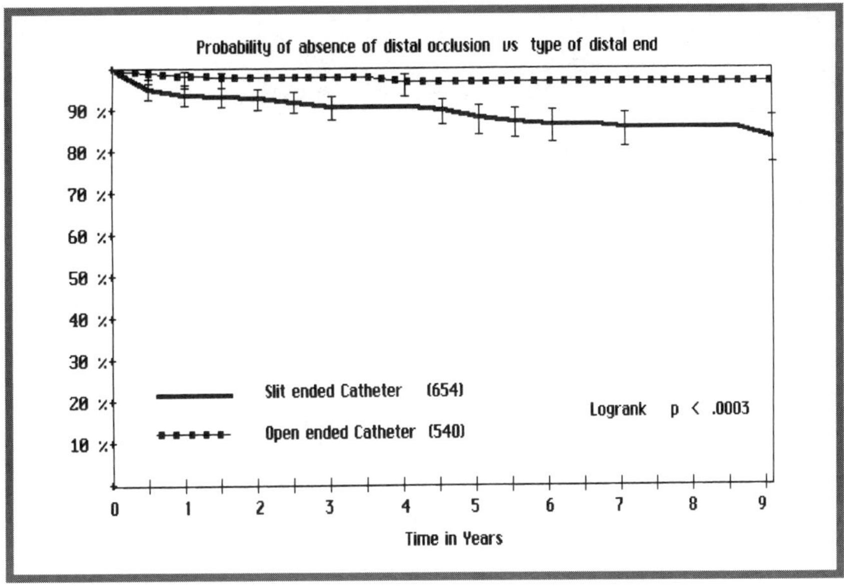

FIGURE 5-9
Correlation between the occurrence of distal occlusion and type of distal catheter end. The majority of distal obstructions are due to slit-ended distal catheters.

drainage catheter migrates out of the right atrium. This is due to thrombus formation. Peritoneal catheters are free from this risk.

Partial distal obstructions may be due to lowering of the absorption capacity of the peritoneal cavity (ascites or abdominal pseudocyst). Most of these phenomena have a clear origin (peritoneal infections, tumor seeding, mucopolysaccharidosis). However, in some cases, despite multiple investigations, the cause of the malabsorption remains unclear (immune reaction to the drainage device?) (42).

In summary, it appears that shunt occlusions can occur in many different circumstances. Ideally, they could be prevented by draining pure CSF, from an uncollapsable cavity, using a shunt system ideally designed and with adequate hydrodynamic properties. Aside from using superlative techniques, the surgeon should attempt to achieve the best compromise regarding the patient's situation and the shunt system. Guidelines for the process are as follows:

(1) Attempt to shunt the purest and the cleanest CSF, which may mean using alternative methods, such as external ventricular drainage or transitory ventricular access port, in patients with evidence of debris in the CSF at the time of diagnosis of hydrocephalus.
(2) Choose a nonflanged ventricular catheter and an open-ended distal catheter.
(3) Locate the tip of the ventricular catheter in the place that is expected to remain the largest after ventricular decompression.

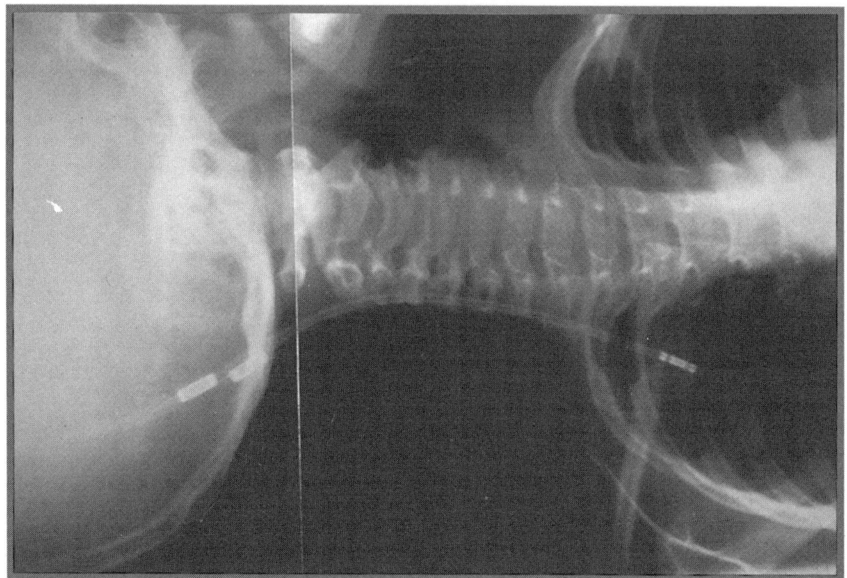

FIGURE 5-10
An example of shunt fracture, migration, and disconnection on the same shunt because of a connector improperly placed at the thoracic level.

(4) Choose appropriate flow-pressure characteristics of the shunt in order to limit as much as possible the phenomenon of chronic overdrainage and to avoid the ventricular catheter being placed in a collapsed cavity.
(5) Check that the shunt and, particularly, the valve, are free of debris or clots and flowing normally prior to inserting the distal end in the drainage cavity.

DISCONNECTION AND FRACTURE

The second most frequent cause of shunt failure in pediatric patients is shunt fracture or disconnection (Figure 5-10). These complications can be observed throughout the follow-up period (Figure 5-4). Factors that predispose to these complications include the design of the shunt, the material itself, and the surgical technique. There are strong interactions between these factors and others related to the patient. For example, younger patients have more potential for growth and, therefore, more risk of fracture or disconnection. As patients grow, the shunt must be free to move under the skin. Any point of fixation creating tension in the material can lead to a fracture. Also, host reaction to foreign material results in degradation and calcification (which is variable from one person to another and from one type of silicone to another) leading to material failure (43-45).

SURGICAL TECHNIQUE

A loose ligature or an absorbable suture at connector sites will lead to disconnection when stress is applied to the shunt system. Rough manipulation, partic-

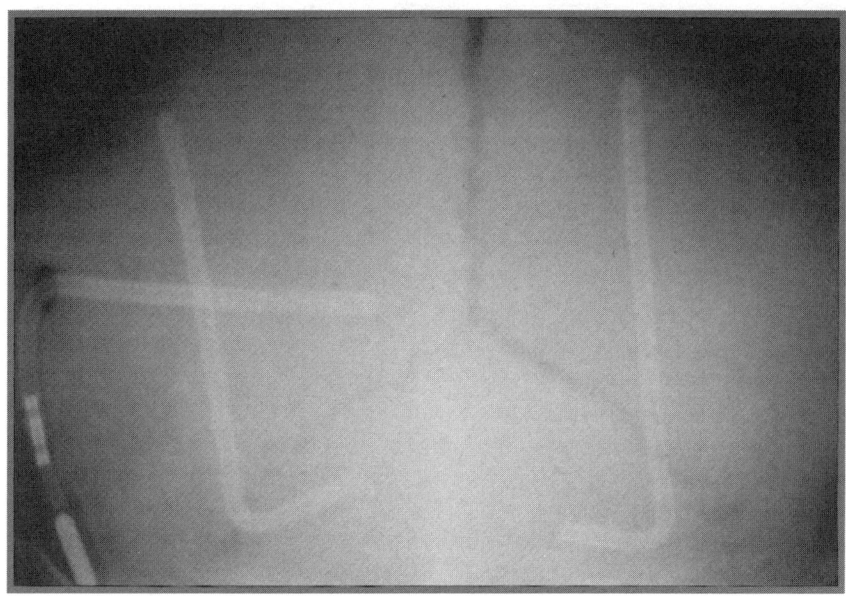

FIGURE 5-11
Disconnection due to improper ligature application at a connector. Three attempts were necessary in this particular case to connect correctly the ventricular catheter and the valve.

ularly with metal instruments, can lead to small cracks or even full-thickness tears in the tubing, which will result in a fracture later on (Figure 5-11).

In the management of a shunt fracture or withdrawn peritoneal catheter, it is important not to place a connector too far distal to the cranial end or in the abdominal or thoracic wall where fixation to the subcutaneous tissues will lead to recurrent fracture or migration. The catheter distal to the valve system must be entirely replaced.

DESIGN OF THE SHUNT

The risk of disconnection exists only with connectors in the shunt system. One-piece shunts, where the components are glued together, avoid this problem (46,47). However, it is important to remember that an attempt to avoid one particular risk can increase risks of another kind. For example, the use of a one-piece system decreases the risk of fracture, but it increases the risk of occlusion at shunt insertion time—a one-piece system being more likely to ingest clot and debris during insertion. Often, risk reduction on shunts involves some form of compromise. As the risk of disconnection proximal to the valve is minimal as compared with distal disconnection, it can be assumed that a two-piece system (a shunt with a separated ventricular catheter) is an acceptable compromise between the risk of disconnection and the risk of fracture. However, it must be stressed that all connections have to be outside of the cranial cavity, and any connection at or deeper than the burr hole level can end in a loss of the

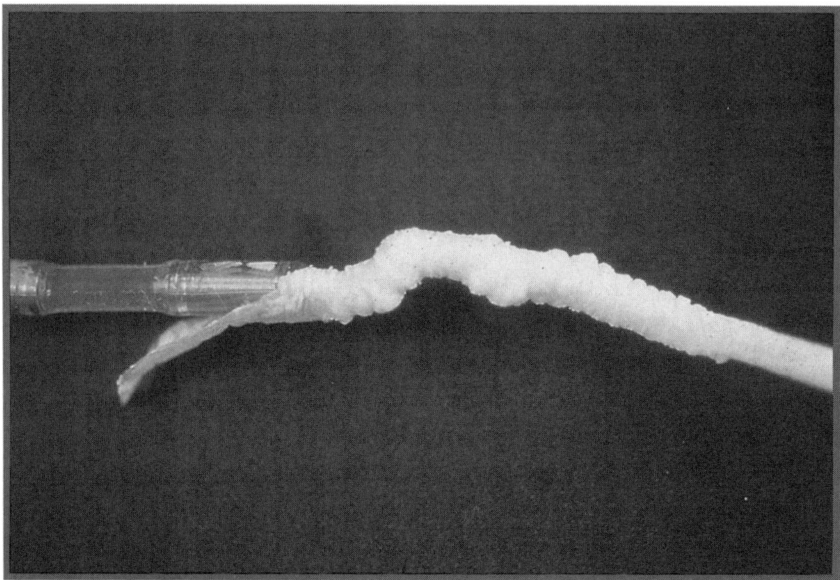

FIGURE 5-12A

Deterioration of the silicone and host reaction result frequently in calcification of the outer wall of the distal tubing; in children, the ensuing shunt fixation in the subcutaneous tissue will inevitably end in migration or fracture of the shunt system. (A) The macroscopic appearance of a "calcified shunt" after five years of implantation in that particular patient; (B) and (C) The electron microscopic images of a calcified distal catheter, the calcium deposit is firmly adherent of the outer wall of the tubing, surrounded by fibrous tissue.

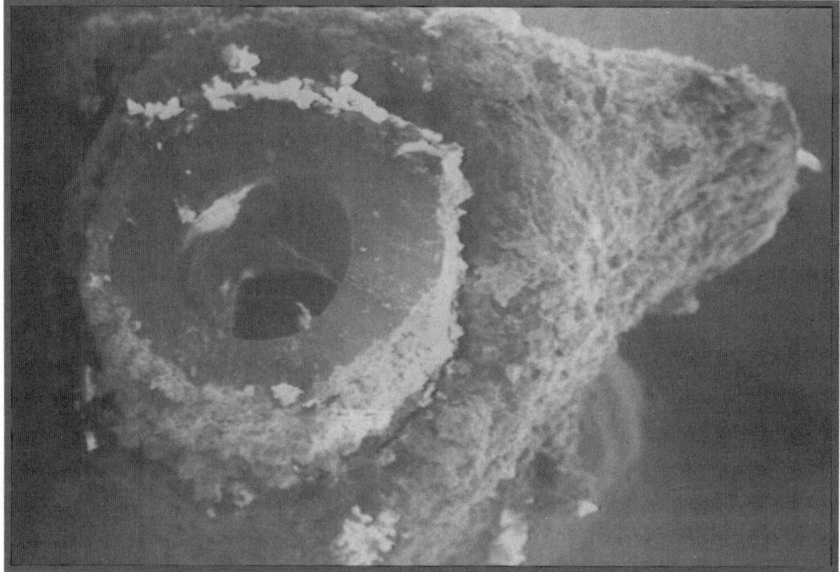

FIGURE 5-12B

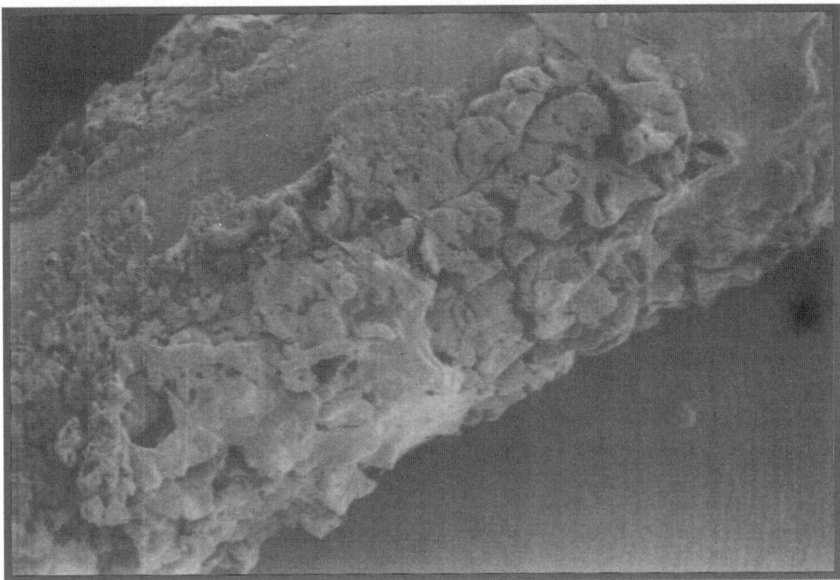

FIGURE 5-12C

ventricular catheter at shunt revision time.

MATERIAL

The approximation association of material of different physical characteristics (steel and silicone) in tubing results in breakage of the silicone (e.g., metal spring peritoneal catheters). Hard nylon connectors tear the silastic tubing with the continual stresses associated with movement.

It has been more recently demonstrated that even pure silicone catheters progressively deteriorate following implantation, altering the mechanical properties of the material (43). In addition, deterioration of the subcutaneously implanted silicone and host reaction induce calcified deposits on the outer wall of the catheter, producing fixation to the subcutaneous tissues (44,45) (Figure 5-12A-C). As children grow, this fixation of the distal tubing stretches the tubing and can cause a disconnection (if there are any connectors), a fracture of the tubing, or a narrowing of the lumen, increasing the resistance of the system. Calcification may take years to develop, preferentially occurs at the neck and the thoracic level, is rarely encountered in fatty tissue or in the abdominal cavity, and is never seen in the CSF. These calcifications are considered by some as caused by the barium impregnation of the tubing, recently leading the manufacturers to propose catheters being coated on their outer wall with pure silicone.

In summary, a distal tubing glued to the valve system, coated on its outer wall with pure silicone and with a proper ligature connecting the ventricule to the valve seems at present the best that can be done to reduce these complications. However, further material research and development is required to understand and avoid calcification of the tubing in the subcutaneous tissue. In addition, some recommendations can be made at the time of reoperation in order to decrease the risk of subsequent fracture, disconnection, or more serious complications:

(1) In case of fracture of the distal tubing or when a lengthening procedure is required, it is safest to replace the entire distal tubing; in all cases, connectors placed far from the valve system must be avoided.
(2) Disconnection or fracture of the distal tubing without evidence of clini cal signs of shunt malfunction, does not necessarily mean that the patient has become shunt-independent; in most cases, the tunnel of fibrous tissue developed around the silicone tube allows the CSF to flow through the gap of the broken catheters. Removing the shunt in such a case without further diagnostic tests could end in serious problems.

MIGRATION

There are important similarities between shunt migrations and fractures. Actually, in many cases, a shunt that is not able to migrate (because of the shape of the valve or fixation of the valve in the subcutaneous tissue or at the burr hole) will fracture later on. To migrate, a shunt needs to be pulled and to be able to move in the subcutaneous tissue. These two requirements indicate the two potential causes of this type of complication: a point of fixation (connector, calcifications, etc.) in the subcutaneous tissue distal to the valve system and a shape of the valve close to that of the tubing (minivalves, cylindrical shape).

Surgical Technique

Valves not fixed in the subcutaneous tissue either by ligature or inherent valve shape will migrate into the distal site or, exceptionally, in a retrograde fashion, in the ventricles (Figure 5-13). Overdissection of the subcutaneous tissue also predisposes to migration.

Design of the Valve

Cylindrical (elliptical) shape is very popular (small size, pumping chamber, etc.) but, unless properly secured, very prone to migration. Large valves located remote from the burr hole (e.g., over the anterior chest wall) will prevent migration but will act as the primary site of fixation and cause catheters above to migrate.

IMPROPER PLACEMENT

The shunt can be improperly placed at the level of the ventricles or at the level of the drainage cavity. This avoidable complication remains unacceptably high.

At Ventricular Level

In most centers, ventricular catheter insertion remains a "blind" procedure. All methods of assisting the ventricular catheter placement increase the cost and complexity of the operation. Increased complexity leads to prolonged operation

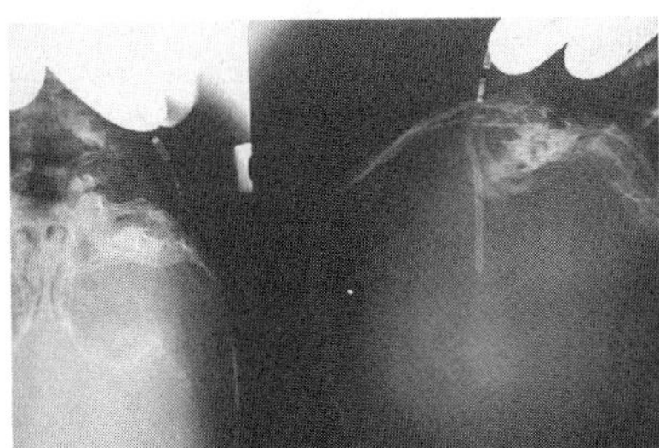

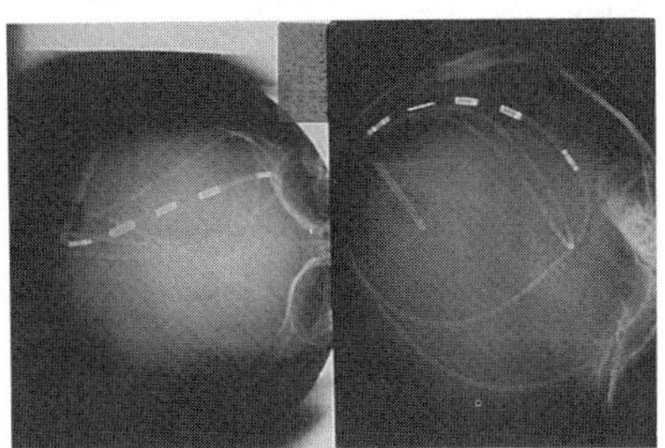

FIGURE 5-13
Small and cylindrical valves are very prone to migration distally when they are not properly secured at the scalp level; exceptionally, this migration can be proximally, into the ventricular system. (A) A downward migration; (B) an upward migration in the same patient because of an improperly secured shunt.

times, increased hardware manipulation, and at least the risk of increased shunt infection rates. Such aids include endoscopes, ultrasound probes, and, on rare occassions, stereotactic frames or guidance systems (see Chapter 4). The original peel away sheath method of introducing ventricular catheters left an opening in the brain larger the the catheter itself, risking pericerebral collections. Newer endoscopes, where the viewing system acts as the catheter introducer, may prove very useful with minimal complexity. Burr hole ultrasound systems are also currently available, and ultimately may be routinely implemented, but are very cumbersome at the moment.

Whether all or some subset of patients will benefit from the routine use of placement aids awaits proper perspective studies. For most routine shunt insertions, careful neurosurgical technique is probably the best insurance for proper catheter placement. For difficult cases, such as slit ventricles, a tripod (see Chapter 4, Figure 4-41) or even a stereotactic frame may be necessary. An alternative technique at the time of shunt revision is to simply place the ventricle catheter without the central stylet down the same tract. Multiple blind passes toward slit ventricles should be avoided; one should get the proper assistance using some kind of aid.

AT DRAINAGE PERITONEAL LEVEL

While the question of whether or not to use a trocar stimulates controversy

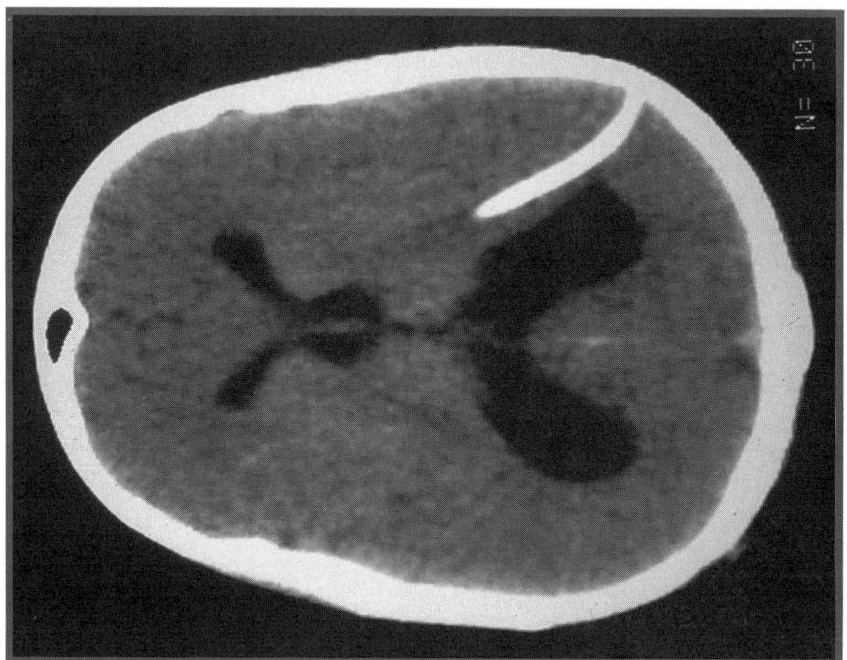

FIGURE 5-14
Improper placement of the ventricular catheter.

among neurosurgeons, one has to admit that there are no reported differences between these two techniques. The answer to the question seems to be common sense. It is dangerous to use a trocar in a peritoneal cavity when there has been previous abdominal surgery; otherwise, it is faster, and safer, to use a trocar. Once again, it is more a question of the skill and experience of the surgeon.

AT RIGHT ATRIUM LEVEL

EKG or fluoroscopy are usually utilized to correctly localize the tip of the catheter in the right atrium (48-50). Percutaneous tapping of the jugular vein, peel-away catheters, and a predetermination of the length make possible the use of a one-piece system without connectors.

SKIN PROBLEMS AND SUBCUTANEOUS CSF EFFUSION

SKIN PROBLEMS

As with other types of shunt complications, skin problems are usually the result of an interaction between the patient, the surgical technique, and the material. The problems can occur at the scar level because of poor surgical technique or as a necrosis of the skin over the shunt. These types of complications carry a major risk of shunt contamination, and all efforts must be made to prevent their occurrence.

Patient

Two factors must be considered: the quality of the skin (e.g., erosion, previous scar, thickness, etc.) and the risk of skin necrosis. A careful evaluation of the local skin condition prior to surgery can help to minimize further problem by choosing the least harmful shunt material and by being particularly attentive in the high-risk patient's group. Prolonged compression of the skin over the shunt (tight bandage, patient lying down on the valve system) must be avoided. Proper patient management at the hospital and parent education are mandatory for bedridden patients, specifically, those who are young or comatose.

Surgery

Ideally, the valve system must be placed in a pocket of an appropriate size under the galea through a small skin incision. This incision must be closed "perfectly" in two layers. In order to achieve this goal, efforts must be directed at preventing skin trauma and excessive retraction at the time of surgery; over or under-subcutaneous dissection must also be avoided. The surgical plane must be subgaleal; it is more difficult to reach the appropriate subgaleal surgical plane with an abdominal to cranial tunnel. In this condition, the tunneler usually ends in the subcutaneous fat over the galea, thus intefering with proper skin closure. Finally, the skin incision should be as small as possible, just large enough to insert the valve under the skin without excessive retraction. The common 10-cm horseshoe skin incision is probably unecessary. The large subcutaneous pocket promotes shunt migration and subcutaneous fluid collection, the incision is more difficult to close, and the blood supply to the skin pedicle may be inadvertantly leading to skin necrosis.

Shunt Design

A large-size valve, sharp edges, and hard plastic promote skin injury and necrosis. At the connectors level, the use of a thick suture with large knot is traumatic to the skin, the knot must be turned down facing the subcutaneous tissue.

Subcutaneous Fluid Collections

Subcutaneous accumulation of CSF is usually due to shunt obstruction. However, this type of complication can also be observed with a well-functioning shunt in certain circumstances. The use of a high or variable resistance valve, large ventricles (CSF close to the dura at insertion site), large dural opening, overdissection of the subcutaneous tissue, and the loose skin of the youngest patients are factors that can predispose to this type of complication even if the shunt is functioning normally. This complication occurs when the resistance opposed to leakage of the CSF around the ventricular catheter is less than the shunt resistance and when the skin can be easily dissected by this CSF to create a pouch around the valve (infants, overdissection). Once started, it is difficult to stop because the movement of the shunt into the pouch of CSF will promote the leak. This problem is avoidable by a small dura opening, minimal trauma to the brain, and by elevating the patient's head in the immediate postoperative period to artificially increase the drainage long enough to get a proper healing.

OVERDRAINAGE

Overdrainage is a constant problem with the existing valves (51,52); for example, the potential drainage capacity of a "low-resistance medium-pressure valve" is well over 200 cc/hr for a 25 cm H_2O differential pressure, while the CSF production is around 21 cc/hr. Increase of the differential pressure applied to the shunt system above the opening pressure of the valve plus the pressure of the drainage cavity may cause overdrainage. This point is reached in many occasions during normal life: postural changes, REM sleep, straining, etc., may induce an overdrainage situation.

The risk of overdrainage can be minimized by increasing the opening pressure of the valve, adding a siphon-resistive device to the system (53), or using a flow-regulating device (23). Even with future development (41, 54), none of these systems are able to provide a flow rate exactly matching the needs of each particular case. In addition, these systems carry their own risks of malfunctions (55,57). The adverse consequences of the overdrainage phenomenon are emphasized by the intraventricular location of the drainage site. Normally, the CSF flows from the ventricles to the subarachnoid spaces; in a shunted patient the flow is in the oppostive direction.

The phenomenon is directly responsible for several types of complications, namely, clinical signs of orthostatic hypotension, subdural CSF collections, slit ventricles syndrome, craniosynostosis, and loculation of the ventricles (24,51,58-62). As the overdrainage phenomenon is partly related to postural changes and patient height, this risk is highest in the oldest patient. Altogether, this complication represents less than 10% of shunt failures in pediatric series and about 30% in adult series (63). Besides these classical complications, overdrainage is also highly correlated with the occurrence of obstruction of the ventricular catheter. As already discussed under "proximal obstruction," occurrence of slit ventricles will promote obstruction of the ventricular catheter.

SUBDURAL COLLECTIONS (63,64) (FIGURE 5-15)

The risk of subdural collection is related to (1) the drainage capacity of the shunt (valve opening pressure, valve resistance, level of differential pressure applied to the shunt) and (2) the size of the ventricles and the compliance of the brain. Most shunted patients demonstrate enlargement of their subarachnoid spaces, which is actually an indirect sign of a well-functioning shunt. In some cases, disruption of the arachnoid or the stretched subarachnoid vessels can end in hygromas or true subdural hematomas, respectively. These complications occur spontaneously in most cases, but they can be produced by a minimal head trauma or surgery (e.g., ventricular tap, ICP sensor, etc.).

At present, prevention of this type of complication can be achieved by avoiding a shunt in the presence of a valid alternative (third ventriculostomy) and the use of overdrainage-limiting devices. Not all subdural collections require

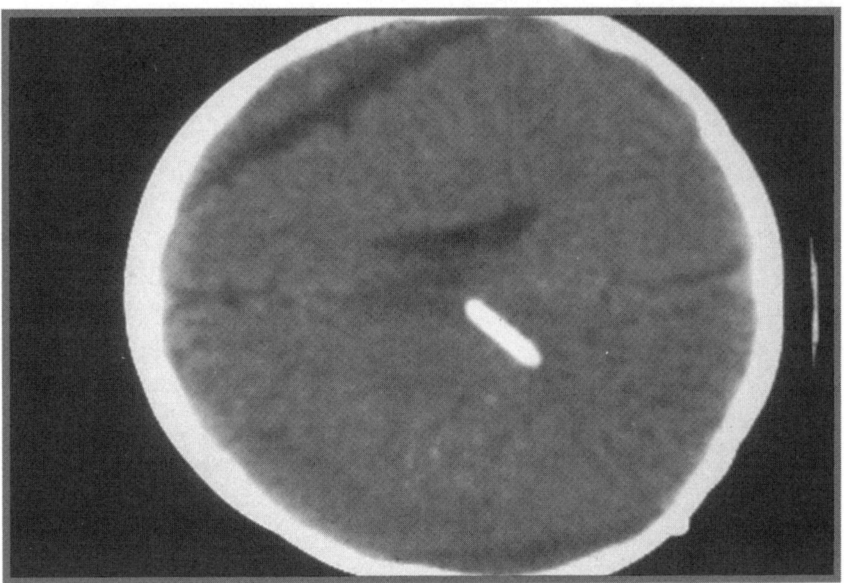

FIGURE 5-15
Bilateral subdural hematomas after shunting.

treatment. Some hygromas in symptom-free patients, can resolve spontaneously. In other cases, drainage limitation by upgrading of the valve opening pressure or use of a drainage flow-rate-limiting system can be successful. Finally, insertion of subdural shunt functioning at a lower pressure than the ventricular system (tubing without interposition of a valve system) will solve the problem in most cases by restoring a pressure gradient between the ventricles and the subarachnoid spaces.

SLIT VENTRICLE SYNDROME (24,40,58,59,65-68) (FIGURE 5-16)

There are numerous definitions of this syndrome in the literature, probably because of a mixture of different types of shunt complications. By strict definition, it is a syndrome of transient intracranial hypertension occurring in patients having a fully patent shunt and slit ventricles. In these patients, a dramatic decrease of the cranial CSF compartment can end in the loss of the CSF-buffering reserve for volumetric modifications of the two other compartments (brain parenchyma and blood); under these conditions, all alterations of this unstable equilibrium (fever, minimal head trauma, etc.), which are usually of no consequence, result in severe intracranial hypertension. Overdrainage limitation and/or skull expansion are the possible strategies for solving this problem.

CRANIOSTENOSIS (69-70) (FIGURE 5-17)

While frequently observed in the shunted pediatric patient because of chronic lowering of ICP below its physiological values, postshunt craniostenosis is

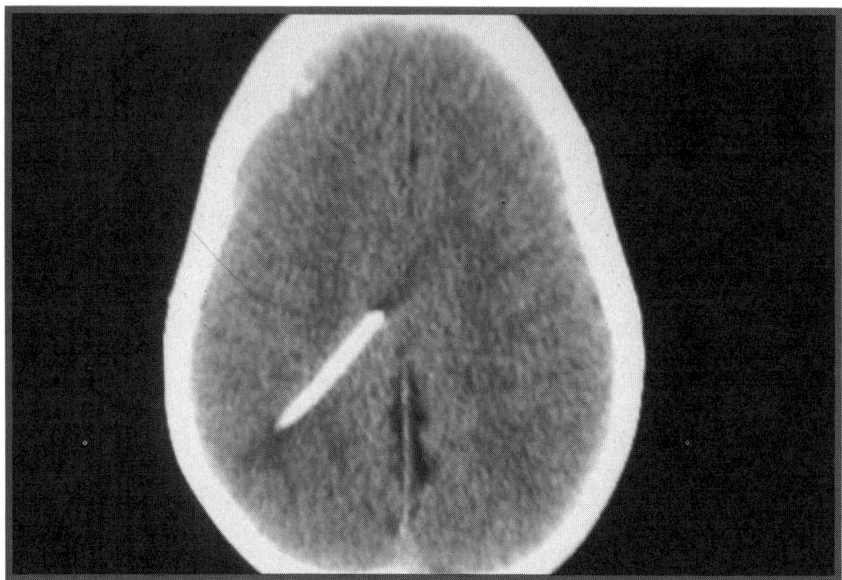

FIGURE 5-16
Slit ventricles syndromes defined by slit ventricles and episodes of intracranial hypertension while the shunt remains fully patent. This condition is difficult to differentiate from proximal obstruction in patients with slit ventricles, which is much more frequent, or from patients suffering from orthostatic hypotension.

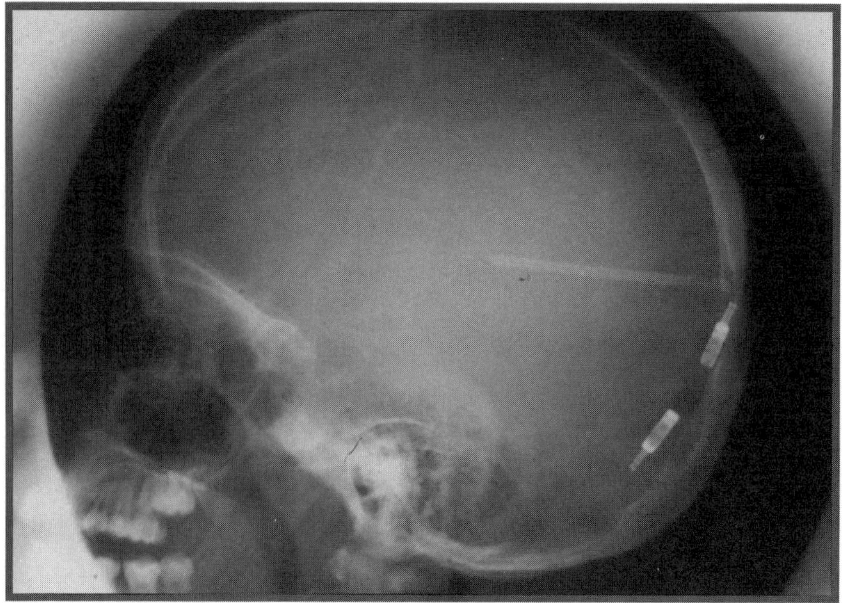

FIGURE 5-17
An example of bilateral coronal synostosis.

rarely, by itself, an indication for reoperation. More often, premature closing of the cranial sutures, in conjunction with chronic overdrainage of the CSF and brain growth in infants, creates slit ventricles with their potential adverse consequences. Patients who really require cranial vault surgical expansion generally have true "craniocephalic disproportion." Subtemporal decompression was once popular but is no longer used. Instead, the cranioplasty techniques currently utilized in craniofacial surgery are recomended. In some patients having very thick cranial vaults, sculpting the inner surface of the bone may provide enough additional cranial volume.

Loculation of the Ventricles (21,62) (Figure 5-18)

Loculated ventricles in hydrocephalic patients are usually observed after an inflammatory process, such as meningitis or hemorrhage. But, in some cases, excessive drainage of the CSF by itself results in loculation of the ventricular system. Asymmetry of the ventricles after shunt insertion is commonly observed, the ventricle where the shunt is located being the smallest. It is probable that in some cases, obstruction can develop at the site of maximum narrowing on the CSF pathways (foramen of Monro or aqueduct of Sylvius). Loculation of the ventricular system can require multiple drainage systems to be treated. To prevent generation of pressure gradients between locuted areas several ventricular catheters are connected to the same valve system instead of using several different shunts. When possible, the most satisfactory solution is to reestablish communication within the ventricles by neuroendoscopic procedures; however, endoscopic surgery generates debris in the ventricles that can obstruct the existing shunt system.

Orthostatic Hypotension (24,51,60,61)

Clinical symptoms of orthostatic hypotension (e.g., headaches, nausea, etc.) are frequently observed in the older patients after shunt insertion. Usually, these symptoms disappear after a short period of time as the patient adapts to the new hydrodynamic conditions. However, in some cases, it is necessary to upgrade the opening pressure of the valve, or to use a higher resistant shunt.

Miscellaneous Causes

Occassionally, shunted patients are reoperated upon wihtout a definite preoperative diagnosis of shunt malfunction. Minor symptoms (e.g., subtle deterioration in intellectual function or episodic headaches) can lead to surgery when both the surgeon and pateint (or the patient's family) can see no other solution to an unrelenting problem. The shunt is generally found to be patent. This shunt can be entirely changed or replaced in the ventricle after being shortened by a few centimeters. Some of these cases are recognized later on as early infection; some are probably related to partial obstruction of the shunt system, and some still remain unclear. In this last group, it is probable that the patient has intercurrent manifestations not related to shunt malfunction. In other words, one has to remember that shunted patients can demonstrate headaches, nausea,

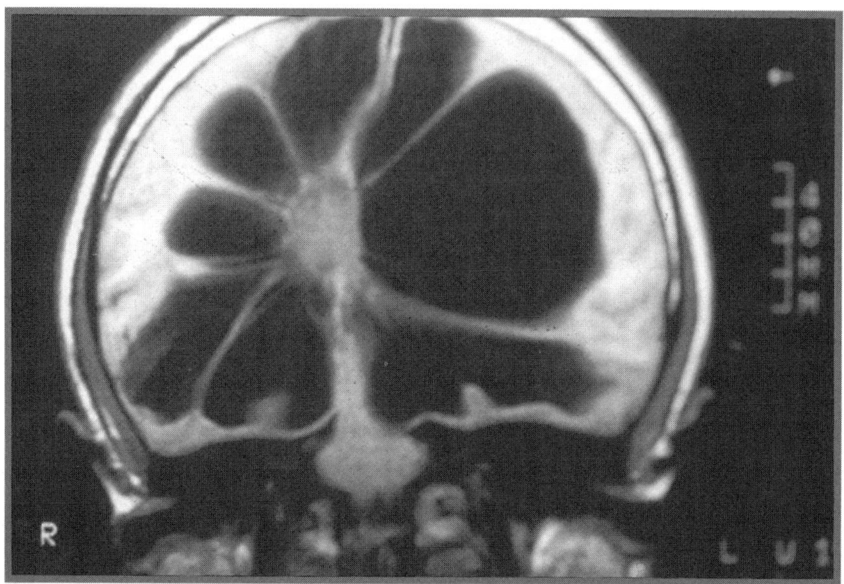

Figure 5-18A
Loculated ventricles. (A) Postinfectious in a shunted patient

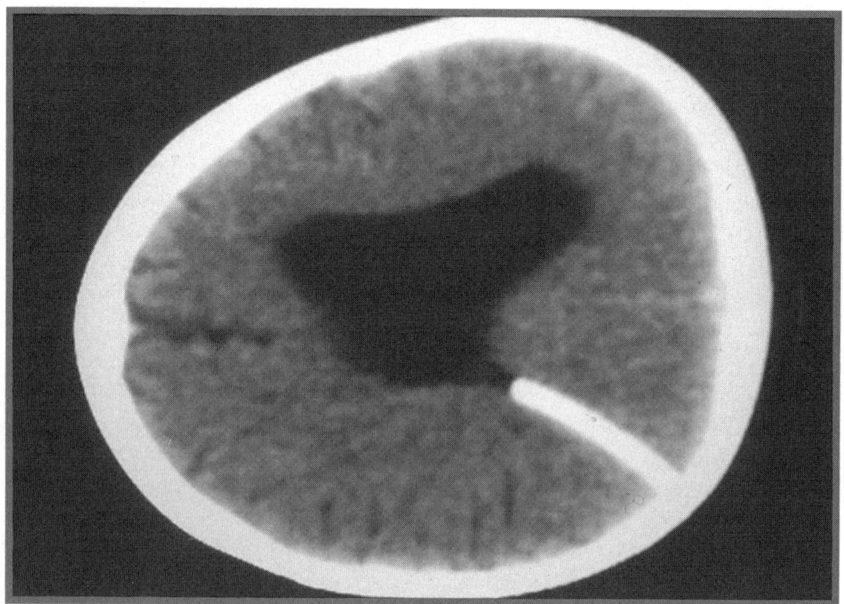

Figure 5-18B
(B) related to overdrainage

vomiting, deteriorations, seizures, etc. not related to improper function of the shunt (25). Instead of performing unecessary surgery, extensive preoperative investigation, including CSF flow measurement and ICP monitoring is recomended in unclear cases (24,71-75).

CONCLUSION

For inherent technical reasons, it is probable that a "shunt forever" is an impossible dream, (76) but delaying shunt malfunction as long as possible is a realistic goal. Even if some problems, like deterioration of the silicone tubing, are still unsolved, several possible causes of shunt malfunction can be easily avoided. Shunt failures are not inevitable, and for a large part they are quite preventable. At present, it seems that far more than shunt manufacturers, the surgeon has the most important role to play in this challenge.

SHUNT FAILURE SPECIFIC TO PARTICULAR SHUNTS AND DEVICES

LUMBOPERITONEAL SHUNTS

Lumboperitoneal (LP) shunts that drain CSF from the lumbar thecal sac to the peritoneal cavity have been used for over 100 years (77). They have several specific advantages (78,79). There is no need to transgress the cerebral mantle with a catheter, avoiding the risk of injury either at the time of insertion or removal; there is no choroid plexus, ependyma, or glial tissue to block the openings of the proximal end; they can be used when the ventricles are very small and would be difficult to cannulate with a ventricular catheter — this makes them the sole shunt of choice in pseudo-tumor cerebri requiring a shunt (80-82); there is generally a lower incidence of infection (78) (for reasons that are not entirely clear); theoretically, migration with growth in children is not as much of an issue as the shunt is not along the main axis of growth; and, finally, they can be placed under local anesthesia in patients at high risk for general anesthesia. A disadvantage of the LP shunts is that they can only be used in communicating hydrocephalus.

LUMBOPERITONEAL SHUNT FAILURE

Because of the specific advantages and the requirement for communicating hydrocephalus, LP shunts are used in a different population of patients from ventriculoperitoneal (VP) shunts (78,81,83-85). Therefore, comparisons between series of LP and VP shunts are not entirely valid. Interestingly, the five-year failure rate in a group of 143 patients retrospectively reviewed at the Hospital for Sick Children between 1974 and 1991 was not that different from that with VP shunts — approximately 50% (79,86) (Figure 5-19). The composition of this pediatric population is shown in Table 5-3.

The most striking feature of this shunt failure rate was the difference between the basic two types of LP shunt (Chapter 4, Figure 4-36), the percuta-

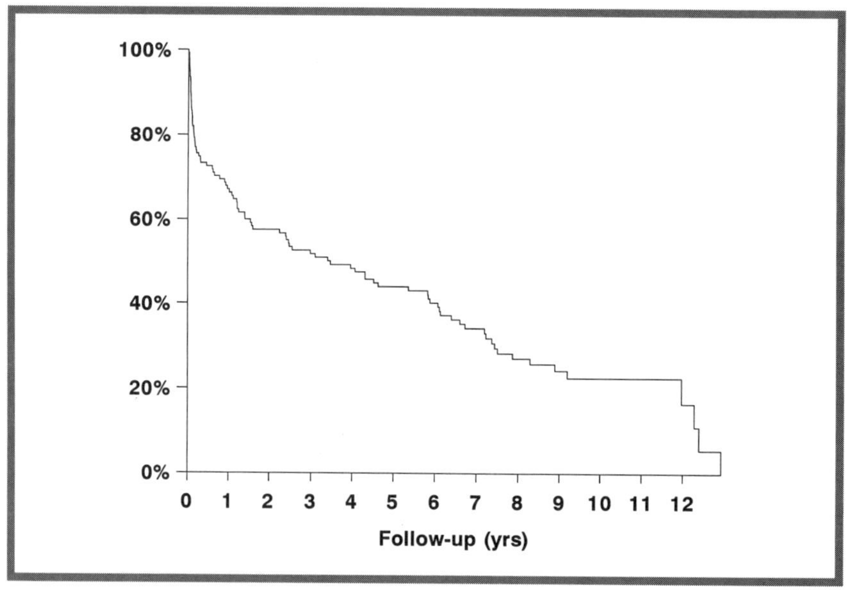

FIGURE 5.19
Complication-free survival of 143 patients with lumboperitoneal shunts. After one year, approximately 70% of shunts have failed. Reproduced by permission from Chumas PD, Kulkarni AV, Drake JM, Hoffman HJ, Humphreys RP, Rutka JT. Lumboperitoneal shunting: a retrospective study in the pediatric population. Neurosurg 1993; 23:376–383.

neous type (87,88), and the T-tube type (89) (Figure 5-20). The T-tube shunt was much more resistant to early failure from migration, presumably because the "T" resists migration through the dura. Eventually, even the T tube shunts did migrate, although at an average time of 6.2 years. The theoretical advantage of protection from the usual causes in proximal obstruction was, in a sense, confirmed in that distal obstruction was more common than proximal obstruction, a dramatic contrast to VP shunts.

LP shunts have two unique complications that are extremely important. The earliest, and particularly severe problem with the polyethylene shunts was arachnoiditis (90-92). This fibrosis of the arachnoid led to a stiff back, loss of range of lumbar flexion, sciatica, and even bladder dysfunction, and ultimately paraplegia. While silastic shunts largely eliminated this problem, it still occurs (Table 5-4).

Perhaps the most disturbing complication of LP shunts is acquired tonsillar herniation, a condition where the cerebellar tonsils descend into the upper cervical canal (93-95). This can lead to severe neck pain and, with increasing severity, upper cervical cord and lower brain stem compression, leading to lower cranial nerve dysfunction and apnea. Obstruction of the normal flow of CSF at the foramen magnum can lead to syringomyelia, leading progressively to scoliosis and loss of neurological function in the arms and legs.

While this problem had been recognized with both LP and VP shunts for some time (95), it was thought to be extremely rare. It was astonishing to learn that the Hospital for Sick Children patients, 38 of 54 (70%) patients in whom there was a CT scan image of the foramen magnum, had a full foramen magnum suggestive of acquired tonsillar herniation (Figure 5-21). This finding was confirmed with MRI where 12 of 17 asymptomatic patients had tonsillar herniation (94) (Figure 5-22). While only 5% of this series of patients were symptomatic to the point of requiring further surgery, the problem may not have been recognized in a number of patients, and one patient died from tonsillar herniation. Furthermore, surgery for this problem was difficult as foramen magnum decompression could lead to further descent of the cerebellar tonsils (96). Conversion to a ventriculoperitoneal shunt is also a possible treatment (97). The other striking finding was that the changes brought about by LP shunts were not restricted to the cerebellar tonsils. Obliteration of the perimesencephalic cisterns, which had been used as evidence of a functioning LP shunt, in fact represented uncal herniation (98) (Figure 5-23). As well, there was often descent of the entire brain stem.

TABLE 5-3 INDICATIONS AND TYPE OF LUMBOPERITONEAL SHUNT INSERTED

Indication for Shunt Insertion	Number of Patients	T-tube Shunt	Percutaneous Shunt
Hydrocephalus	116 (81.1%)	93 (80%)	23 (20%)
Cerebrospinal fluid fistula	17 (11.9%)	8 (47%)	9 (53%)
Pseudotumour cerebri	10 (7.0%)	0	10 (100%)
Total	143	101	42

TABLE 5-4 UNIQUE COMPLICATIONS ASSOCIATED WITH LUMBOPERITO

Scoliosis and hyperlordosis	18/126 (14.3%)
Limited spinal flexion	19/139 (13.7%)
Transcient back pain	14/139 (10.1%)
Sciatica	14/139 (10.1%)
Transient neck pain	12/135 (8.9%)
Lower limb neurological changes	8/126 (6.3%)
Symptomatic tonsillar herniation	6/143 (4.2%)

ANTISIPHON DEVICES

Antisiphon devices prevent overdrainage in the upright position by means of a flexible diaphragm that responds to atmospheric pressure (Chapter 2, Figure 2-9). However, proper function of these devices demands that the diaphragm is freely mobile and that atmospheric pressure is transmitted through the intact skin (99-102).

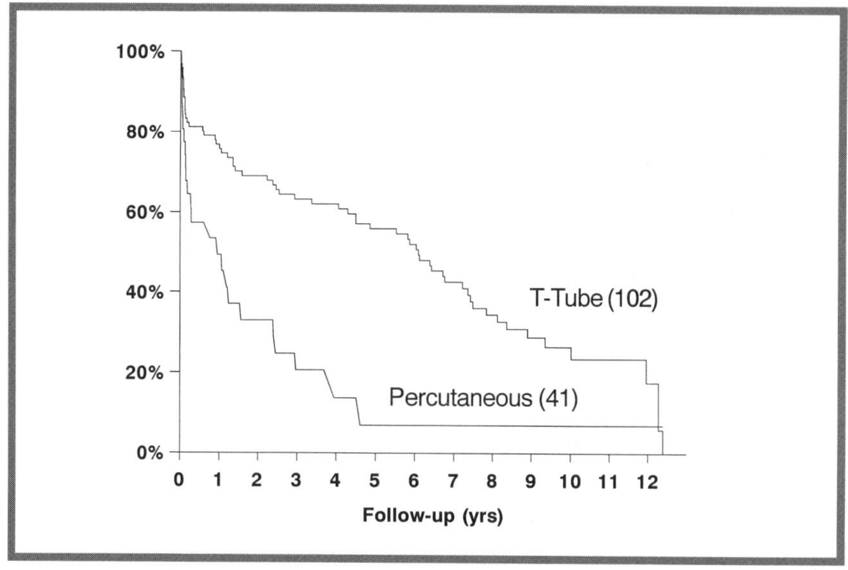

FIGURE 5-20
Comparison of complication-free survival between T-tube and percutaneous lumboperitoneal shunts. Percutaneous shunts have a much higher failure rate, usually due to migration. Reproduced, with permission, from Chumas PD, Kulkarni AV, Drake JM, Hoffman HJ, Humphreys RP, Rutka JT. Lumboperitoneal shunting: a retrospective study in the pediatric population. Neurosurg 1993;23:376–383.

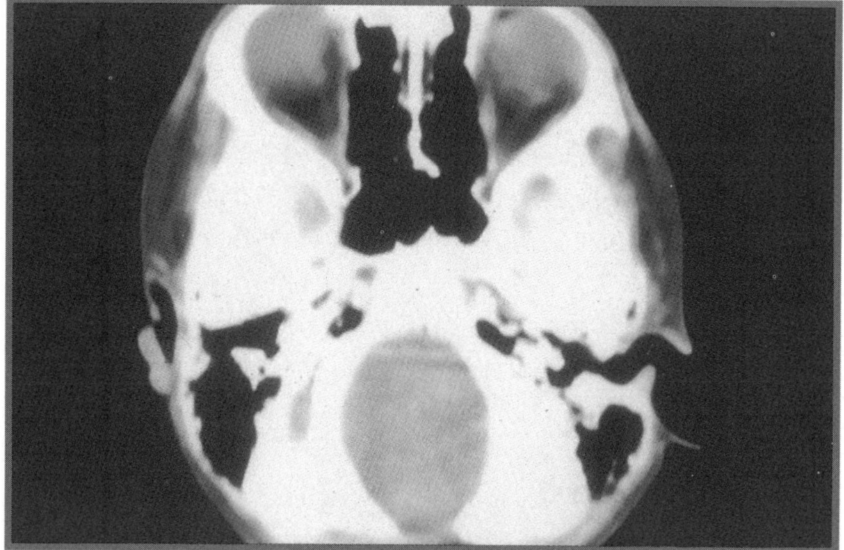

FIGURE 5-21
Axial CT scan at the level of the foramen magnum of a patient with a lumboperitoneal shunt, demonstrating a "full" foramen magnum that is suggestive of tonsillar herniation.

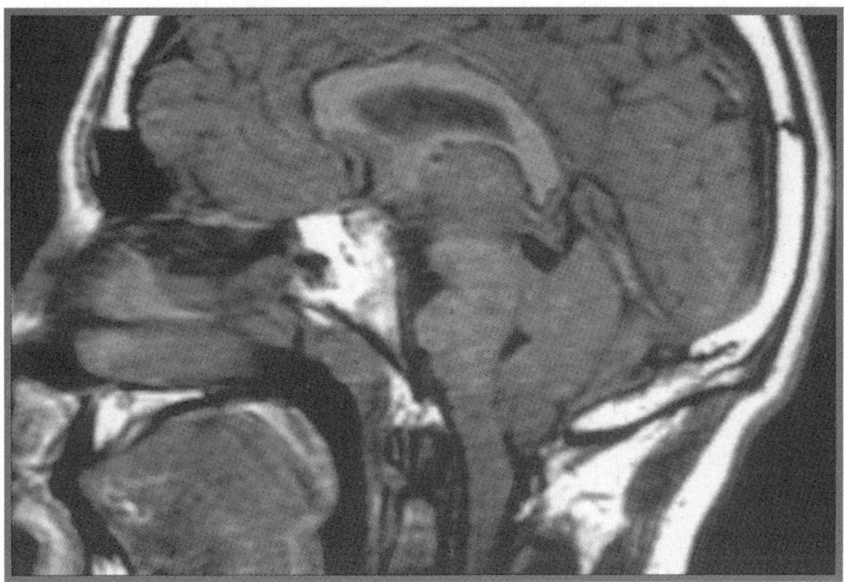

FIGURE 5-22
Sagittal MR image at the craniocervical junction, demonstrating tonsillar herniation in an asymptomatic patient with a lumboperitoneal shunt.

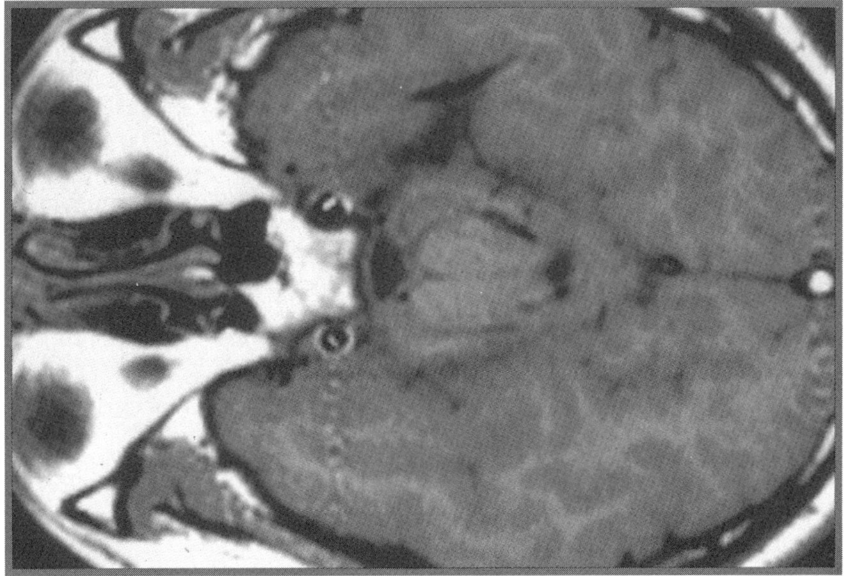

FIGURE 5-23
Axial RM image at the level of the incisura, demonstrating obliteration of the perimesencephalic cisterns and uncal herniation in an asymptomatic patient with a lumboperitoneal shunt.

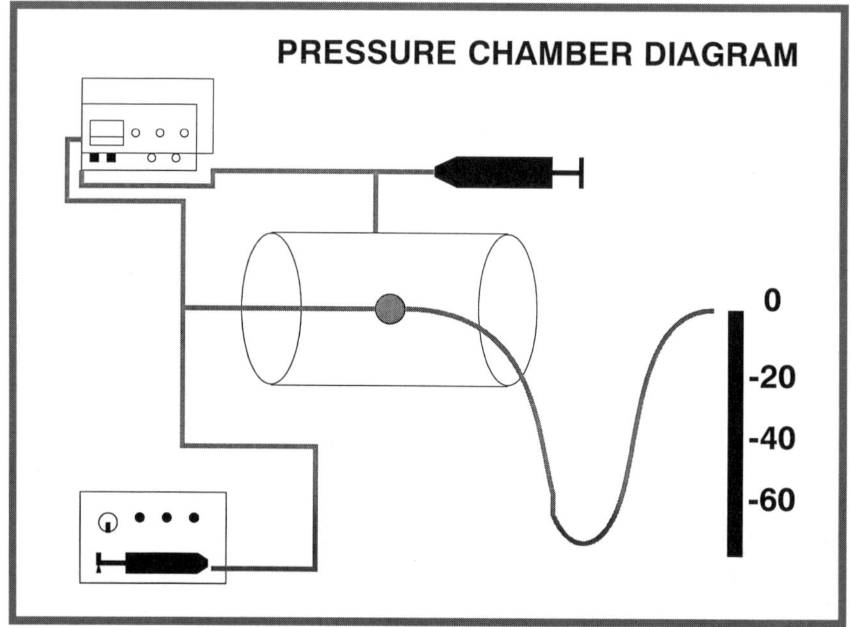

FIGURE 5-24A
Schematic for testing antisiphon devices in a barometric chamber. Shunt flow and pressure are measured as a function of the height of the distal catheter and the pressure surrounding the antisiphon device.

Just how sensitive these devices are to changes in external pressure can be demonstrated by placing them in a barometric waterbath at 37° C (Figure 5-24A,B). There is a linear relationship between the increase in external pressure and the increase in the resistance of the device (99). This is true for all antisiphon devices, including the Heyer-Shulte ASD, PS Medical SCD, and Delta valve. For completeness, exposing the membrane to a negative pressure abolishes the anti-siphoning effect.

As all implanted silicone devices are encased in a fibrous tissue capsule, it is reasonable to wonder if, in fact, the flexible membrane is always exposed to atmospheric pressure. When the Heyer-Shulte ASD and the PS Medical SCD were implanted subcutaneously in pigs for a period of four weeks, there was a sustained increase in resistance of the devices until the external capsule surrounding them was cut (99) (Figure 5-25A,B).

Does the same process happen in patients? While the same caution about comparing different populations of shunted patients applies, when the complication-free survival of patients with a Heyer-Shulte ASD was examined, it was extremely poor (103) (Figure 5-26A,B). Ten of the 24 patients requiring reoperation had a functional obstruction — the shunt clinically was obstructed, but radiologically and at surgery it was patent (Figure 5-27). Several patients were

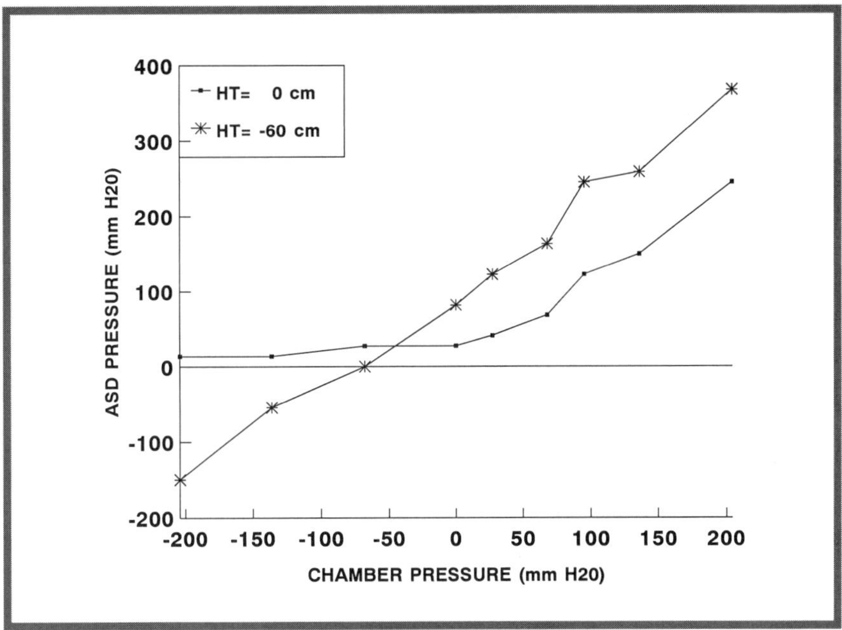

Figure 5-24B
Results of the pressure measurements from Figure 5-24A. Pressure in the shunt system rises linearly with extreme barometric pressure. The flexible membrane of the antisiphon device moves against the internal orifice, increasing the resistance, as the pressure rises above atmospheric pressure. Negative external barometric pressure has no effect with the distal shunt catheter at a height of zero (there is no tendency to siphon). Negative external barometric pressure removes the antisiphoning effect of the antisiphon device, with the distal shunt catheter at –60 cm, by preventing the flexible membrane moving against the resistive orifice. Reproduced by permission from da Silva MC, Drake JM, Effect of subcutaneous implantation of antisiphon devices on CFS shunt function. Pediatr Neurosurg 1990–91;16:197–202.

unconscious until the ASD was removed. This same finding was reported by Mc Cullough (101). Proof of this phenomenon was provided in a patient who developed progressive ventricular enlargement with an Heyer-Shulte ASD in place and had pressure measurements performed before and after incision of the tissue capsule surrounding the ASD (104) (Figure 5-27). The ASD was functionally obstructed.

Should antisiphon devices still be used? Capsule contraction and functional obstruction is unpredictable and does not happen in all patients. It has been claimed by proponents of the PS Medical SCD and Delta valve that the recessed diaphragm is not susceptible to tissue capusule effects. While that was not the experience when the SCD was implanted in pigs, proof will only come from following these patients carefully with clinical trials.

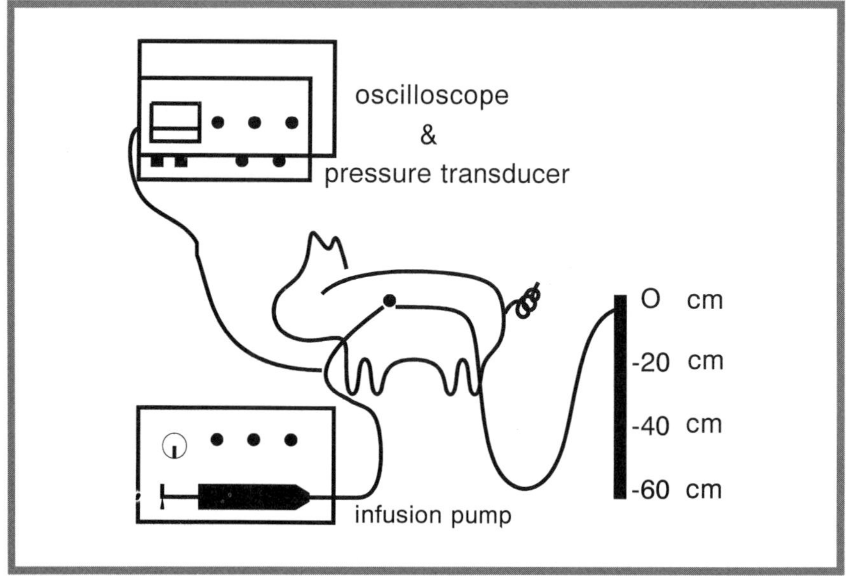

FIGURE 5-25A
Schematic diagram of experimental set-up for measuring pressure and flow characteristics of implanted antisiphon devices.

SHUNT INFECTION

Shunt infection remains an important and distressing cause of shunt failure (105). Shunt infection puts the patient at increased risk of intellectual impairment (106), the development of loculated CSF compartments, and even death (107-110). Despite intensive efforts to prevent shunt infection for decades, most centers report infection rates on the order of 5%. Recently, a report of a consistently much lower rate of infection, less than 1% (110), has stimulated the neurosurgical community to match these results. Although the mechanism of shunt contamination seems relatively straightforward, the exact intervention that has led to lower rates in some centers remains elusive. In this section, we will discuss the mechanism, diagnosis and treatment of shunt infection, and, perhaps most importantly, how shunt infections might be prevented.

DEFINITION AND CLASSIFICATION OF CSF SHUNT INFECTION

Shunt infection remains remarkably difficult to establish in some cases, even in retrospect. Perhaps a simple working definition is unequivocal evidence of infection of the shunt equipment, the overlying wound, the CSF, or distal drainage site related to the shunt. Unequivocal evidence requires demonstration of the organism on Gram stain or culture from material in, on, or around the shunt or from fluid withdrawn from the shunt. Shunt infection is probably best classified defined in terms of site: (1) wound infection — an incision or shunt track with signs of inflammation, purulent discharge, and organisms seen on Gram stain or culture; (2) meningitis — fever, meningismus, CSF leukocytosis,

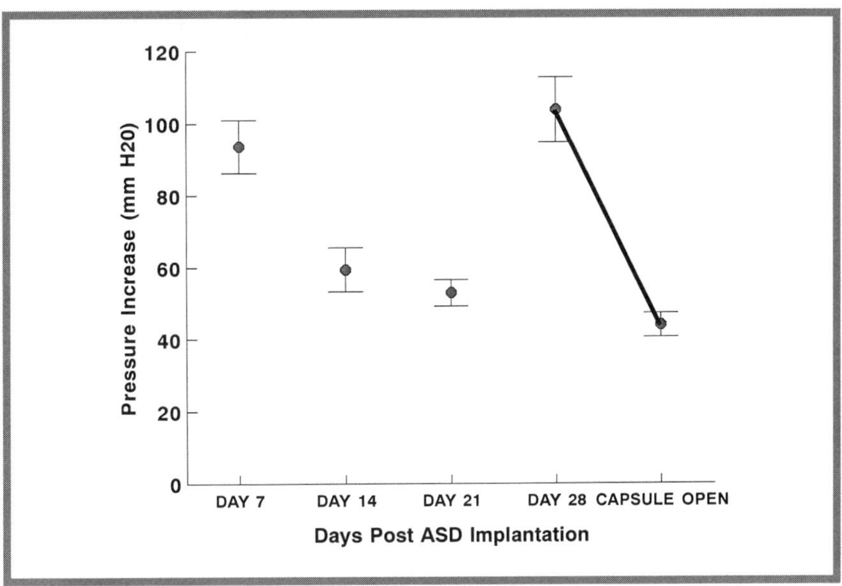

FIGURE 5-25B

Results of the pressure measurements from Figure 5-25A. Subcutaneous implantation raises the pressure in the shunt system through the four-week implantation period. Cutting the capsule causes an immediate fall in pressure, indicating that the capsule has a constrictive effect on the antisiphon device. Pressure does not fall to zero, as weight of skin is sufficient to cause an increase in pressure. Reproduced by permission from da Silva MC, Drake JM, Effect of subcutaneous implantation of antisiphon devices on CFS shunt function. Pediatr Neurosurg 1990–91;16:197–202.

and organisms seen on Gram stain or culture; (3) peritonitis — fever, abdominal tenderness (abdominal pseudocyst, and abdominal abscess may present with mass with or without fever), and organisms seen on Gram stain or culture. For vascular shunts, fever, leukocytosis, positive blood culture, with or without evidence of shunt nephritis or cor pulmonale; or (4) infected shunt apparatus — minimal signs of CSF contamination with bacteria recovered from purulent exudate in or on shunt material, Gram stain of CSF withdrawn from the shunt, or positive culture on fluid aspirated from the shunt under sterile conditions (111). Organisms that only grow from the shunt equipment or CSF on broth culture are probably contaminants.

Although most shunt infections appear within two months of surgery, including shunt revisions, confirmation that a shunt infection is cured requires longer follow-up. No specific time period can be claimed as delayed infections, with skin commensal organisms, are possible (110,111); however, at least six months, and preferably one year, following treatment is probably necessary. In cases where there is some doubt, particularly if the shunt apparatus is not removed, demonstration that the CSF is sterile by repeat aspiration of fluid from the shunt with the patient off antibiotics is necessary.

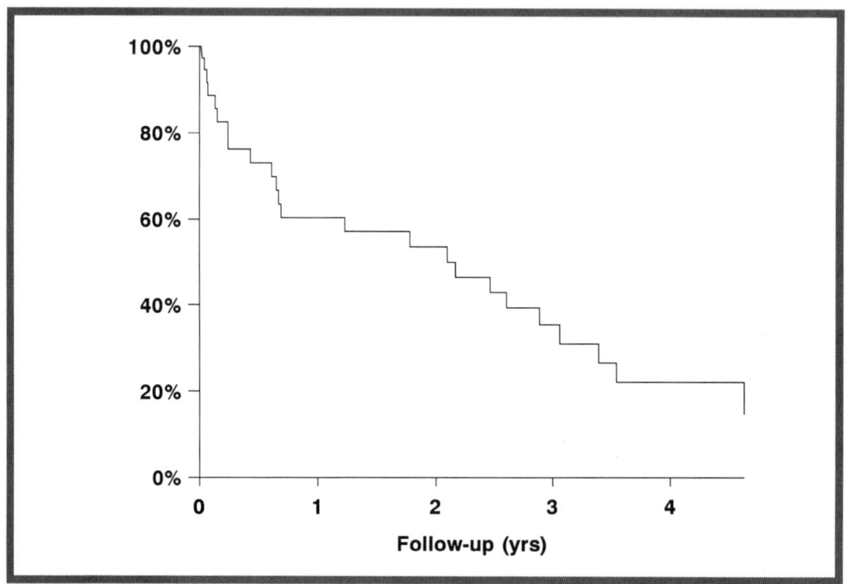

FIGURE 5-26A
Complication-free survival of 38 patients with implanted antisiphon devices. The one-year failure rate is approximately 40%

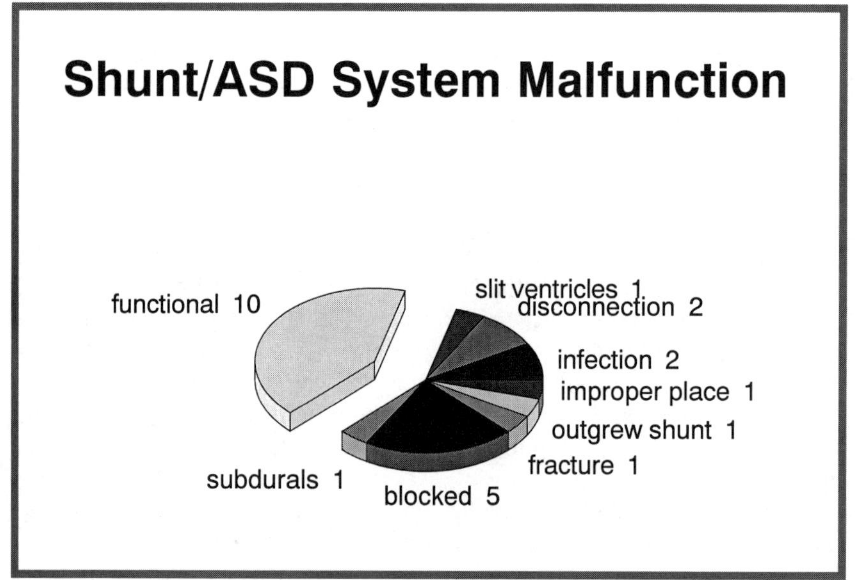

FIGURE 5-26B
Pie daigram of etiology fo shunt failure from Figure 5-26A. A large proportion of failures are due to functional obstruction, believed in retrospect to be due to tissue capsule effects. Reproduced by permission from da Silva MC, Drake JM. Complications of cerebrospinal fluid shunt antisiphon devices. Pediatr Neurosurg 1991–92;16:304–309.

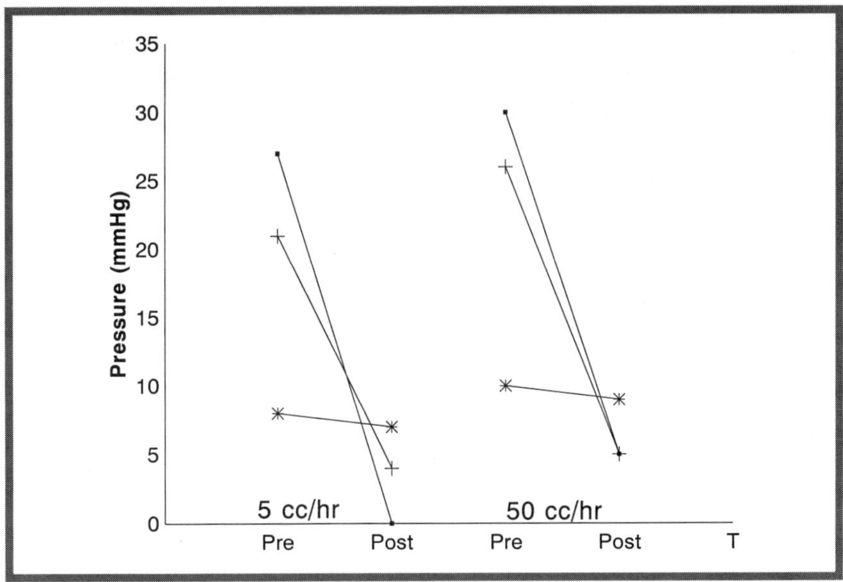

FIGURE 5-27

Pressure measurements in three patients with antisiphon devices undergoing shunt revision. Measurements were made at flow rates of 5 and 50 cc/hr. Lines connect pressure before and after incision of the tissue capsule around the antisiphon device. Two patients had functional obstruction due to the capsule, characterized by a marked reduction in pressure when the capsule was incised. In the third patient the tissue capsule had no effect. Reproduced by permission from Drake JM, da Silva MC, Rutka JT. Functional obstruction of an antisiphon device by raised tissue capsule pressure. Neurosurg 1993;32:13–139.

PATHOGENESIS OF INFECTION

SOURCE OF INFECTING ORGANISMS

The most common organisms infecting CSF shunts are staphylococci — approximately 40% of shunt infections are caused by *S. epidermidis* infections and 20% by *S. aureus* (108-110,112-115). Other species isolated from infected shunts include the coryneforms, streptococci, enterococci, aerobic Gram-negative rods, and yeasts (116). As these organisms are commonly part of the normal skin flora and shunt infection usually occurs within two months of surgery, endogenous spread from the patient or surgical staff would be the logical route of infection. Various studies have, indeed, shown this to be the case.

Bayston and Lari (117), in a study of 100 shunt operations, found that in 58 cases, the surgical wound was found to be contaminated with organisms just before closure. In 32 of these cases, the identical organism had been found in the patient's nose, ear, or scalp preoperatively. The remaining 26 cases were presumably from aerial origin but were present in much lower quantities within the wound. Of the nine shunt infections that arose in their series, in seven cases the organism that was isolated from the infected shunt was identical to the strain that had been isolated preoperatively from the patient. In the remaining two cases, involving a coryneform infection and a *Streptococcus viridans* infection, laboratory techniques could not discern whether or not the two species were of the same strain as that of the patient's preoperative flora. The authors concluded that in most shunt infections, the organism is spread to the surgical wound either directly from the adjacent skin or by contamination of gloves or instruments with the patient's flora.

Pople et al. (114) reported that during shunt insertion, there was significantly higher pre-operative skin-surface bacterial density in those patients in whom the surgical wound became contaminated and in those who developed shunt infection. Shapiro et al. (115) found that of 20 shunt infections studied, 20% were caused by organisms identical to those recovered from the skin incision sites, 20% were due to different strains, and 60% may or may not have originated from the patient's skin. They acknowledged that while the majority of shunt infections are caused by typical skin organisms, the relative importance of other sources of contamination, such as the patient's nasopharynx, operative personnel, or the hospital environment, had yet to be determined.

Various studies have attempted to determine the contribution of the operating room aerial environment to the rate of wound infections (118-120). While these demonstrated some benefit after the implementation of improved ventilation, in each case, other changes in protocol were also introduced, and, as a result, one could not determine with certainty how much of the improved infection rate was attributable to better ventilation. In one study, in which the patients were operated upon using a surgical isolator in which airborne contamination was eliminated, the infection rate was still 7.9% (108).

Late shunt infections usually demonstrate a very different bacteriological profile, involving predominantly Gram-negative bacilli, and there is usually also an attributable cause. Shapiro et al. (115) found that, in their series, all shunt infections involving Gram-negative bacilli had an associated predisposing factor, including bowel erosion by the distal shunt catheter, *Haemophilus influenza* meningitis, postlaparotomy infection, and pressure necrosis of the skin exposing shunt tubing. In fact, whenever a Gram-negative organism is implicated in a shunt infection, a primary cause should always be considered and sought out.

Mechanism of Shunt Colonization

The detailed mechanisms by which CSF shunts become colonized with microorganisms is important for the understanding of many the issues surrounding prevention and treatment of shunt infection. Many of the details of shunt colonization apply equally to other implantable biomaterials, and, in fact, much of the research in this field has come from work in urology, orthopedics, and other surgical disciplines.

The implanted shunt is almost immediately coated with a glycoproteinaceous conditioning film (121) derived from serum and extracellular matrix proteins providing potential receptor sites for bacterial or tissue adhesion (122).

The shunt material's surface properties determine the sequence and layering of the deposited proteins. It is at this stage that there is competition for shunt surface adhesion between the host tissue cells and whatever bacteria exist in the vicinity. This competition for adhesion has been termed the "race for surface" (121). The relative success of either the bacteria or the host cells in this "race" will determine, in large part, the ultimate clinical scenario associated with the implanted shunt.

If tissue cells are the first to adhere and integrate with the shunt surface, this eukaryotic cell surface will provide resistance to any further attempts at bacterial colonization. Tissue integration with the shunt surface, however, is limited to that portion of the shunt that lies within the subcutaneous tissue and generally does not occur on the distal portion that lies within the peritoneal cavity. It is during this crucial stage of surface adhesion that maintaining a sterile shunt system is of paramount importance in order to eliminate any bacterial competition to tissue integration.

Bacterial adhesion is a complicated process that involves both physical and chemical interactions (121). As it approaches the shunt surface, the bacteria, like any particle, acts under the influence of van der Waals forces and attractive hydrophobic interactions between its surface and that of the shunt. Such forces may place the bacteria within a close enough range of the shunt surface (usually less than 1 nm) to allow for irreversible adhesion. This irreversible binding occurs as a result of interaction between specific fimbrial adhesins and/or bacterial exopolysaccharides and the conditioning film receptors on the shunt surface. Initially, cell division within the bacterial microcolonies and then, later, recruitment and aggregation of bacteria from the surrounding environment, produce a continuous biofilm on the shunt surface (Figure 5-28). This biofilm is composed of bacterial cells, either singly or in microcolonies, all embedded in an anionic matrix of bacterial exopolymers and trapped macromolecules (123). This will eventually produce a clinical shunt infection, although it may take up to several months to manifest.

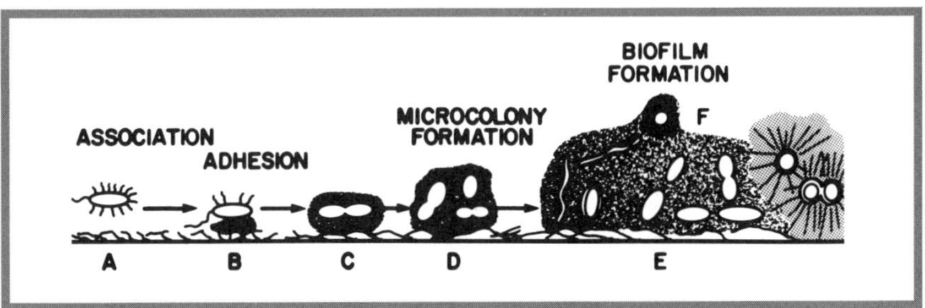

FIGURE 5-28
Sequential steps in the formation of the bacterial biolayer on an implanted prosthesis. Reprinted by permission from Costerton JW, Cheng KJ, Geesey GG, Ladd TI, Nickel JC, Dasgupta M, Marrie TJ: Bacterial biofilms in nature and disease. Ann Rev Microbiol 1987;41:435–464.

The existence of bacteria in the form of a biofilm is one of the most important properties of bacterial colonization of biomaterials. This mode of growth has been shown to be associated with an appreciable measure of protection against many common antibacterial agents, including antibodies (124), white blood cells (125,126), surfactants (127), and antibiotics (128,129). Obviously, those bacterial strains that possess a greater ability to adhere to the shunt surface have a definite survival advantage in their new environment. These particular strains are the most successful in surviving beyond the initial stages of contamination and are primarily responsible for shunt infection.

The protective effects of the biofilm provide an explanation for the relative lack of success associated with the treatment of shunt infections by the exclusive use of systemic and/or intraventricular antibiotics (106,130-132). Aggressive antimicrobial chemotherapy may clear the acute inflammation, but the organisms within the surface biofilm will only be reduced in number and rarely eradicated. Therefore, since the source of the bacteria remains, the biofilm is free to shed more organisms, resulting in recurrent acute inflammation once antibiotic administration is discontinued (128,129). It has not yet been determined whether the lack of sensitivity to antibiotics is a result of limited penetration of the biofilm by the antibiotics or is due to physiological alterations of bacteria in the biofilm environment (133).

The biofilm mode of growth may explain the different clinical scenarios that are commonly associated with the different infecting organisms (116). Organisms that lack the ability to adhere to the shunt surface, such as *S. aureus*, are more likely to be associated with a wound infection of the surrounding tissue that secondarily infects the shunt. However, those organisms that can produce extracellular slime, particularily *S. epidermidis* (134), possess an enhanced ability to bind to the shunt material. Therefore, they are able to form a biofilm on the luminal shunt surface and then present as a true shunt colonization, not as a wound infection.

Risk Factors for Shunt Infection

Despite the information available on the pathogenesis of shunt infection, few factors have been identified as clear risks for shunt infection. Young age has represented a higher risk in a number of studies (108,135-137). This may relate to immaturity of the immune system, vulnerability of the thin skin, or other factors. Poor condition of the skin or other intercurrent sites of infection have been shown to increase risk of shunt infection while other factors that also might be thought to promote infection, such as duration of operation or presence of CSF leak or drain, have not clearly been shown to be causative (108). The experience of the surgeon in one study did influence infection rate (136), but in another larger study had no effect (108). The risk for each shunt procedure also appears to be approximately the same (108), but with additional procedures, the cumulative risk to the individual patient rises.

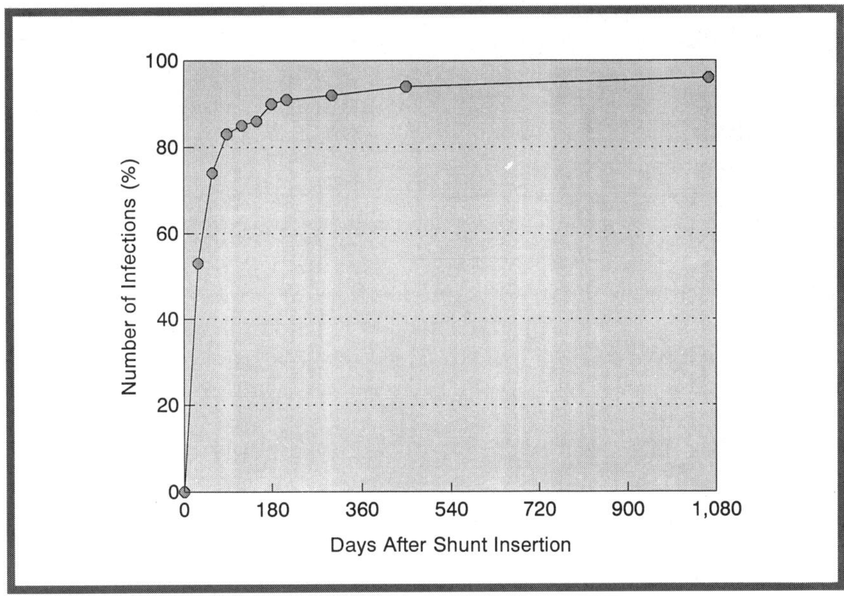

FIGURE 5-29
Time of occurrence of shunt infection following surgery, expressed as accumulation of all shunt infections versus time following surgery. Reprinted by permission from George R. Librock L, Epstein M: Long-term analysis of cerebrospinal fluid shunt infections: a 25-year experience. J Neurosurg 1979;51:804–811.

DIAGNOSIS OF SHUNT INFECTION

Clinical Features

Most shunt infections present within two months of shunt insertion (108-110,112,136,138) (Figure 5-29). The clinical features depend on the site of infection. Wound infections are usually manifested as fever, reddening of the incision site or shunt tract, and, with progression, discharge of pus from the incision. In chronic wound infections, the shunt may actually become exposed as the wound breaks down. Erosion of the thin skin in infants, particularly premature infants, from pressure also results in wound infection. Any leak of CSF from the incision because of a high resistance valve, poor distal flow, etc., also often results in contamination of the shunt and subsequent infection.

Patients with meningitis or ventriculitis usually present with fever, headache, or irritability and often with some neck stiffness, if not nuchal rigidity. Peritonitis is less common, although in one series seven of 21 patients presented with signs of peritoneal irritation (138). The patients typically present with fever, anorexia or vomiting, and abdominal tenderness. The severity of the symptoms depend to some extent on the infecting organism. Patients infected with *S. epidermidis* may look remarkably well and may have intermittent fever or irritability only. They may also present with signs of a typical shunt obstruction (110), without fever or leukocytosis. Patients with abdominal pseudocysts (which are invariably infected) may present with a mass only. Small pseudocysts may be difficult to detect on abdominal exam. Historically, patients with ventriculoatrial shunts, in addition to presenting with signs of a septicemia, could manifest shunt nephritis or cor pulmonale.

The infection often involves more than one compartment or progresses to multiple compartments as in a patient who develops a wound infection that progresses to meningitis. Shunts have been demonstrated to be impervious to bacterial migration across the shunt wall (139), so that spread occurs along the inside or outside of the shunt. Although the possibility of retrograde bacterial movement up the lumen of the shunt has been disputed (140,141), clear evidence of spread of infection from the peritoneal cavity to the brain has been reported (142).

In terms of differential diagnosis, all patients with suspected shunt infection should have a thorough history and physical exam to rule out other possible infections or identify possible sources of infection. This is particularly important in children, where any of the common child febrile illnesses can look like a shunt infection, otitis media and particularly in myelomeningocele patients, urinary tract infection. Patients with an uninfected shunt obstruction can have nuchal rigidity due to tonsillar herniation and occasionally, a low-grade fever.

Diagnostic Tests

Routine blood work will frequently reveal a polymorphonuculear leukocytosis (109-138). Blood culture is perhaps less important in patients with ventriculoperitoneal shunts but should be performed in febrile patients. Culture of the urine or other obvious sites of infections, for example, the wound, should also be taken. Plain film examination of the shunt system will reveal whether the shunt system is still intact, whether an abdominal viscus may have been perforated, and whether or not there are any extraneous pieces of shunt equipment from previous revisions that may also be contaminated. A CT or MRI scan of the head is also important to display the size of the ventricles as part of determining whether or not the shunt is obstructed, but also how the size and configuration of the ventricles may influence decisions to remove the shunt and insert extaventricular drainage (EVD). Placing an EVD in a patient with a functioning but infected shunt with slit ventricles may be quite difficult. Rarely, evidence of ventriculitis or, even more uncommonly, brain abscess may be revealed on cerebral images (142). Abdominal ultrasound should be performed in any patient with abdominal pain or tenderness or a mass. In patients with a suspected shunt infection, particularly if there is suggestion of incomplete shunt obstruction, abdominal ultrasound should be performed.

Probably all patients without obvious wound infection or cutaneously extruded hardware should have the shunt system aspirated through an existing reservoir. Examination of the CSF for cell count, Gram stain, and culture will confirm the diagnosis of shunt infection and quickly give an index of the probable infecting organism. Needless to say, shunt aspiration should be done with meticulous aseptic technique so as not to contaminate a shunt system that is, in fact, sterile or to introduce a second organism in shunts that are already infected. Shunt aspiration provides a high diagnostic yield of shunt infection of approximately 95% (109), and is quite safe (143). Lumbar puncture or ventricular puncture give a much lower yield (7% to 26%). Although CSF leukocytosis, of 50 to 200 cells per cc, is common (138), a normal CSF count may not rule out a colonized shunt, and CSF protein and glucose are often normal (108). Repeat aspiration may be necessary in some cases where shunt infection is suspected, particularly if antibiotics were being used during the first negative aspiration. In patients with a wound infection, care should be taken not to contaminate the interior of the shunt when aspirating the collection surrounding the shunt system.

Sustained elevation of serum levels of C-reactive protein following shunt insertion also correlates strongly with the presence of shunt infection (116). CSF eosinophilia, defined as greater than 7% of total CSF white blood cell count, also correlates with CSF shunt infection (144).

At the time of surgery, ventricular CSF should be resampled. All removed hardware should be sent to the microbiology laboratory. The manner in which the shunt material is handled, however, is important. Simply placing the shunt material in broth culture probably leads to overdiagnosis of shunt infection from growth of organisms that contaminated the shunt at the time of removal (111). As discussed previously, clean surgical wounds are known to harbor skin commensal organisms, and the shunt usually comes into contact with at least the wound edges during removal. Bayston (111) recommended that any purulent material on the shunt be swabbed for microscopy and culture. Subsequently, a local area of the shunt should be swabbed with alcohol and fluid aspirated from the lumen of the shunt with a sterile syringe and needle. If no aspirate is obtained, then the shunt component should be irrigated with sterile saline. Comparing this technique (A) to simply immersing the shunt in broth media (technique B), he found that eight of nine clinically apparent infections were correctly identified with technique A, whereas technique B overdiagnosed shunt infection in 24 of 31 patients (Table 5-5).

Treatment of CSF Shunt Infections

The number of combinations and permutations in the treatment of shunt infection is almost as great as the variety of shunt equipment and techniques of shunt placement in the original operation. There has been one randomized controlled trial that examined the efficacy of three different treatment options (131), and this had only 10 patients in each group, not enough to establish any statistically valid conclusions. All other studies examining shunt infection treatment are hampered by their retrospective nature and frequent lack of strict definition of shunt infection and shunt infection cure.

The main treatment options essentially encompass whether or not the shunt hardware is removed, whether or not interval external drainage is established, and whether or not intraventricular antibiotics are administered. In the sole randomized trial, James (131) compared shunt removal combined with external

TABLE 5-5 CULTURE TECHNIQUES IN DETERMINING CSF SHUNT INFECTION

Method	Total Positive	Clinically Infected
A	9	8
B	31	7
A alone	1	1
B alone	23	0

In method A, purulent material on the shunt is swabbed and cultured. Flid from inside the shunt is aspirated after the outside of the tubing has been swabbed with alcohol. In method B, the whole shunt is immersed in culture media. Method B grossly overestimates the incidence of shunt infection. Reprinted with permission by Bayston R, Leung TSM, Wilkins BM, Hodges B. Bacteriological examination of removed cerebrospinal fluid shunts. J Clin Pathol 1983;36:987-990.

ventricular drainage (EVD) or ventricular taps (Group A) to shunt removal and immediate shunt replacement (Group B) to antibiotics alone (Group C). All patients received intravenous and intraventricular antibiotics, Group A for a minimum of seven days; Groups B and C had intravenous antibiotics for a minimum of three weeks and intraventricular antibiotics for two weeks. All 10 patients in Group A were cured of shunt infection, nine of 10 patients in Group B were cured of shunt infection, and three of 10 patients in Group C were cured of shunt infection. Group A also had the shortest hospital stay, Group C the longest. Two Group C patients died.

Although the patient numbers were too small to draw any conclusions regarding efficacy, the results, in general, reflected what has been identified in a number of other retrospective studies with much larger numbers of patients. CSF shunt removal with interval antibiotic treatment (usually with external ventricular drainage) carries the highest shunt infection cure rate and the lowest mortality rate (110,145,146). CSF shunt removal with immediate replacement carries an almost equal shunt infection cure rate with a higher morbidity and mortality rate. Antibiotic treatment alone has the lowest cure rate and the highest mortality rate.

It is of interest to examine these general treatment options in greater detail. Given the production of a biolayer by the most common infecting organism, and the accompanying resistance to antibiotics that this confers, it seems logical that any treatment short of removal of the shunt hardware would be less successful. While removal of equipment along with interval EVD and subsequent drainage carries the highest chance of eradication of the infection, it also is the most burdensome in terms of surgical procedures for the patient. Two operations are necessary and may involve three surgical sites — the original incision, a new EVD location, and a new shunt site. Normally, the EVD is left in place for approximately one week. This provides an opportunity to examine the CSF daily, to verify that the CSF has become sterile and that the antibiotics in use are appropriate, given the organisms' antibiotic sensitivity. Intraventricular antibiotic injection and antibiotic level measurement is routine with EVD.

However, the EVD largely restricts the patient to bed, is at risk of being dislodged, particularly by children, and can lead to recontamination of the CSF either by the same or a different organism. EVDs can also become obstructed or overdrain, leading to subdural collections. EVDs may be difficult to insert in patients with slit ventricles so that externalization of the peritioneal catheter is an option to establish interval drainage.

Intermittent ventricular puncture and antibiotic instillation is an alternative to an EVD; however, it never provides as good control of the hydrocephalus as the EVD, and there is the risk of injury to the brain by the repeated brain cannulations and development of porencephaly (147). Patients with Gram-negative infections in particular may have very low CSF output (148), however, and not require much CSF drainage.

Immediate shunt insertion, usually at an alternative site, is an attractive option as it saves the patient a subsequent surgical procedure. There is, however, no guarantee that the CSF is sterile at the time of immediate reinsertion. Subsequent treatment with intraventricular antibiotics involves puncture of the reservoir in the region of a fresh incision, and depending on the architecture of the valve system, it may not be possible to inject antibiotics in a retrograde fashion into the ventricle.

Treatment with antibiotics alone can save the patient any subsequent procedures. It has the same difficulties regarding retrograde injection of antibiotics into the ventricles as immediate shunt replacement. While some series have had good success in using antibiotics alone (107,132,145), most series have found an unacceptable morbidity and mortality rate (110-146).

The concentration of intraventricular antibiotics is somewhat unpredictable following both intravenous and intraventricular instillation. Although many antibiotics will cross the blood brain barrier in the presence of inflammation, CSF levels are frequently below mean inhibitory concentration (MIC) levels following intravenous injection (147). CSF levels following intraventricular injection are frequently above MIC concentration, but there is often little correlation between either the weight of the patient or the size of the ventricles and CSF levels (145,147). For this reason, measurement of at least trough levels is advisable during intraventricular administration. It should be borne in mind that MIC levels may not eradicate bacteria in a biolayer as established on shunt equipment.

At the time of shunt reinsertion following an interval EVD, the EVD is usually clamped for eight to 12 hours (providing the patient can tolerate it) to allow the ventricles to expand, and facilitate ventricular cannulation with the new shunt. Whether the EVD should be removed prior to shunt reinsertion is unknown. Removal of the EVD ensures that there is no potentially contaminated hardware in place at the time of reinsertion. However, EVD removal may vent a sufficient amount of CSF to make ventricular cannulation difficult.

Important Exceptions for Antibiotic Alone Treatment

Organisms that cause meningitis in the general population and infect patients with shunts or cause hydrocephalus and are discovered at time of shunt insertion can usually be treated with antibiotics alone. There are a number of patients with *H. influenzae* who have been successfully treated with antibiotics alone (149-152). Successful treatment of meningococcal meningitis and even gonnococcal meningitis in the presence of a shunt has also been reported (153). Although not well documented in the literature, patients presenting with hydrocephalus and unsuspected pneumococcal meningitis can also be successfully treated with antibiotics alone (154). Incumbent in this form of treatment is that the CSF be resampled to verify sterilization. Failure to clear the CSF within 48 to 72 hours should prompt removal of the shunt equipment.

Prevention of Shunt Infection

Given the considerable morbidity, let alone financial cost, of shunt infections, prevention is the leading consideration for the future. Several studies have instituted a number of procedures aimed at risk reduction (such as restricting operating room personnel, operating early in the day, soaking the shunt in antibiotics, and using prophylactic antibiotics) and reported a reduction in shunt infection from 7.75% to .17% (155) in one series and from 12.9% to 3.8% (156) in another, using historical controls from the same institution. Unfortunately, this leaves doubt as to which of the deliberately altered factors is important.

Table 5-6 Results of different types of treatment of CSF shunt infection.

Trial (reference)	Placebo (Y/N)	Sample Size Control	Exp	Outcome Event Rate (%) Control	Exp	Risk ratio	p value	Age range	Follow-up period
Bayston, 1975 112	N	78	54	9.0	1.9	0.36	0.648	NR	NR
Haines & Taylor 1982 137	Y	39	35	12.8	5.7	0.45	0.435	3 days-17 yrs.	6 mos.
Yogev. et.al., 1983 176			48	7.1	1.9	0.26	0.142	Pediatric	6 mos.
	Y	84	58						
Lambert et. al., 1984 171	Y	44	24	18.0	4.4	0.23	0.144	Pediatric	6 mos.
Odio et. al., 1984 172	Y	17	18	24.0	17.0	0.71	0.691	2 days-15 yrs.	7-12 mos.
Wang et. al., 1984 175	Y	65	55	7.7	7.3	0.95	1.00	Pediatric	1-28 mos.
Blomstead, 1985 163	Y	60	62	23.0	6.5	0.28	0.0086*	NR	6 wks.
Schmidt et. al., 1985 173	N	73	79	5.5	9.7	1.62	0.421	<1-14 yrs.	6 mos.
Djindjian et. al., 1986 170	N	30	30	20.0	3.3	0.17	0.103	<6-60 yrs.	6 mos.
Rieder et. al., 1987 168	Y	32	31	9.4	6.5	0.69	1.00	1 wk.-9 yrs.	3 mos.
Blum et. al.,1989 169	N	50	50	14.0	6.0	0.43	0.182	0-14 yrs.	8 wks.
Walters et. al., 1992 174	Y	113	190	19.0	12.0	0.63	0.125	Pediatric	2 yrs.

NR not reported; Exp, experiment group; Y, yes; N, no. Reprinted with permission from Langley JM, LeBlanc JC, Drake JM, Milner R.. Efficacy of antimicrobial prophylaxis in cerebrospinal fluid shunt placement: a meta-analysis. Clin. Infect Dis 1993;17;98-103.
* Statistically significant result by two-tailed test.

TFN Reprinted by permission from Walters BC, Hoffman HJ, Hendrick EB, Humphreys RP. Cerebrospinal fluid shunt infection. Influences on initial management and subsequent outcome. J Neurosurg 1984;60:1014-1021.

Surgical Asepsis

Preoperative skin preparation with iodine-based agents tends to remove transient skin flora and reduce, but not eliminate, resident flora that remain viable in the portals of sweat and sebaceous glands and hair follicles (117,157). These organisms reemerge as the operation proceeds. Shaving with a razor more than a few hours prior to surgery has been clearly related to an increased incidence of infection (158,159). Safety razors invariably produce skin cuts that are visible on scanning electron microscopy (160), so razor shaving should be done just prior to surgery. Chemical depilation, which would remove the hair shafts but leave the epidermal layers intact, may be less traumatic (32). A recent studuy concluded that forgoing shaving did not increase the risk of any neurosurgical procedure, including shunts (161).

While adhesive drapes prevent the shunt from coming in contact with exposed skin remote from the incisions, they do not appear to lower the bacterial density of wounds (162) or the postoperative wound infection rate (158,163,164) . Adhesive drapes may also permit accumulation of sweat under the drapes leading to spillage and contamination of the incision (165). Wound edge barriers, such as those soaked in antiseptic, also do not appear to lower the incidence of wound contamination or shunt infection (164).

Antimicrobial Prophylaxis

Perhaps nothing has aroused as much controversy in the quest for reduced shunt infection as the use of prophylactic antibiotics. While of demonstrated benefit in certain surgical procedures, including surgical implants (166), no clinical trial has convincingly proven efficacy for shunt surgery. The way in which prophylactic antibiotics might work is also debatable since systemic antibiotic prophylaxis did not reduce the number of wounds that were contaminated before skin closure, nor was there any reduction in the rate of shunt colonization (165). As well, bacteria that have contaminated the interior lumen of the shunt apparatus are protected from relatively lower antibiotic concentrations in the CSF and from the host's own immune system. This has led some to recommend administration of antibiotic directly into the shunt at the time of insertion (167).

A number of randomized controlled trials comparing the effects of antibiotic prophylaxis have been reported (113,137,165,168-176) (Table 5-1). Only one detected a significant reduction in infection with antibiotics, and there was a 23% infection rate, which is very high, in the control group (113). All trials suffered from a lack of sufficient number of patients to detect a difference, if one existed. To get around this problem, the trials can be combined and a meta-analysis performed. Langley et al. (177), combining the 12 trials listed in Table 5-6 for a total of 1359 patients, found a significant risk reduction of 50% in the patients treated with prophylactic antibiotics. Haines (178) combined the results of nine controlled studies and also found that antibiotic prophylaxis use resulted in a significant decline in infection rates. This result was restricted to centers in which the baseline infection rate was greater than 15%. Proving that centers that experience an infection rate of 5% would find a significant reduction in infection with prophylactic antibiotics would require thousands of patients. As most of the centers now are reporting very low rates of infection with prophylactic antibiotics and as there is evidence of meta-analysis of the previous reported trials that prophylactic antibiotics are efficacious, it seems reasonable to use them.

In order to be of any effect, the antibiotic must be present in the tissue before contamination occurs (179). Stone et al. (109) reported that if antibiotics were started postoperatively, the infection rate was not significantly different than if no antibiotics were given at all. Experimental dermal incisions in which antibiotic was administered after contamination of the incision were no different than the controls, while the use of antibiotics prior to contamination resulted in a significant difference (180). Therefore, the drug should be given as close to the beginning of the operation as possible while ensuring adequate tissue levels. The overall duration of antibiotic administration should be kept to a relatively short period (usually less than 24 hours) as there is no evidence of benefit after prolonged administration (181), and to prevent superinfection and the development of resistant organisms, it is best to use relatively narrow spectrum drugs that are effective against the most likely infecting organisms. In the case of shunt surgery, the chosen antibiotic should have efficacy against staphylococci.

Modified Shunt Properties

Silastic is relatively biocompatible, and, thus, induces minimal inflammation to the host tissue, thereby enhancing early tissue colonization of the surface and maintaining local tissue resistance (133). Silastic does, however, contain surface imperfections and crevices that can harbor bacterial colonies (139). Smoother surfaces or electrically charged surfaces might be more resistant to colonization. A further modification to the shunt material has been the incorporation of antibacterial substances, including antibiotics. Bayston (182), through a series of experiments, has demonstrated that antibiotics can be incorporated into silastic shunt material and confer long-lasting resistance to colonization by *S. epidermidis* in the laboratory. A combination of rifampin and clindamycin appears to be the most efficacious. A clinical trial evaluating the effects of antibiotic incorporation in reducing shunt infection is underway.

INVESTIGATING SHUNT COMPLICATIONS

DIAGNOSIS

Clinical Evaluation

Shunt mechanical complications may occur at any time from in the recovery room immediately following the shunt operation, to years and years later, when the patient and the family may have all but forgotten about the shunt or falsely believed that the shunt is no longer necessary and the patient is shunt-independent.

Common to most mechanical complications is the obstruction of CSF shunt flow and the accompanying rise in intracranial pressure. This leads most commonly to headache, nausea, and vomiting. The onset of symptoms may be quite variable, ranging from sudden and severe, to slow and insidious. A rapid and severe rise in intracranial pressure will lead to lethargy and, ultimately, unconsciousness. Less obvious signs of shunt mechanical malfunction include irritability, deterioration in school performance, or delay in achievement of developmental milestones. Occasionally, new or increased seizure frequency may be a symptom of mechanical shunt dysfunction. Patients may also complain of double vision or families notice loss of conjugate gaze with sixth nerve palsies. Loss of vision from chronic papilledema may be insidious, particularly in small children. The only sign may be the child moving closer and closer to the television and subsequently "bumping into things."

Signs of mechanical dysfunction relate to the clinical manifestations of raised intracranial pressure as well as abnormalities of the performance of the shunt hardware. Examination of the mental status of the patient will vary from subtle intellectual deterioration to coma. On physical exam, infants often present with a bulging fontanelle, split sutures, and abnormally increased head circumference. Despite the absence of infection, nuchal rigidity may be present from herniation of the tonsils through the foramen magnum. Papilledema will appear in patients with closed sutures. Sixth nerve palsy, which may be bilateral, often accompanies papilledema. Loss of vertical gaze is also common. With impending brain herniation, decerebrate posturing, apnea, bradycardia and pupillary dilatation ensue.

Examination of the site of the shunt equipment implantation may provide confirmatory evidence of shunt dysfunction. While pumping of the shunt reservoir is a time-honored shunt functional assessment technique, in fact, it is often misleading. A patient in whom a reservoir fills very slowly may simply have small ventricles. However, shunts whose reservoirs remain umbilicated for prolonged periods of time, or even permanently, are often blocked proximally. A reservoir that is very difficult to depress or refills apparently instantaneously frequently indicates a distal obstruction. Some shunt reservoirs contain proximal and distal occluders (or, less satisfactory, two valveless reservoirs). By occluding the distal reservoir and depressing and allowing the reservoir to refill, one can imply that the proximal catheter is patent. Similarly, by occluding the proximal reservoir and flushing distally, one can infer patency of the distal catheter. In this situation, the reservoir should remain umbilicated if the occluder is working properly.

Fluid collecting around the shunt, particularly if it firmly distends the skin, is progressive, and tracks along the distal catheter is often a sign of shunt occlusion. When shunts fracture, CSF often continues to track along the fibrous sheath. In this scenario, one can often feel a small amount of fluid and a space where the shunt has come apart. It may be difficult, however, to distinguish an empty sheath from the sheath containing shunt tubing, particularly if the shunt has been implanted for some years or the tract is calcified. A fluid thrill can sometimes be felt at the site of a distal catheter disruption, with pumping a proximal reservoir.

Patients with shunt overdrainage may complain of postural headache -- headache that commences with the assumption of the upright posture and disappears with recumbency. Patients with subdural hematoma may present with signs of raised intracranial pressure, but there may be some true localizing signs, such as hemiparesis. Patients with loculated CSF compartments also tend to present with signs of increased pressure. Patients with loculated fourth ventricles may present specifically with bulbar paralysis and apnea. Sometimes symptoms and signs of syringomyelia, particularly in shunted myelomeningocele patients, may be a manifestation of shunt obstruction. The clinical features of shunt mechanical dysfunction may also be intermittent. This occurs both in the slit ventricles syndrome, and with partially occluded proximal or distal catheters.

Diagnostic Tests

Imaging studies are normally the first investigation undertaken. Plain anteroposterior and lateral films of the skull, chest, and abdomen will demonstrate whether the shunt is in continuity or has come apart or fractured. For this reason alone, all shunt tubing, housing, etc., should be easily seen on x-ray. These x-rays may also demonstrate a peritoneal catheter that has migrated out of the abdomen with growth or obvious misplacement of the ventricular or pertioneal catheter. The films must often be scrutinized quite closely to detect small separations at connectors or along tubing. Calcification along the tubing is common in long implanted shunts, which are prone to fracture. Common sites of shunt fracture are at connectors between the valve and the peritoneal catheter, where the hard connector repeatedly stresses the soft tubing, and in the neck, where it is presumably related to movement. Distal slit valves, which fill with debris and occlude, may be distended on plain abdominal films (183).

CT, MRI, or ultrasound imaging will determine the size and shape of the ventricles as well as any other collections or loculated compartments. The position and course of the shunt can also be seen, best on CT. Dilation of the ventricles, compared to a previous image when the shunted patient was well, is the simplest and clearest evidence of shunt dysfunction. Some patients, however, may have small ventricles or demonstrate minimal enlargement in the presence of shunt obstruction, and the ventricle size alone, in the absence of previous images, may be quite misleading in terms of shunt function. This is true particularly in children where growth and development of the brain and congenital malformations alter one's notions of what normal ventricular size is. Uncertainty about the status of the shunt in a patient with symptoms compatible with shunt obstruction often leads to other diagnostic tests. Perhaps the simplest is the shunt tap. Under sterile conditions, the reservoir can be punctured with a 25-gauge butterfly needle catheter. Free flow of fluid indicates patency of the proximal catheter. The tubing can be used as a manometer to measure the pressure in the ventricular system. If the reservoir is distal to the proximal valve, flow of CSF back into the shunt gives an indication of the patency of the distal

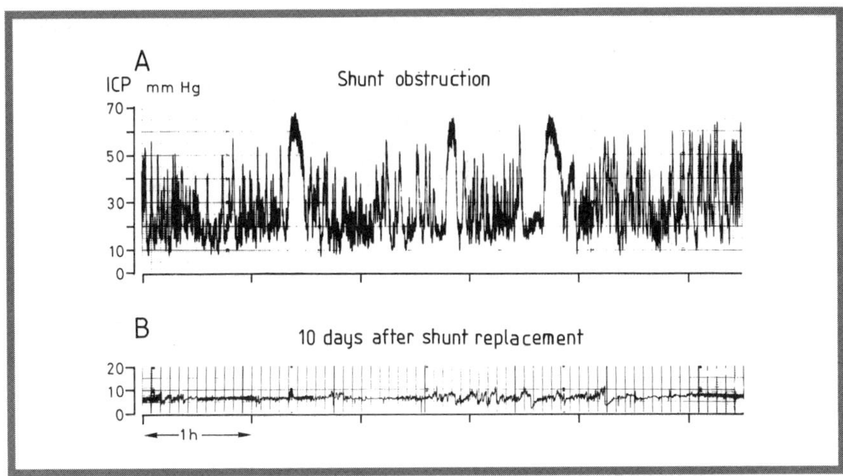

FIGURE 5-30
Pressure tracing in patient with blocked shunt. Note intermittent pressure waves over 60 mm Hg. Immediate resolution following revision of the shunt.

catheter. A shunt tap can also be therapeutic and life-saving in critically ill shunted patients. Aspiration of five of 10 cc of fluid will frequently dramatically improve a deteriorating shunted patient while preparations for surgery are made. In life-threatening situations, when the proximal catheter is blocked and no CSF can be aspirated, passing a lumbar puncture needle through the shunt, burr hole, and brain into the ventricle may be life-saving. This will often destroy the proximal portion of the shunt but is of little consequence given the gravity of the situation and the forthcoming shunt revision.

In patients with headache in whom there is doubt about the functional status of the shunt, intracranial pressure (ICP) monitoring may often resolve the nature of a headache, whether low or high pressure or whether or not there is any relation between the onset of headache and ICP. Monitors may be placed extradural, subdural, intraparenchymal, or intraventricular or in the lumbar theca. In patients in whom low pressure headache is a strong possibility, it is important to measure the pressure in both the recumbent and upright position and encourage activity as normal as possible. In measuring negative pressure, some fiber-optic transducers may not behave linearly at large negative pressures.

In valve systems with a reservoir proximal to the valve and in which the ventricular catheter is known to be patent, a #25 butterfly can be inserted into the reservoir under strict aseptic conditions and connected to a pressure transducer for 24 to 48 hours. The risk of infecting the valve with this type of monitoring has reported to be quite low (184). There are also two implantable pressure transducers, as described in Chapter 4 (185). The pressure can be measured transcutaneously (and noninvasively) with reasonable accuracy. The site for pressure monitoring is not critical as long as it is a true reflection of the intracranial pressure. Figure 5-30 shows the change in pressure following revision of a

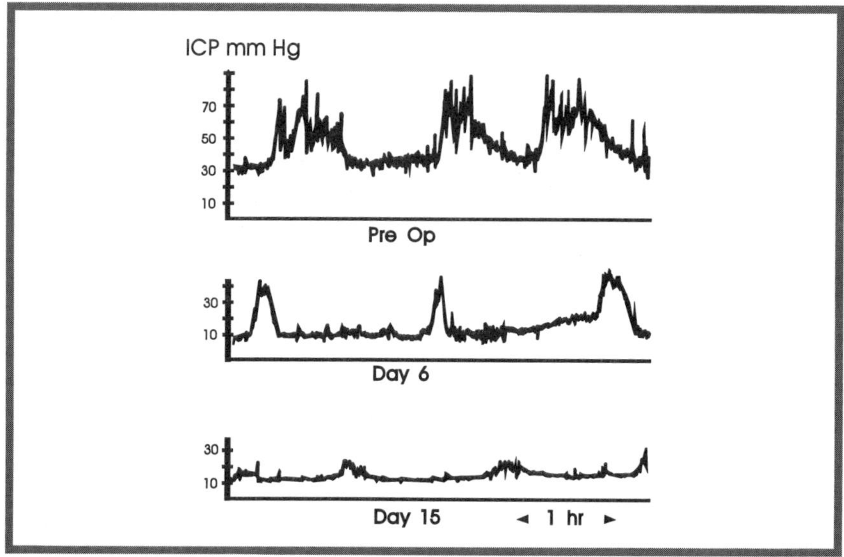

FIGURE 5-31
Pressure tracing in patient with slit ventricles and a functioning standard differential pressure shunt. Similar periodic elevations in pressure. Progressive decrease in pressure following revision of valve to Orbis Sigma.

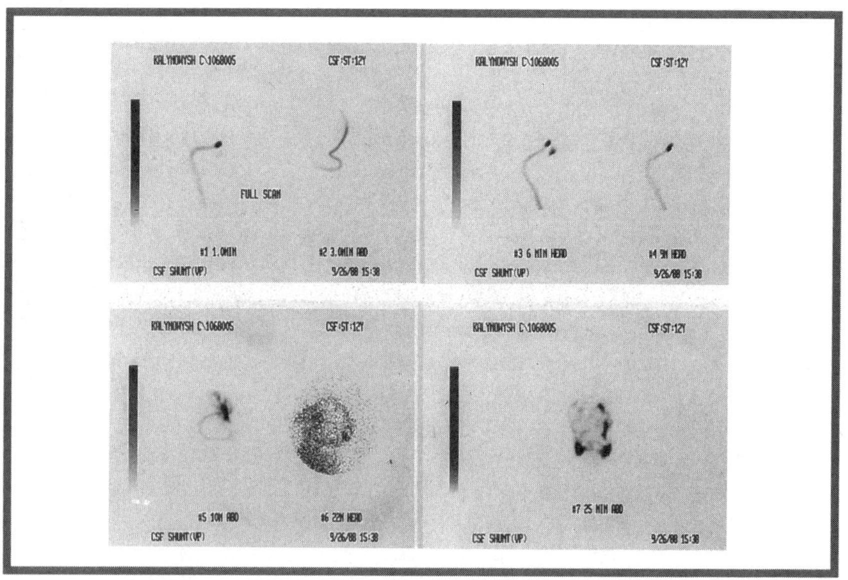

FIGURE 5-32
Radioisotope injection into shunt system. Flow is seen in shunt reservoir, and passes quickly into abdominal cavity where it freely diffuses. A normal study in a functioning shunt.

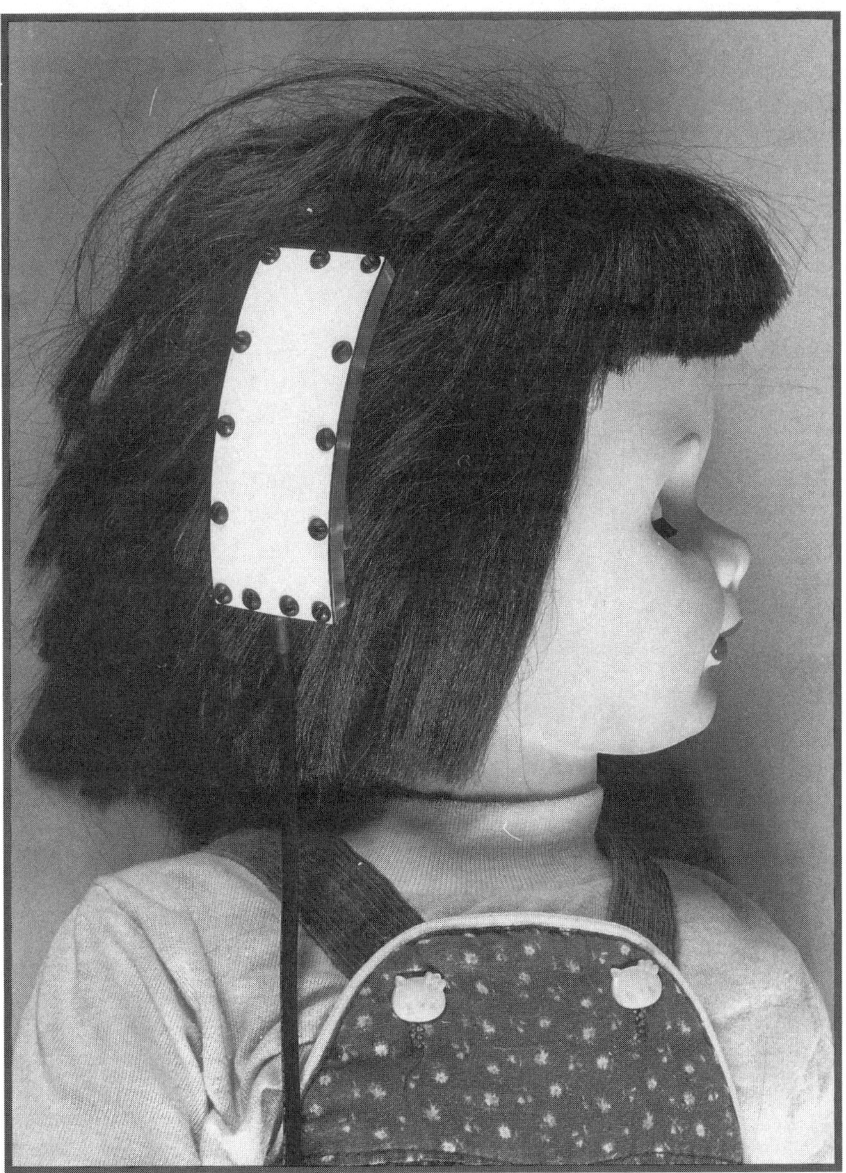

FIGURE 5-33
Special shunt-imaging surface coil. The coil is placed along the course of the shunt over the scalp just distal to the reservoir. Metal components in the near vicinity and patient motion may produce uninterpretable images.

patient with a blocked shunt. Occasionally, a monitor may have to be left in place for some time, particularly if it is critical to measure the response to a particular treatment. Figure 5-31 shows the change in pressure in a patient with slit ventricles syndrome following revision of the shunt.

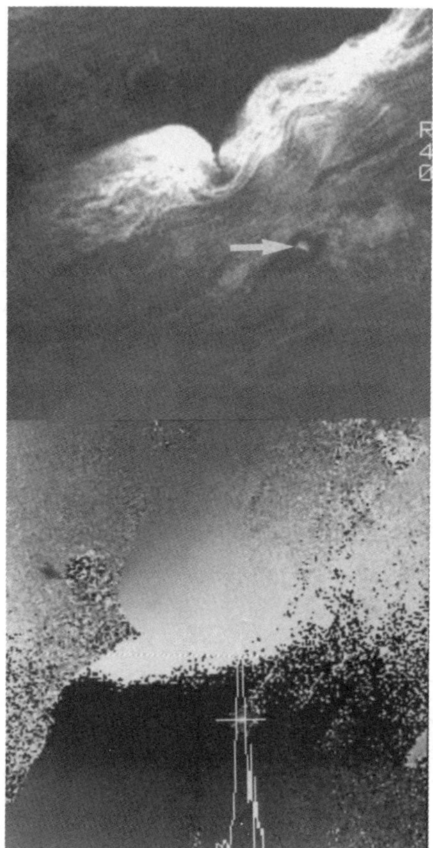

FIGURE 5-34
Magnitude (upper) and phase images (lower) in a patient with a functioning shunt (right). The lumen of the shunt is partially obscured in the flowing shunt due to flow artefact (arrows). In the phase images, the horizontal line crosses the shunt lumen. The corresponding velocity profile is shown below. In the flowing shunt there is a parabolic flow profile corresponding to a flow rate of 6 cc/hr.

Occasionally, it is necessary to establish absolutely whether or not the shunt is patent and tests of shunt flow are a direct method of determining this. The most widely used techniques employ injections of isotope or radopgraphic contrast. Injection of isotope, typically technetium^{99} into the reservoir, allows one to follow qualitatively the flow of radioactive tracer along the shunt tube (Figure 5-32). If the reservoir is above the valve, then reflux into the ventricles will confirm that the upper end is patent. Otherwise, it may be more difficult to decide which end is blocked. Sitting the patient up or pumping the reservoir helps to see what effect these manipulations have on the shunt system. Collection of contrast in a localized cyst in the abdomen can also be seen with this technique and confirmed with ultrasound. A quantitative shunt flow rate can be measured using isotope and an external detector placed over the injected reservoir if the whole system has been calibrated for that particular shunt system (186). From the observed decay in intensity, a flow rate is determined. This is only really useful if the same shunt system is implanted routinely. Injection of iodinated contrast, or the "shuntogram," gives essentially the same information (187). The problem with both of these techniques is that there is always the low but attendant risk of infecting the shunt. The reservoir or its contained valve can be damaged by the needle. Neither of these techniques is fool-proof. False negatives and false positives occur. Extravasated contrast from a disconnected shunt may track along the narrow shunt sheath, at least as far as the abdominal wall, and give the appearance of flow. Very sluggish flow may be a feature of a partially blocked shunt, or simply indicate a patient who is not that shunt-dependent.

The problems with the aforementioned invasive tests have led to the quest for other ways for measuring shunt flow. Some of these techniques have been very ingenious. Leading the way in technical complexity has been the implantation of an electrolysis unit in line with the shunt system (188,189). The movement of the generated gas bubble is then measured with either ultrasound or electrical impedance. A similar but noninvasive concept involves cooling the shunt tubing upstream with ice and detecting the passage of the cooled CSF below with a thermistor (190). While an appealing concept, one can just imagine melting ice cubes, screaming children, etc. Skin thickness also affects the measurements so that it ends up being a detection of patency. Simplest of all is determination of shunt patency by placing an ultrasound probe over the shunt and pumping the reservoir (191).

Recently, we have used MRI to measure shunt flow experimentally and in a few clinical situations (192). MRI is intrinsically sensitive to flow and can be made more so by using specialized pulse sequences. The difficulties surround visualizing the shunt tubing (1.2 mm inside diameter) and detecting the flow, which may be on the order of a few cc an hour. Using a curved surface coil (Figure 5-33), a flow-sensitive pulse sequence, and high resolution images perpendicular to the shunt tubing, shunt flow was measured and used to determine shunt patency (Figure 5-34). The advantage of the technique is that it is noninvasive. Disadvantages relate to artefacts produced by patient motion or metallic components.

An indirect indication of the patency of the shunt may be determined by measuring the cerebral blood flow velocity in the major basal arteries using transcranial Doppler (193). This method measures the velocity, but not the actual blood flow, since the caliber of the arteries is not known. Various indices can be calculated, including the pulsatility index, which relates the systolic to diastolic velocity. In hydrocephalic patients, there is a substantial fall in the pulsatility index. This is restored following implantation of a CSF shunt. Shunt obstruction produces a subsequent fall in the index. As there is considerable overlap between normal and hydrocephalic patients in terms of the absolute index, the test is most reliable when baseline measurements are made when the shunted patient is well.

REFERENCES

1. Choux M. Shunts and problems in shunts. Basel/New York: Karger, 1982: 1-6.
2. Griebel R, Khan M, Tan L. CSF shunt complications: an analysis of contributory factors. Child's Nerv Syst 1985;1:77-80.
3. Hayden PW, Shurtleff DB, Stuntz TJ. A longitudinal study of shunt function in 360 patients with hydrocephalus. Dev Med Child Neurol 1983;25:334-337.
4. Olsen L, Frykberg T. Complications in the treatment of hydrocephalus in children. Acta Paediatr Scand 1983;72:385-390.
5. Piatt JH Jr., Carlson CV. A search for determinants of cerebrospinal fluid shunt survival: retrospective analysis of a 14-year institutional experience. Pediatr Neurosurg 1993;19:233-242.
6. Sainte-Rose C, Piatt JH, Renier D, Pierre-Kahn A, Hirsch JF, Hoffman HJ, Humphreys RP, Hendrick EB. Mechanical complications in shunts. Pediatr Neurosurg 1991-92;17:2-9.
7. Sayers MP. Shunt complications. Clinical Neurosurg 1976;28:393-400.
8. Sekhar LN, Moosy J, Guthkelch N. Malfunctioning ventriculoperitoneal shunts. J Neurosurg 1982;56:411-416.
9. McLaurin RL. Shunt complications. In: Pediatric neurosurgery: surgery of the developing nervous system. New York: Grune & Stratton, 1982:243-253.
10. Johnson DL, Fitz C, McCullough DC, et al. Perimesencephalic cistern obliteration: a CT sign of life-threatening shunt failure. J Neurosurg 1986;386-389.
11. Post EM. Currently available shunt systems: a review. Neurosurgery 1985;16:257-260.
12. Sainte-Rose C. Third ventriculostomy. In: Manwaring KH, Crone KR, eds. Neuroendoscopy. Volume 1. New York: Mary Ann Liebert, 1992:47-62.
13. Epstein F, Murali R. Pediatric posterior fossa tumors: hazards of the "preoperative" shunt. Neurosurgery 1978;3:348-350.
14. Gurtner P, Bass T, Gudeman SK, Penix JO, Philput CB, Schinco FP. Surgical management of posthemorrhagic hydrocephalus in 22 low-birth-weight infants. Child's Nerv Syst 1992;8:198-202.
15. James HE, Bejar R, Meritt A, et al. Management of hydrocephalus secondary to intracranial hemorrhage in the high risk newborn. Neurosurgery 1984;14:612-618.

16. James HE, Boynton BR, Boynton CA. Severe intracranial hemorrhage and hydrocephalus in low-brithweight infants treated with CSF shunts. Child's Nerv Syst 1987;3:110-111.

17. Pezzotta S, Locatelli D, Bonfanti N. Shunt in high-risk newborns. Child's Nerv Syst 1987;3:114-116.

18. Albanese V, Tomasello F, Sampaolo S, et al. Neuroradiological findings in multiloculated hydrocephalus. Acta Neurochir 1982;60:297-311.

19. Hirsch JF, Pierre-Kahn A, Renier D, et al. The Dandy-Walker malformation. A review of 40 cases. J Neurosurg 1984;61:515-522.

20. Kalsbeck JE, DeSousa AL, Kleiman MB, et al. Compartmentalization of the cerebral ventricles as a sequela of neonatal meningitis. J Neurosurg 1980;52:547-552.

21. Lourie H, Shende MC, Krawchenko J, Steward OH. Trapped fourth ventricle as delayed complication of ventricular shunting. Report of two unusual cases. Neurosurgery 1980;7:279-282.

22. Collins P, Hockley AD, Woollam DHM. Surface ultrastructure of tissues occluding ventricular catheters. J Neurosurg 1978;48:609-613.

23. Sainte-Rose C, Hooven MD, Hirsch JF. A new approach in the treatment of hydrocephalus. J Neurosurg 1987;66:213-226.

24. Abbott R, Epstein FJ, Wisoff JH. Chronic headache associated with a functioning shunt: usefulness of pressure monitoring. Neurosurg 1991;28:72-77.

25. Nowak TP, James HE. Migraine headaches in hydrocephalic children: a diagnosis dilemma. Childís Nerve Syst 1989:5:310-314.

26. Bierbrauer KS, Storrs BB, McLone DG, Tomita T, Dauser R. A prospective, randomized study of shunt function and infections as a function of shunt placement. Pediatr Neurosurg 1990-91;16:287-291.

27. Giuffre' R. Choroidal and ependymal reactions. J Neurosurg Sci 1976;20:123-129.

28. Noetzel MJ, Baker RP. Shunt fluid examination: risks and benefits in the evaluation of shunt malfunction and infection. J Neurosurg 1984;61:328-332.

29. Gower DJ, Lewis JC, Kelly DL. Sterile shunt malfunction. A scanning electron microscopic perspective. J Neurosurg 1984;61:1079-1084.

30. Bigio MRD, Bruni E. Reaction of rabbit lateral periventricular tissue to shunt tubing implants. J Neurosurg 1986;64:932-940.

31. Walters BL, Hoffman HJ, Hendrick EB, et al. Cerebrospinal fluid shunt infections. Influences on initial management and subsequent outcome. J Neurosurg 1984;60:1014-1021.

32. Albright AL, Haines SJ, Taylor FH. Function of parietal and frontal shunts in childhood hydrocephalus. J Neurosurg 1988;69:883-886.

33. Reeder JD, Kaude JV, Setzer ES. The occipital horn of the lateral ventricles in premature infants. An ultrasonographic study. Eur J Radiol 1983;3:148-150.

34. Rubin R, Hochwald GM, Tiell M, et al. Reconstitution of the cerebral cortical mantle in shunt-corrected hydrocephalus. Dev Med Child Neurol 1975;17:(Suppl 35):151-156.

35. Rubin RC, Hochwald GM, Tiell M, et al. Hydrocephalus. III. Reconstruction of the cerebral cortical mantle following ventricular shunting. Surg Neurol 1976;5:179-183.

36. Shkolnik A, McLone DC. Intraoperative real-time ultrasonic guidance of ventricular shunt placement in infants. Radiology 1981;141:515-517.

37. Vries JK. Endoscopy as an adjunct to shunting for hydrocephalus. Surg Neurol 1980;13:69-72.

38. Haase J, Weeth R. Multiflanged ventricular catheter for hydrocephalic shunts. Acta Neurochir (Wien) 1976;33:213-218.

39. Go KG, Ebels EJ, VAn Woerden H. Experiences with recurring ventriuclar catheter obstructions. Clin Neurol Neurosurg 1981;83:47-56.

40. Rekate HL. Classification of slit-ventricle syndromes using intracranial pressure monitoring. Pediatr Neurosurg 1993;19:15-20.

41. Sainte-Rose C. Shunt obstruction: a preventable complication? Pediatr Neurosurg 1993:19:156-164.

42. Agha MD, Amendola MA, Shirazi KK, et al. Abdominal complications of ventriculoperitoneal shunts with emphasis on the role of imaging methods. Surg Gynecol Obstet 1983;156:473-478.

43. Echizenya K, Satoh M, Mural H. Mineralization and biodegradation of CSF shunting systems. J Neurosurg 1987;67:584-591.

44. Griebel RW, Hoffman HJ, Becker L. Calcium deposit on CSF shunts. Clinical observations and ultrastructural analysis. Child's Nerv Syst 1987;3:180-182.

45. Sugar O, Bailey OT. Subcutaneous reaction to silicone in ventriculoperitoneal shunts. Long-term results. J Neurosurg 1974;41:367-371.

46. Haase J, Bang F, Tange M. Danish experience with the one-piece shunt. A long-term follow-up. Child's Nerv Syst 1987;3:93-96.

47. Raimondi AJ, Robinson JS, Kuwamura K. Complications of ventriculoperitoneal shunting and a critical comparison of the three-piece and one-piece systems. Child's Brain 1977;3:321-342.

48. Cantu RC, Mark VH, Austen WG. Accurate placement of the distal end of a

ventriculoatrial shunt catheter using vascular pressure changes. J Neurosurg 1967;27:584-596.

49. Pritz MB. A simple method for distal catheter lengthening of ventriculoatrial shunts. Report of eight cases. J Neurosurg 1980;53:229-232.

50. Robertson JT, Schick RW, Morgan F, et al. Accurate placement of ventriculoatrial shunt for hydrocephalus under electrocardiographic control. J Neurosurg 1961;18:255-257.

51. Gruber R. The problem of chronic overdrainage of the ventricular-peritoneal shunt in congenital hydrocephalus. Z Kinderchir 1980;31:362-369.

52. Gruber R. Should 'normalization' of the ventricles be the goal of hydrocephalus therapy? Z Kinderchir 1983;38(Suppl. 2):80-83.

53. Portnoy HD, Schulte RR, Fox JL, et al. Anti-siphon and reversible occlusion valves for shunting in hydrocephalus and preventing postshunt subdural hematomas. J Neurosurg 1973;38:729-738.

54. Gruber R, Jenny P, Herzog B. Experiences with the anti-siphon device (ASD) in shunt therapy of pediatric hydrocephalus. J Neurosurg 1984;61:156-162.

55. Da Silva MC, Drake JM. Effect of subcutaneous implantation of antisiphon devices on CSF shunt function. Pediatr Neurosurg 1990-91;16:197-202.

56. McCullough DC, Wells M. Complications with antisiphon devices in hydrocephalics with ventriculoperitoneal shunts. In: Concepts in pediatric neurosurgery/American Society for Pediatric Neurosurgery. Basel/New York: Karger, 1982:63-75.

57. McCullough DC. Symptomatic progressive ventriculomegaly in hydrocephalics with patent shunts and anti-siphon devices. Neurosurgery 1986;19:617-621.

58. Epstein F. Increased intracranial pressure in hydrocephalic children with functioning shunts: a complication of shunt dependency. In: Shapiro K, Marmarou A, Portnoy H, eds. Hydrocephalus. New York: Raven Press, 1984:315-321b.

59. Epstein F, Marlin AE, Wald A. Chronic headache in the shunt-dependent adolescent with nearly normal ventricular volume: diagnosis and treatment. Neurosurgery 1978;3:351-355.

60. Faulhauer K, Schmitz P. Overdrainage phenomena in shunt-treated hydrocephalus. Acta Neurochir 1978;45:89-101.

61. Foltz EL, Blanks JP. Symptomatic low intracranial pressure in shunted hydrocephalus. J Neurosurg 1988;68:401-408.

62. Foltz EL, Shurtleff DB. Conversion of communicating hydrocephalus to stenosis or occlusion of the aqueduct during ventricular shunt. J Neurosurg 1966;24:520-529.

63. Hoppe-Hirsch E, Sainte-Rose C, Renier D. Pericerebral collections after shunting. Childs Nerv Syst 1987;3:97-102.

64. Sivalingam S, Corkill G. Treatment of hydrocephalus and bilateral subdural effusions in a patient with closed sutures. Case report. J Neurosurg 1976;45:447-448.

65. Engel M, Carmel PW, Chutorian AM. Increased intraventricular pressure without ventriculomegaly in children with shunts: "normal volume" hydrocephalus. Neurosurgery 1979;5:549-552.

66. Holness RO, Hoffman HJ, Hendrick EB. Subtemporal decompression for the slit-ventricle syndrome after shunting in hydrocephalic children. Child's Brain 1979;55:137-144.

67. Hyde-Rowan MD, Rekate HL, Nulsen FE. Reexpansion of previously collapsed ventricles: the slit ventricle syndrome. J Neurosurg 1982;556:536-539.

68. Kiekens R, Mortier W, Pothmann R, et al. The slit-ventricle syndrome after shunting in hydrocephalic children. Neuropediatrics 1982;13:190-194.

69. Andersson H. Craniosynostosis as a complication after operation for hydrocephalus. Acta Paediatr Scand 1966;55:192-196.

70. Kloss JL. Craniosynostosis secondary to ventricular shunt. Am J Dis Child 1968;116:315-317.

71. Chapman PH, Griebel R, Cosman ER, et al. Telemetric ICP measurement in normal and shunted hydrocephalus patients. In: Chapman PH, ed. Concepts in pediatric neurosurgery. Volume 6. Basel/New York: Karger, 1985:115-132.

72. Chiba Y, Ishiwata Y, Suzuki N, et al. Thermosensitive determination of obstructed sites in ventriculoperitoneal shunts. J Neurosurg 1985;62:363-366.

73. Cosman ER, Zervas NT, Chapman PH, et al. A telemetric pressure sensor for ventricular shunt systems. Surg Neurol 1979;11:287-294.

74. Savoiardo M, Solero CL, Passerini A, et al. Determination of cerebrospinal fluid shunt function with water-soluble contrast medium. J Neurosurg 1978;49:398-407.

75. Stein SC, Apfel S. A noninvasive approach to quantitative measurement of flow through CSF shunts. Technical note. J Neurosurg 1981;556-558.

76. Epstein F. How to keep shunts functioning, or "The Impossible Dream." Clin Neurosurg 1984a;32:608-631.

77. Ferguson AH. Intraperitoneal diversion of the cerebrospinal fluid in cases of hydrocephalus. NY Med J 1898;67:902.

78. Aoki N. Lumboperitoneal shunt: clinical applications, complications and comparison with ventriculoperitoneal shunt. Neurosurgery 1990;26: 998-1004.

79. Chumas PD, Kulkarni AV, Drake JM, Hoffman HJ, Humphreys RP, Rutka JT. Lumboperitoneal shunting: a retrospective study in the pediatric population. Neurosurgery 1993;32:376-383.

80. Guy J, Johnston PK, Corbett JJ, Day AL, Glaser JS. Treatment of visual loss in pseudotumor cerebri associated with uremia. Neurology 1990;40:28-32.

81. James HE, Tibbs PA. Diverse clinical applications of percutaneous lumboperitoneal shunts. Neurosurgery 1981;8:39-42.

82. Johnston I, Besser M, Morgan MK. Cerebrospinal fluid diversion in the treatment of benign intracranial hypertension. J Neurosurg 1988;69:195-202.

83. Eisenberg HM, Davidson RI, Shillito J. Lumboperitoneal shunts. Review of 34 cases. J Neurosurg 1971;35:427-431.

84. Kuwana N, Kuwabara. Lumbar subarachnoid-peritoneal shunt: follow-up study on 158 cases. Neurol Med Chir (Tokyo) 1984;24:485-489.

85. Selman WR, Spetzler RF, Wilson CB, Grollmus JW. Percutaneous lumboperitoneal shunt : Review of 130 Cases. Neurosurgery 1980;6:255-257.

86. Sainte-Rose C, Hoffman HJ, Hirsh JF. Shunt failure. In: Marlin AE, ed. Concepts Pediatr Neurosurg. Basel: Karger, 1989;9:7-20.

87. Selman WR, Spetzler RF. New lumboperitoneal shunt catheter. Surg Neurol 1984;21:58-60.

88. Spetzler R, Wilson C, Grollmus J. Percutaneous lumboperitoneal shunt. J Neurosurg 1975;43:770-773.

89. Hoffman HJ, Hendrick EB, Humphreys RP. New lumboperitoneal shunt for communicating hydrocephalus. J Neurosurg 1976;44:258-261.

90. Kushner J, Alexander E, Davis CH, Kelly DL. Kyphoscoliosis following lumbar subarachnoid shunts. J Neurosurg 1971;34:783-791.

91. McIvor J, Krajbich JI, Hoffman HJ. Orthopaedic Complications of lumboperitoneal shunts. J Pediatric Orthopaedics 1988;8:687-689.

92. Steel HH, Adams DJ. Hyperlordosis caused by the lumboperitoneal shunt procedure for hydrocephalus. J Bone Joint Surg 1972;54:1537-1542.

93. Chumas PD, Drake JM, del Bigio M. Death from unsuspected tonsillar herniation in a patient with Crouzon's disease and a lumboperitoneal shunt: a case report. Br J Neurosurg 1992;6:593-598.

94. Chumas PD, Armstrong DC, Drake JM, Kulkarni AV, Hoffman HJ, Humphreys RP, Rutka JT, Hendrick EB. Tonsillar herniation-- the rule rather than the exception after lumboperitoneal shunting in the pediatric population. J Neurosurg 1993;78:568-573.

95. Hoffman HJ, Tucker WS. Cephalocranial disproportion: a complication of the treatment of hydrocephalus in children. Child's Brain 1976;2:167-176.

96. Duddy MJ, Williams B. Hindbrain migration after decompression for hindbrain hernia: a quantitative assessment using MRI. Br J Neurosurg 1991;5:141-152.

97. Sullivan LP, Stears JC, Ringel SP. Resolution of syringomyelia and Chiari malformation by ventriculoatrial shunting in a patient with pseudotumor cerebri and a lumboperitoneal shunt. Neurosurgery 1988;22:744-747.

98. Chuang S, Hochhauser L, Fitz C, et al. Lumboperitoneal shunt malfunction: a new, reliable CT sign. Acta Neuroradiologica 1986;10(Suppl 369):645-648.

99. da Silva MC, Drake JM. Effect of subcutaneous implantation of anti-siphon devices on CSF function. Pediatr Neurosurg 1990-91:16;197-202.

100. Fox JL, Portnoy HD, Shulte RR. Cerebrospinal fluid shunts: an experimental evaluation of flow rates and pressure values in the anti-siphon valve. Surg Neurol 1973:1;299-302.

101. McCullough DC. Symptomatic progressive ventriculomegaly in hydrocephalics with patent shunts and anti-siphon devices. Neurosurgery 1986;19:617-621.

102. Portnoy HD, Schulte RR, Fox JL, Croissant PD, Tripp L. Anti-siphon and reversible occlusion valves for shunting in hydrocephalus and preventing postshunt subdural haematomas. J Neurosurg 1973;38:729-738.

103. da Silva MC, Drake JM. Complications of CSF shunt anti-siphon devices. Pediatr Neurosurg 1991-92;17:304-309.

104. Drake JM, da Silva MC, Rutka JT. Functional obstruction of an anti-siphon device by raised tissue capsule pressure. Neurosurgery, 1993;32:137-139.

105. Drake JM, Kulkarni AV. CSF shunt infections. Neurosurgical Quarterly 1993;3:283-294.

106. Luthardt TH. Bacterial infections in ventriculoauricular shunt systems. Dev Med Child Neurol 1970;22(Suppl)105-107.

107. O'Brien M, Parent A, Davis B. Management of ventricular shunt infections. Child's Brain 1979;5:304-309.

108. Renier D, Lacombe J, Pierre-Kahn A, Sainte-Rose C, Hirsch JF. Factors causing acute shunt infection. J Neurosurg 1984;61:1072-1078.

109. Schoenbaum SC, Gardner P, Shillito J. Infections of cerebrospinal fluid shunts: epidemiology, clinical manifestations, and therapy. J Infect Dis 1975;131:543-552.

110. Walters BC, Hoffman HJ, Hendrick EB, Humphreys RP. Cerebrospinal fluid shunt infection. Influences on initial management and subsequent outcome. J Neurosurg 1984;60:1014-1021.

111. Bayston R, Leung TSM, Wilkins BM, Hodges. Bacteriological examination of removed cerebrospinal fluid shunts. J Clin Pathol 1983;36:987-990.

112. Bayston R. A prospective randomised controlled trial of antimicrobial prophylaxis in hydrocephalus shunt surgery. Z Kinderchir 1990;45(Suppl I):5-7.

113. Blomstedt GC. Results of trimethoprim-sulfamethoxazole prophylaxis in ventriculostomy and shunting procedures. J Neurosurg 1985;62:694-697.

114. Pople IK, Bayston R, Hayward RD. Infection of cerebrospinal fluid shunts in infants: a study of etiological factors. J Neurosurg 1992;77:29-36.

115. Shapiro S, Boaz J, Kleiman M, Kalsbeck J, Mealey J. Origin of organisms infecting ventricular shunts. Neurosurgery 1988;22:868-872.

116. Bayston R. Hydrocephalus shunt infections. London: Chapman & Hall, 1989:12-57.

117. Bayston R, Lari J. A study of the sources of infection in colonized shunts. Dev Med Child Neuro 1974;16(Suppl):17-22.

118. Blowers R, Mason GA, Wallace KR, Walton M. Control of wound infection in a thoracic surgery unit. Lancet 1955;ii:786-794.

119. Charnley J, Eftekhar N. Postoperative infection in total prosthetic replacement arthroplasty of the hip joint, with special reference to the bacterial content of the air of the operating room. Br J Surg 1969;56:641-649.

120. Lidwell OM, Lowbury EJL, Whyte W, Blowers R, Stanley SJ, Lowe D. Effect of ultraclean air in operating rooms on deep sepsis in the joint after total hip or knee replacement. Br Med J 1982;285:10-14.

121. Gristina AG. Biomaterial-centered infection: microbial adhesion versus tissue integration. Science 1987;237:1588-1595.

122. Vercelloti GM, McCarthy JB, Lindholm P, Peterson PK, Jacobs HS, Furcht LT. Extracellular matrix proteins (fibronectin, laminin and type IV collagen) bind and aggregate bacteria. Am J Pathol 1985;120:13-21.

123. Costerton JW, Cheng KJ, Geesey GG, Ladd TI, Nickel JC, Dasgupta M, Marrie TJ. Bacterial biofilms in nature and disease. Ann Rev Microbiol 1987;41:435-464.

124. Baltimore RS, Mitchell M: Immunological investigations of mucoid strains of Pseudomonas aeruginosa: comparison of susceptibility by opsonic antibody in mucoid and nonmucoid strains. J Infect Dis 1980;141:238-247.

125. Peterson PK, Wilkinson BJ, Kim Y, Schmeling D, Quie PG. Influence of encapsulation on staphylococcal opsonization and phagocytosis by human polymorphonuclear leukocytes. Infect Immun 1978;19:943-949.

126. Whitnak E, Bisno AL, Beachey EH: Hyaluronate capsule prevents attachment of Group A streptococci to mouse peritoneal macrophages. Infect Immun 1981;31:985-991.

127. Govan JRW. Mucoid strains of Pseudomonas aeruginosa: the influence of culture medium on the stability of mucus production. J Med Microbiol 1975;8:513-522.

128. Nickel JC, Ruseska I, Costerton JW. Tobramycin resistance of cells of Pseudomonas aeruginosa growing as a biofilm on urinary catheter material. Antimicrob Agents Chemother 1985;27:619-624.

129. Nickel JC, Ruseska I, Whitfield C, Marrie TJ, Costerton JW. Antibiotic resistance of Pseudomonas aeruginosa colonizing a urinary catheter in vivo. Eur J Clin Microbiol 1985;4:213-218.

130. Diaz-Mitoma F, Harding GKM, Hoban DJ, Roberts RS, Low DE. Clinical significance of a test for slime production in ventriculoperitoneal shunt infections caused by coagulase-negative staphylococci. J Infect Dis 1987;156(4):555-560.

131. James HE, Walsh JW, Wilson HD, et al. Prospective randomised study of therapy in cerebrospinal fluid shunt infection. Neurosurg 1980;7:459-463.

132. Shurtleff DB, Foltz EL, Weeks RD, Loesser J. Therapy of Staphylococcus epidermidis: infections associated with cerebrospinal fluid shunts. Pediatr 1974;53:55-62.

133. Khoury AE, Lamb K, Ellis B, Costerton JW. Prevention and control of bacterial infections associated with medical devices. A SAIO J 1992;38:174-178.

134. Bayston R, Penny SR. Excessive production of mucoid substance by Staphylococcus SIIA: a possible factor in colonisation of Holter shunts. Dev Med Child Neuro 1972;14(Suppl27):25-28.

135. Ammirati M, Raimondi AJ. Cerebrospinal fluid shunt infections in children. A study on the relationship between the etiology of hydrocephalus, age at the time of shunt placement, and infection rate. Child's Nerv Syst 1987;3:106-109.

136. George R, Librock L, Epstein M. Long-term analysis of cerebrospinal fluid shunt infections: a 25-year experience. J Neurosurg 1979;51:804-811.

137. Haines SJ, Taylor F. Prophylactic methicillin for shunt operations: effects on incidence of shunt malfunction and infection. Child Brain 1982;9:10-22.

138. Forward KR, Fewer D, Stiver HG. Cerebrospinal fluid shunt infections. A review of 35 infections in 32 patients. J Neurosurg 1983;59:389-394.

139. Guevara JA, Zuccaro G, Trevisan A, Denoya CD. Bacterial adhesion to cerebrospinal fluid shunts. J Neurosurg 1987;67:438-445.

140. Bayston R, Spitz L. The role of retrograde movement of bacteria in ventriculoatrial shunt colonisation. Z Kinderchir 1978;25:352-356.

141. Holt RJ. Bacteriological studies on colonized ventriculoatrial shunts. Dev Med Child Neuro 1970;12(Suppl 22):83-87.

142. Gower DJ, Horton D, Pollay M. Shunt-related brain abscess and ascending shunt infection. J Child Neurol 1990;5:318-320.

143. Noetzel MJ, Baker RP. Shunt fluid examination: risks and benefits in the evaluation of shunt malfunction and infection. J Neurosurg 1984;61:328-332.

144. Tung H, Raffel C, McComb JG. Ventricular cerebrospinal fluid eosinophilia in children with ventriculoperitoneal shunts. J Neurosurg 1991;75(4):541-544.

145. Wald SL, McLaurin RL. Cerebrospinal fluid antibiotic levels during treatment of shunt infections. J Neurosurg 1980;52:41-46.

146. Yogev R. Cerebrospinal fluid shunt infections: a personal view. Pediatr Infect Dis J 1985;4:113-118.

147. James HE, Wilson HD, Connor JD, Walsh JW. Intraventricular cerebrospinal fluid antibiotic concentrations in patients with intraventricular infections. Neurosurg 1982;10(1):50-54.

148. Drake JM, Sainte-Rose C, da Silva MC, Hirsch JF. Cerebrospinal fluid flow dynamics in children with external ventricular drains. Neurosurg 1991;28:242-250.

149. Lerman SJ. Haemophilus influenzae infections of cerebrospinal fluid shunts. Report of two cases. J Neurosurg 1981;54:261-263.

150. Patriarca PA, Lauer BA. Ventriculoperitoneal shunt-associated infection due to haemophilus influenzae. Pediatr 1980;65(5):1007-1009153.
Leggiadro RJ, Atluru, Katz SP. Meningococcal meningitis associated with cerebrospinal fluid shunts. Pediatr Infect Dis J 1984;3:489-490.

151. Petrak RM, Pottage JC Jr, Harris AA, et al. Haemophilus influenzae meningitis in the presence of a cerebrospinal fluid shunt. Neurosurg 1986;18:79-81.

152. Rennels MB, Wald ER. Treatment of haemophilus influenzae type B meningitis in children with cerebrospinal fluid shunts. J Pediatr 1980;97:424-426.

154. Klein DM: Shunt infections. In: Scott RM, ed. Hydrocephalus: concepts in neurosurgery. Baltimore: Williams and Wilkins, 1990:88.

155. Choux M, Genitori L, Lang D, Lena G. Shunt implantation: reducing the incidence of shunt infection. J Neurosurg 1992;77:875-880.

156. Hoffman HJ, Soloniuk D, Humphreys RP, Drake JM, Hendrick EB. A concerted effort to prevent shunt infection. In: Matsumoto S, Tamaki N, eds: Hydrocephalus: pathogenesis and treatment. Toyko: Springer-Verlag, 1991:510-514..

157. Saggers BA, Stewart GT. Polyvinylpyrolidone iodine: an assessment of antibacterial activity. J Hyg (Camb) 1964;62:509-518.

158. Cruse PJE, Foord. The epidemiology of wound infection. Surg Clin North Amer 1980;60:27-40.

159. Seropian R, Reynolds BM. Wound infections after preoperative depilatory versus razor preparation. Am J Surg 1971;121:251-254.

160. Hamilton HW, Hamilton KR, Lone FJ. Preoperative hair removal. Can J Surg 1977;20:269-275.

161. Winston KR. Hair and neurosurgery. Neurosurg 1992;2:320-329.

162. Raahave D. Effect of plastic skin and wound drapes on the density of bacteria in operation wounds. Br J Surg 1976;63:421-426.

163. Jackson DW, Pollock AV, Tindal DS. The value of a plastic adhesive drape in the prevention of wound infection. Br J Surg 1971;58:340-342.

164. Tabara Z, Forrest D. Colonisation of CSF shunts: preventive measures. Z Kinderchir 1982;37:156-157.

165. Bayston R. Antibiotic prophylaxis in shunt surgery. Dev Med Child Neuro 1975;17{Suppl 35):99-103.

166. Sandusky WR. Use of prophylactic antibiotics in surgical patients. Surg Clin North Amer 1980;60:83-92.

167. Welch K: The prevention of shunt infection. Z Kinderchir 1977;22:465-475.

168. Blum J, Schwartz M, Voth D. Antibiotic single-dose prophylaxis of shunt infections. Neurosurg Rev 1989;12:239-244.

169. Djindjian M, Fevrier MJ, Otterbein G, Soussy JC. Oxacillin prophylaxis in cerebrospinal fluid shunt procedures: results of a randomized open study in 60 hydrocephalic patients. Surg Neurol 1986;25:178-180.

170. Lambert M, MacKinnon AE, Vaishnav A. Comparison of two methods of prophylaxis against CSF shunt infection. Z Kinderchir 1984:39(Suppl 2):109-110.

171. Odio C, Mohs E, Sklar FH, et al. Adverse reactions to vancomycin used as prophylaxis for CSF shunt procedures. Am J Dis Child 1984;138:17-19.

172. Reider, MJ, Frewen TC, Del Maestro RF. The effects of cephalothin phophylaxix in postoperative ventriculoperitoneal shunt infections. Can Med Assoc J 1987;136:935-938.

173. Schmidt K, Gjerris F, Osgaard O, et al. Antibiotic prophylaxis in cerebral fluid shunting: a prospective randomized trial in 152 hydrocephalic patients. Neurosurg 1985;17:1-5.

174. Walters BC, Goumnerova L, Hoffman HJ, et al. A randomized controlled trial of perioperative rifampin/trimethoprim in cerebrospinal fluid shunt surgery. Child's Nerv Syst 1992;8:253-257.

175. Wang EEL, Prober CG, Hendrick EB, et al. Prophylactic sulfamethoxazole and trimethoprim in ventriculoperitoneal shunt surgery. A double-blind, randomized, placebo-controlled trial. J Amer Med Assoc 1984;251:1174-1177.

176. Yogev R, Shinco F, McLone D. Prophylaxis for ventriculo-peritoneal shunt surgery with nafcillin alone or in combination with rifampin. [Abstract no. 664]. In: Program and Abstracts of the 23rd Interscience Conference on Antimicrobial Agents and Chemotherapy. Las Vegas, Nevada: American Society for Microbiology, 1983.

177. Langley JM, LeBlanc JC, Drake JM, Milner R. Efficacy of antimicrobial prophylaxis in cerebrospinal fluid shunt placement: a meta-analysis. Clin Infect Dis 1993;17:98-103.

178. Haines SJ. Do antibiotics prevent shunt infections? A meta-analysis. (Abstract) Pediatric Section of AANS, 1991.

179. Haines SJ, Walters BC. Antibiotic prophylaxis for cerebrospinal fluid shunt. Neurosurgery 1994;34:87-92.

180. Burke JF. The effective period of preventive antibiotic action in experimental incisions and dermal lesions. Surgery 1961;50:161-168.

181. Stone HH, Haney BB, Kolb LD, et al. Prophylactic and preventive antibiotic therapy: timing, duration, and economics. Ann Surg 1979;189:691-698.

182. Bayston R, Grove N, Siegel J, Lawellin D, Barsham S. Prevention of hydrocephalus shunt catheter colonization in vitro by impregnation with antimicrobials. J Neurol Neurosurg Psych 1989;52:605-609.

183. Le roux P, Berger M, Benjamin D. Abdominal x-ray and pathological findings in distal unishunt obstruction. Neurosurgery 1988;23:749-752.

184. Abbot R, Epstein FJ, Wisoff JH. Chronic headache associated with a functioning shunt: usefulness of pressure monitoring. Neurosurgery 1991;28:72-77.

185. Chapman PH, Griebel R, Cosman ER, et al. Telemetric ICP measurement in normal and shunted, hydrocephalic patients. In: Chapman, PH, ed. Concepts in pediatric neurosurgery. Volume 6. Basel/New York: Karger, 1985:115-132.

186. Chervu S, Chervu LR, Vallabhajosyula B, Milstein DM, Shapiro KM, Shulman K, Blaufox MD. Quantitative evaluation of cerebrospinal fluid shunt flow. J Nucl Med 1984;25:91-95.

187. French BN, Swanson M. Radionuclide-imaging shuntography for the evaluation of shunt patency. Surg Neurol 1981;16:173-182.

188. Seppanen U, Serlo W, Saukkonen AL: Valvography in the assessment of hydrocephalus shunt function in children. Neuroradiology 29:53-57,1987.

189. Hara M, Kadowaki C, Konishi Y, Ogashiwa M, Numoto M, Takeuchi K. A new method for measuring cerebrospinal fluid flow in shunts. J Neurosurg 1983;58:557-561.

190. Numoto M, Hara M, Tatsuo S, Kadowaki C, Takeuchi K. A noninvasive CSF flowmeter. J Med Eng Technol 1984;8:218-220.

191. Chiba Y, Yuda K. Thermosensitive determination of CSF shunt patency with a pair of small disc thermistors. J Neurosurg 1980;52:700-704.

192. Flitter MA, Bucheit WA, Murtagh F, Lapayowker MS. Ultrasound determination of cerebrospinal fluid shunt patency. J Neurosurg 1975;42:728-730.

193. Drake JM, Martin AJ, Henkelman RM. Determination of CSF shunt obstruction with MR phase imaging. J Neurosurg 1991;75:535-540.

194. Chadduck WM, Crabtree HM, Blankenship JB, Adametz J. Transcranial Doppler ultrasonography for the evaluation of shunt malfunction in pediatric patients. Child's Nerv Syst 1991;7:27-30.

Chapter 6

CHOOSING AND INSERTING A SHUNT

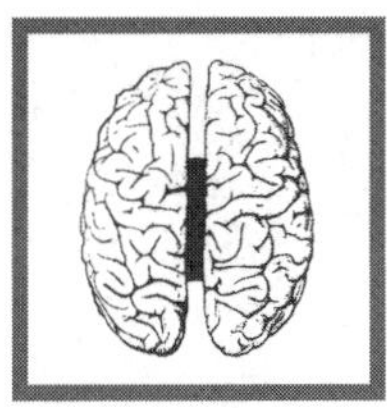

6 Choosing and Inserting a Shunt

It should be emphasized at the outset that this chapter is not meant to endorse any manufacturer's product; however, while the authors are not prepared to recommend a particular type of shunt, nor do they think one particular shunt will be appropriate for all patients, they do offer some guidelines: (1) since a shunt insertion is a lifetime commitment to an imperfect device, all attempts to avoid a shunt should be made; (2) shunt selection should be based as much as possible on a scientific data, and (3) a good surgical technique is the best insurance against shunt complications.

ALTERNATIVES TO SHUNT

Alternatives to shunting exist in hydrocephalus due to an obstacle within the ventricles including the outlets of the fourth ventricle (e.g., aqueductal stenosis and posterior fossa arachnoid cyst), and in conditions where the alteration of the hydrodynamics of the cerebrospinal fluid could be transient (e.g., hemorrhage and tumoral hydrocephalus). These alternative treatments must be considered first, even if they are less evident than simple shunt insertion. The restoration of a normal CSF circulation will always be better than any artificial drainage. However, in some cases these alternative treatments are not sufficient. Their results must be carefully assessed, and the surgeon should not rule out a shunt device.

MEMBRANE FENESTRATION

In cases of aqueduct stenosis, fenestration of the floor of the third ventricle establishes an alternative route for the CSF flow toward the subarachnoid spaces (1). This treatment is of particular interest due to the morbidity and even mortality related to shunt failure in this type of hydrocephalus. In shunted patients, drainage of the lateral and third ventricles is assured by the shunt while drainage of the fourth ventricle is done through normal CSF pathways. Alteration of this fragile equilibrium can induce severe clinical consequences. The obstacle created by aqueduct stenosis on the midline is responsible for the development of a pressure gradient at a very vulnerable site. In addition to restoration of a pseudonormal CSF circulation, third ventriculostomy reestab-

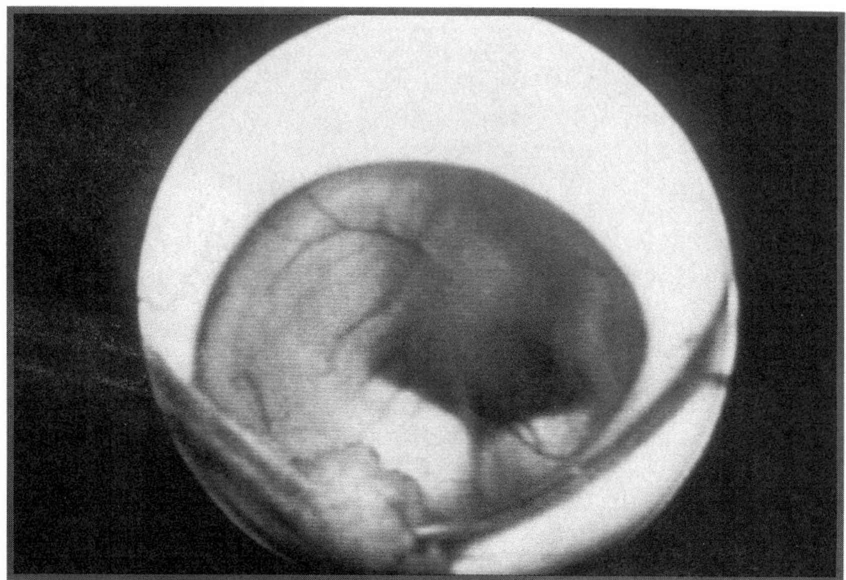

FIGURE 6-1
Endoscopic view of the right foramen of Monro in a patient selected for third ventriculostomy. The choroid plexus and the septal vein are well identifiable. The mamillary bodies, and the thin part of the floor of the third ventricle in front of them, are visible trough the enlarged foramen of Monro.

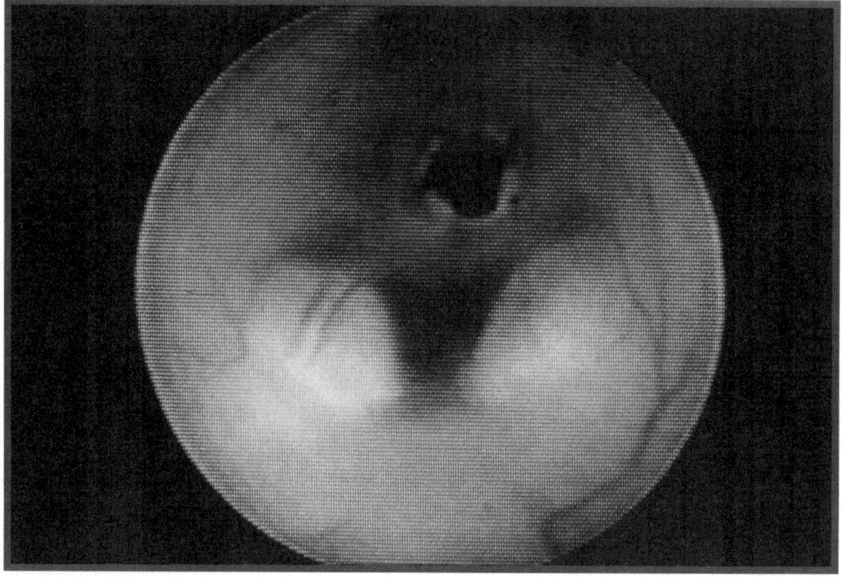

FIGURE 6-2
Appearance of the orifice of third ventriculostomy in front of the mamillary bodies. This orifice allows communication between the third ventricle and the interpeduncular cistern.

lishes a uniform hydrostatic pressure regimen in the whole central nervous system. Magnetic resonance imagery and particularly phase contrast studies have greatly improved the diagnosis of this type of hydrocephalus patient, showing the aqueduct stenosis, and its causes, but also giving semi-quantitative information on the CSF flow alteration. At present, perforation of the floor of the third ventricle to bypass the blocked aqueduct is essentially assured by endoscopic surgery. A neuroendoscope, rigid or steerable, is introduced in the lateral ventricle through a coronal burr hole 2 to 3 cm from the midline. The foramen of Monro is located through identification of the choroid plexus and the septal and thalamostriate veins (Figure 6-1). The endoscope is then passed into the third ventricle. Landmarks in the third ventricle, posterior to anterior, are the mamillary bodies, the dome of the division of the basilar artery often visible through the stretched floor, the dorsum sellae, and the infundibulum recess. An orifice is created in front of the division of the basilar artery, putting into communication the third ventricle and the prepeduncular cistern (Figure 6-2). Several methods, namely, laser, monopolar wire coagulator, "saline torch", and balloon catheter, may be used to perforate the ventricular floor. For safety reasons, the authors prefer to make an initial inframillimetric hole using a coagulation wire or a laser beam or by passing a blunt instrument such as a closed biposy forceps through the transparent floor of the third ventricle. This hole is then dilated with a balloon catheter. One must be aware that the decrease of the ventricular size after an efficient third ventriculostomy is less significant than after shunting. Evidence of a flow at the level of the ventriculostomy orifice by phase contrast magnetic resonance imaging (Figure 6-3), and normalization of the clinical symptoms take priority over the size of the ventricles in evaluating the benefit of the treatment.

Arachnoid cysts impairing the CSF circulation may be treated by endoscopic fenestration in many cases. However, it is necessary not only to establish communication between the cyst and the nearest ventricle, but also between the cyst and the subarachnoid spaces. In other words, the proximal and distal walls of the cyst have to be perforated. Cysts located in the suprasellar region, the foramen magnum, the posterior fossa, and within the ventricles are potential indications for this method of treatment.

TUMORAL HYDROCEPHALUS

The most common brain tumors in childhood are located in the posterior fossa and are responsible for various degrees of ventricular enlargement in the majority of the cases (2). Hydrocephalus will be cured by tumor removal in a significant number of patients, up to 80%. There is a general consensus to admit that a preoperative shunt must be avoided, except in very particular conditions. The old habit to shunt these patients routinely prior to tumor removal is no longer valid since it may induce shunt dependency in patients who are no longer hydrocephalic after tumor surgery and do not need a shunt.

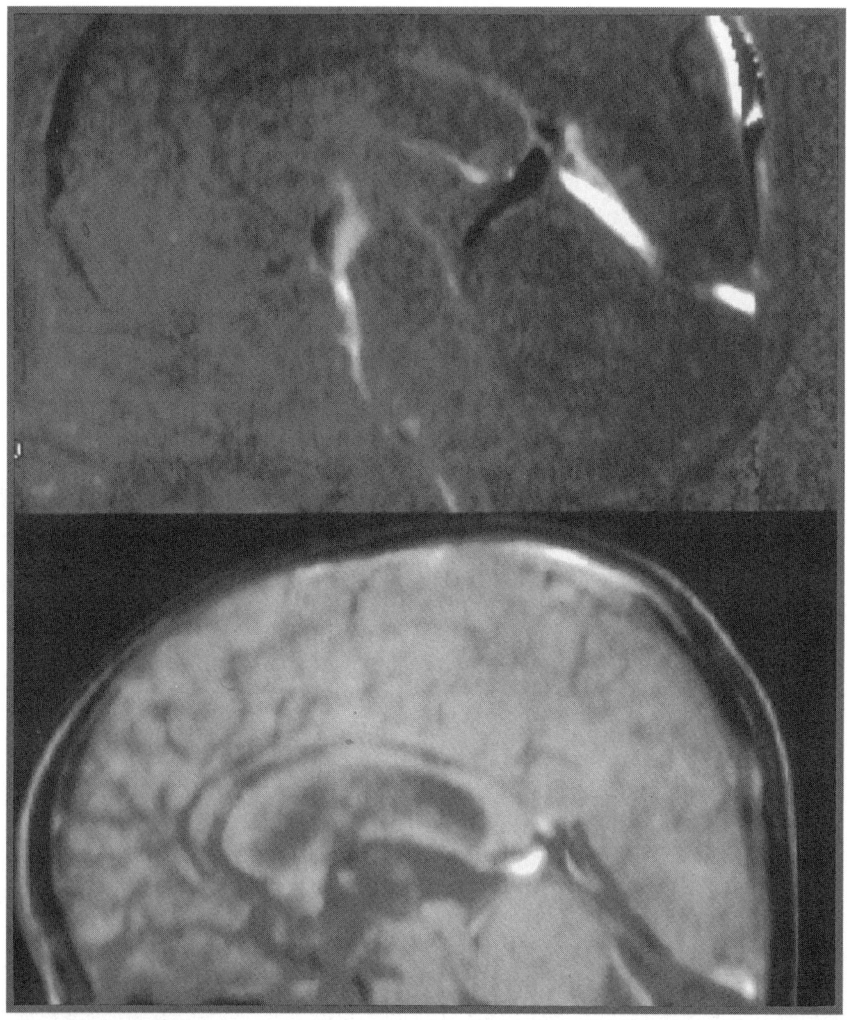

FIGURE 6-3
The patency of the orifice of third ventriculostomy is demonstrated on phase contrast magnetic resonnance imaging.

HEMORRHAGE

If the causes of hemorrhage may vary (prematurity, head injury, rupture of a vascular malformation), the consequences for CSF hydrodynamics are similar. At an acute stage, clots generated by the bleeding create mechanical obstacles to CSF flow in the narrowest parts of its pathways (aqueduct of Sylvius, cisternae, subarachnoid spaces, arachnoid villi); an increased CSF viscosity following bleeding is insufficient to induce hydrocephalus. At a chronic stage, leptomeningeal fibrosis may develop in some cases, leading to a permanent increased resistance to CSF flow. This two-step evolution must be taken into account for the treatment, because not all of these patients will become permanently hydrocephalic. Treatment of the acute phase of the ventricular enlargement using a temporary method of drainage (e.g., external ventricular drainage or access port to the CSF), or medical treatment save a significant number of patients from a permanent shunt (3,4). In addition, these methods allow clearing of the CSF from the debris that it may contain prior to shunting, if needed.

HOW TO CHOOSE A SHUNT

The perfect shunt does not exist. However, the wide number of available devices may allow an acceptable compromise in most cases (5). But, as Fred Epstein pointed out, the selection of a particular shunt is very often "more subjective than scientific." In addition, if shunts differ in their design, from the hydrodynamic standpoint they can be classified in two or three categories only. Prior to selecting a shunt system, the surgeon must consider several factors. The problem is not only the shunt, but also proper patient management and good surgical technique (6-9).

PATIENT MANAGEMENT

Patient considerations such as age, weight, skin thickness, and head size may influence the choice of the design of the shunt to prevent occurrence of skin problems. The size of ventricles, the patient's size, the patient's status (e.g., vegetative, normal, etc.), the pathogenesis of hydrocephalus, and the acuteness of the illness may influence the choice of the hydrodynamic properties of the system. Clinical status (e.g., internal lines, gastrostomy, tracheotomy, laparotomy, augmented bladder, and so forth) may influence the type of surgery to ensure an adequate drainage of the CSF and to reduce the risk of shunt contamination. Status of the CSF, for example, debris from a recent hemorrhage, may require postponement shunt insertion and use of an alternative method of treatment until the CSF is cleared up in order to avoid an early shunt obstruction. Loculation of the ventricles may require an endoscopic surgery prior to shunting in order to use only one shunt system. When a shunt is inevitable, the goal is to try to get a unique cavity fill with normal CSF drains with a simple system, having adequate design and hydrodynamic properties, in a cavity able to resorb the amount of CSF drained.

SHUNT

As already said, the perfect shunt does not exist, but it is probably possible to agree on some items, and necessary to get more information for others. The situation today is such that probably no two neurosurgeons agree on which are the best shunts to implant in hydrocephalic patients. This is a result of the lack of knowledge of hydrocephalus and the lack of scientific data supporting different designs. The range of shunts used is probably a combination of "what one was brought up on", personal experience, the shunt equipment available or in use in an institution, what one has seen or heard at recent meetings with colleagues, including scientific presentation, informal discussions, presentations by companies, and visits by sales representatives, and financial contraints. While one should, above all, use a shunt system with which one is comfortable, one should also be prepared to change or try different designs, especially if there is evidence that the complication rate may be less. One should also be aware of the internal design of the shunt, the design of the entire drainage system, including its accessories, and the flow pressure characteristics of the system. It seems important to examine an unsterile sample of the shunt before implanting it. In this way one will ensure awareness of all its components and physical characteristics. The three basic elements of a shunt--a proximal catheter, a valve system, and a distal catheter--were discussed in Chapter 4 . In addition, several components can be added to the shunt line. As the large number of devices is mainly the consequence of commercial competition, it is interesting to try to evaluate them one by one in an attempt to determine their problems or weaknesses.

Basic materials

As discussed in Chapter 3, most shunts are made from the same components, i.e., silicone elastomer, polycarbonte, polyethylene, polysulfone, metals, and barium impregnation. At present, pure silicone without barium in contact with the subcutaneous tissue appears to be the most appropriate material to achieve biocompatibility. However, there have been several reports implicating silicone as a causative agent for host reactions and suggesting a need for a more biologically inert material (10-12). Several available valve systems incorporate metallic components or even magnets, which may produce artefacts on MR imaging; these systems must be avoided when for some reason the patient has to be followed using MRI.

Ventricular catheters

- Size: It appears that so-called small or ultra-small catheters were designed to be less traumatic in infants or premature babies. It could be interesting to collect data about the risk of proximal occlusions versus catheters diameters on one hand and the risk of neurological consequences (epilepsy) and skin problems versus catheter diameters on the other hand, because if there is no correlation reported in the literature, it makes no sense (except for commercial purposes) to have several different diameters.
- Stiffness: The stiffness of the catheters is a function of the grade of the silicone on one hand and the thickness of the tubing (external diameter to internal diameter on the other hand. This parameter is a compromise between two risks (for straight ventricular catheters): To be soft enough to prevent an injury of the ventricular wall and a subsequent migration into the brain parenchyma and be firm enough to be kink-resistant.
- Length: The length of ventricular catheters is directly related to the surgical technique and, at present, everyone is convinced that his or her own technique is the best. There is a clear need for randomized prospective study.
- Shape (straight, right angle): Because of elasticity, straight has the advantage,

when not used with a right-angle clip, of going naturally up, away from the choroid plexus. It is interesting to note that the aim of the so-called right-angle clip or sleeves is to direct the tubing and not to prevent an exceptional kink (if it exists). A right-angle catheter has the advantage of staying where it was located at shunt insertion time and avoiding extra volume under the skin as realized by right-angle sleeves. It is, however, limited to certain incremental lengths that cannot be altered, and requires carrying a considerable inventory of ventricular catheters.

- Tip (flanged or not flanged): Flanged catheters of various design were proposed either to prevent obstruction by choroid plexus or to prevent debris from going into the valve at shunt insertion time (13). There are enough reported data to conclude that they do not achieve these goals; even more, these devices seem to favor firm choroid plexus attachment on the ventricular catheter. At present, the safest choice seems to be a nonflanged ventricular catheter.

Burr hole

- Preshaped Catheters: The simplest way to contour the burr hole is to use a preshaped right-angle ventricular catheter. However, because of the predetermined length of the catheter, it is necessary to have in stock several catheters of different length to match the needs of each particular case.
- Straight Catheters: They can be cut to the desired length for each case. At the burr hole, this type of catheter can be either bent without accessories, the risk of kinking with the existing material being minimum, or maintained right-angled with some additional device. These right angle clips may be aggressive for the skin when made in hard plastic.
- Burr Hole Reservoir: A straight ventricular catheter may be connected to a reservoir that fits in the burr hole. Both catheter and reservoir must form a one-piece element. No ligature is needed at or under the skull level, thus avoiding eventual disconnection resulting in the loss of the catheter in the ventricle, especially during shunt revision. In addition, the use of a burr hole reservoir needs a longer skin incision to avoid having the device under the scar.
- Right-Angle Connectors (metal or plastic): This device requires a ligature under the skull, with the risk just mentioned of lost catheter. It should be avoided.

Reservoir (shape, size, location, tap)

This device is generally considered an essential element of any shunt system; however, one of the authors followed more than 2,000 patients shunted without reservoir and is still not convinced of its usefulness. The rationale for using this device is to have an easy access to the system for fluid sampling (but the advantages have to be balanced with the low risk of contamination related to this technique and the risk of mechanical problems related to the reservoir), patency testing (but the results are often unreliable), drug injection (but most shunt infections require the removal of all the contaminated system to be cured), and pressure recording (but it carries a low risk of shunt contamination). If considered necessary, the reservoir must present certain characteristics. It must be thick enough to avoid leakage but be soft enough and thus not agressive for the skin. The reservoir must be of a size compatible with pediatric use, but be palpable under the skin of an adult. This device may be located at the burr hole level, in line with the valve proximal to it, or integrated in the valve system. In any case, it increases the total volume of the valve system and requires a larger subcutaneous dissection to be properly inserted compared with a valve without reservoir.

Valve

- Location: Except for distal slit valves, which must be avoided because it is almost the unique cause of distal obstruction, the valves are located proximal in the shunt system. It is up to the surgeon to locate the valve more or less far from the burr hole; most recommend to implant it at the skull level, others in the upper part of the neck, at least in infants, still others recommend the prethoracic region. One must remember that the valve is a point of inherent fixation of the system.
- Design: The valve must not be too big and its shape not too aggressive for the skin to be implantable in infants. But, why do we have pediatric and adult models? Hopefully, a child will grow, and physiology of the CSF is not that different in adults and in children. The shape of the valve seems more important. Some devices have a cylindrical form close to that of the tubing and may migrate easily under the skin if they are not properly secured by a nonabsorbable ligature in the subcutaneous tissue.
- Pumping Device: Pumping devices may be unreliable, and parents should be discouraged from manipulating them. However, they can give some indication of shunt patency and access for CSF sampling.
- Hydrodynamic Characteristics (5,14,15): From the hydrodynamic standpoint, there are three classes of shunt: pressure-regulating devices (externally adjustable or not), siphon-resistive devices, and flow-regulating devices. Most valves act as pressure-regulating devices. A one-way valve mechanism, calibrated at a certain opening pressure, tries to maintain a constant pressure across the valve (differential pressure) regardless of the drainage flow. As shown in Chapter 2, several mechanisms can be used to achieve this. Although they differ in their mechanical construction, they all achieve the same result: when the differential pressure across the valve increases, the valve opens and CSF flows freely. An ideal pressure regulator would give a horizontal pressure/flow curve. By definition, the drainage flow of these valves is very sensitive to the variances in differential pressure. The wide range of pressure induced by postural changes, REM sleep, and physical exertion are known to generate an overdrainage several times higher than CSF secretion. However, two complementary mechanisms enable these derivations to effectively treat hydrocephalus: (1) the choice of an opening pressure limiting overdrainage, but at the expense of some underdrainage when

the differential pressure is low (supine position); and (2) the resilience of a biological system, the patient, capable of adapting to conditions far from normal physiology. However, several complications are recognized to be directly or indirectly linked to the inadequacy of the CSF drainage observed with these shunts. To try and remedy these drawbacks, alternatives have been proposed in the past 15 years: valves with externally adjustable opening pressures, siphon resistive systems, and flow-regulating devices.

- Valves with externally adjustable opening pressures (Sophy, Medos) are derived from conventional systems. They allow a fine tuning in vivo of the balance between under- and overdrainage without surgery. The hydrodynamic characteristics of these shunts are the same as those of traditional valves. The adjustable function is obtained with the use of magnets built in the valve mechanism. They tend to compensate for reduced negative pressure in the upright posture by increased pressure in the recumbent position (see Chapter 3).
- Siphon-Resistive Devices (anti-siphon device, siphon control device, Delta valve): A system reacting to the hydrostatic pressure, equal to the distance between the two ends of the distal catheter, increases the valve opening pressure when the patient leaves the recumbent position. This type of device would react only to the pressure variations upstream of the valve; it would tend to maintain the intracranial pressure always positive, including in standing position. In addition, the function of this device is directly related to atmospheric pressure, which is not always the case in the scarred tissue around the valve (see Chapter 5).
- Flow-Regulating Device (Orbis-Sigma valve): Contrary to a pressure regulator, a flow regulator tries to maintain a constant flow at different pressures. This flow-regulating function is achieved by increasing the valve resistance as the differential pressure increases. The pressure/flow curve of a perfect flow regulator would be a straight vertical line. The flow regulation of the existing system is close to the CSF secretion rate (18 to 30 ml/hr). These characteristics explain why a certain residual overdrainage may still be observed in patients who have retained some physiological CSF resorption capacity. In addition, the very significant flow restriction built into the system requires that specific precautions be taken (elimination of debris, positioning of bedridden patients).

  Ideal flow-pressure characteristics must match the needs, in term of pressure, of an infant as well as an adult, and prevent overdrainage as much as possible. Additional prospective studies are required to evaluate the usefulness of the different categories of valves.
- One-Way Function: Every valve has a one-way function, which is considered mandatory, while the majority of surgeons agree that a subdural collection may be treated successfully with subduroperitoneal shunt made of tubing without any valve added to the system. With ventriculoperitoneal shunts, it is physiologically impossible to get a retrograde flow from the abdominal cavity.

Distal tubing (size, length, types of ends)

Although not proved scientifically, silicone tubing having an outer wall coated with pure silicone seems less prone to promote calcification than barium-impregnated tubing directly in contact with the subcutaneous tissue. As already said, there is no rationale for distal slit-ended catheters (with valve function or not). This type of end does not improve the function of the system and is highly correlated with occurrence of distal obstruction. There are no problems reported in the literature related to the length of tubing introduced into the peritoneal cavity. It can be assumed than at least 25 cm have to be inserted to allow for growth and to avoid a lengthening procedure.

Miscellaneous accessories

The existing accessories, which can be added to the shunt system, have induced numerous shunt complications without any proof of their effectiveness and usefulness. Millipore filters will invariably induce a shunt obstruction, on-off devices may be inadvertently turned off, and telemetric pressure sensors are not widely used at the present time (16).

Connections of the different elements (one-piece, two-pieces, three-piece, multipiece system) (17).

Any connection is a weak point in a shunt system. It carries a risk of disconnection in case of improper ligature, a risk of fracture due to the different physical properties of the two materials, and a risk of migration because, when located on the distal tubing, it creates a point fixation of the shunt, which is no longer able to move freely in the subcutaneous tissue. For these reasons, it is safer to avoid the use of connectors distal to the valve system and to prefer a "two-piece system" where the distal tubing is joined with the valve. What happens at the proximal end of the valve system is more questionable. On one hand, disconnection at this level is quite rare and influenced essentially by the surgical technique; on the other hand, a one-piece system requires a stylet placed out of the catheter to be introduced in the ventricle and is more traumatic for the brain and the dura, leading to a higher risk of CSF leak around the ventricular catheter. In addition clots and debris entering the catheter at insertion time come directly into the valve and increase the risk of shunt obstruction. Above all, we must avoid using multiple-shunt systems, which can easily become a nightmare for the patient and the surgeon.

In conclusion, the authors recommend a two-piece system, composed of a preshaped right-angle nonflanged ventricular catheter, connected to a valve with an appropriate design, without metallic components and able to reduce overdrainage, joined to an open-ended pure silicone-bonded distal tubing.

HOW TO INSERT A SHUNT

Even if the perfect shunt existed, it would rapidly become useless by an inappropriate surgical technique. The purpose of this section is not to legislate on shunt surgery, but to describe the operation the author performs at his medical center, only to serve as a model that demonstrates general principles that apply to the insertion of most of the available shunts. Only ventriculoperitoneal and ventriculoatrial insertion will be described. Problems related to lumboperitoneal shunts are analyzed in Chapter 5. General measures such as the role of the number of people in the operating room, the timing of shunt surgery, and the number of procedures per day have been recently underlined by M. Choux, who reported a series of 1197 procedures in 600 patients with an infection rate of 0.33% (18).

The surgical procedure is described step by step, in the sequence that it is performed at the author's institution.

PREOPERATIVE PREPARATION

Unless the operation is an emergency, the preparation of the patient begins the night before surgery. One scrub of the abdomen and the scalp is performed using a slow-release iodine soap solution. This scrub is repeated in the morning just before surgery. The hair is not shaved. Clipping, if suitable to make the skin incision and closure easier, is achieved by the surgeon.

ANESTHESIA

Prior to anesthesia, it is important to verify that at least two sets of the equipment that the surgeon intends to insert are available. The patient will be operated under general anesthesia with orotracheal intubation. Electrodes for EKG must not be placed on the anterior chest wall that will be included in the surgical field in case of ventriculoperitoneal shunt. The bladder is emptied by Crede' maneuver in anesthetized children or by bladder catheterization if there is a doubt about a full bladder. Peri-operative antibiotics are administered intravenously at the induction of the anesthesia and continued until the end of the surgery. The authors prefer either Cefotaxime 100 mg/K and fosfomycin 100 mg/K or cloxcillin 50 mg/kg alone.

POSITIONING OF THE PATIENT

Positioning the patient is an important stage. When correctly performed, so that the line joining the cranial incision and the abdominal one is straight, it avoids extra skin incisions at the neck or thoracic level. The patient is operated in the supine position, the head rotated contralaterally to the side selected for shunt insertion. The neck is extended as much as possible by building up the sheets under it with linen rolls (Figure 6-4). As already said, a nearly flat plane between the retroauricular region and the abdomen is the best guarantee of avoiding problems with the shunt tunneler at the neck level and of reducing the risk of pleural perforation if passing the peritoneal catheter from above downward.

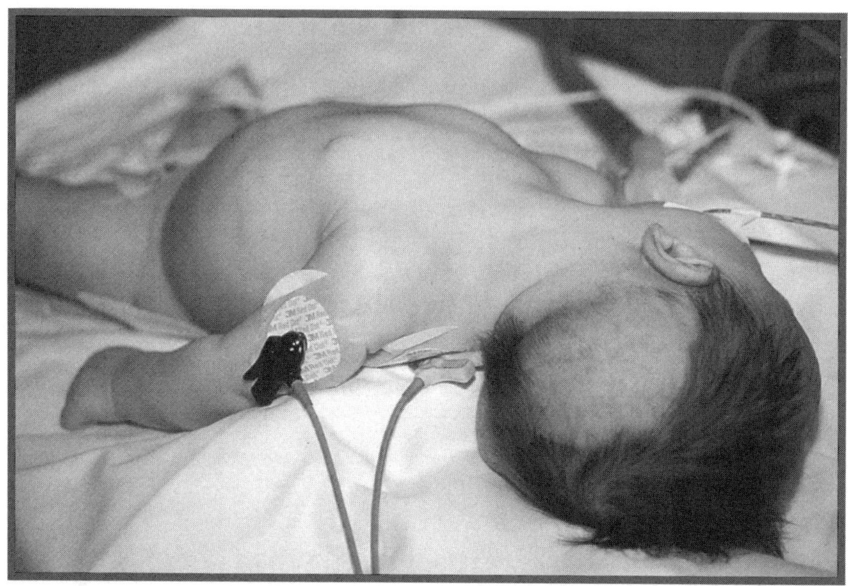

FIGURE 6-4
The head is rotated contralaterally to the side of the skin incision. The line from the cranial incision to the abdominal incision should be as straight as possible.

PREPPING AND DRAPING

The hair is then clipped on a small surface in order to make the skin closure easier. The skin is meticulously prepped with a slow-release iodine solution. Disposable adhesive drapes are used to cover entirely the patient and the operatinge table, except for a 4-cm skin band from the burr hole site to the umbilicus in case of ventriculoperitoneal shunt (Figure 6-5), or to the teat for ventricloatrial insertion.

SKIN INCISION

The skin incision must be small; a 2- to 3-cm long straight skin incision is enough to insert any of the available shunt systems. There is no rationale for the classical half-moon flap (of various size) other than to favor occurrence of skin problems. With a straight incision, it is possible with a gentle downward retraction not to place the burr hole under the scar. A small autostatic retractor is placed (Figure 6-6).

BURR HOLE PLACEMENT

The ideal placement for the burr hole is very controversial and is still a matter of discussion among neurosurgeons (19,20). The choice between the frontal and the occipital burr hole is essentially the result of both local habits and surgeon's conviction. The author prefers the posterior placement for two main reasons: (1) it allows insertion of a shunt with only two skin incisions; an additional incision in the retroauricular region is necessary with frontal place-

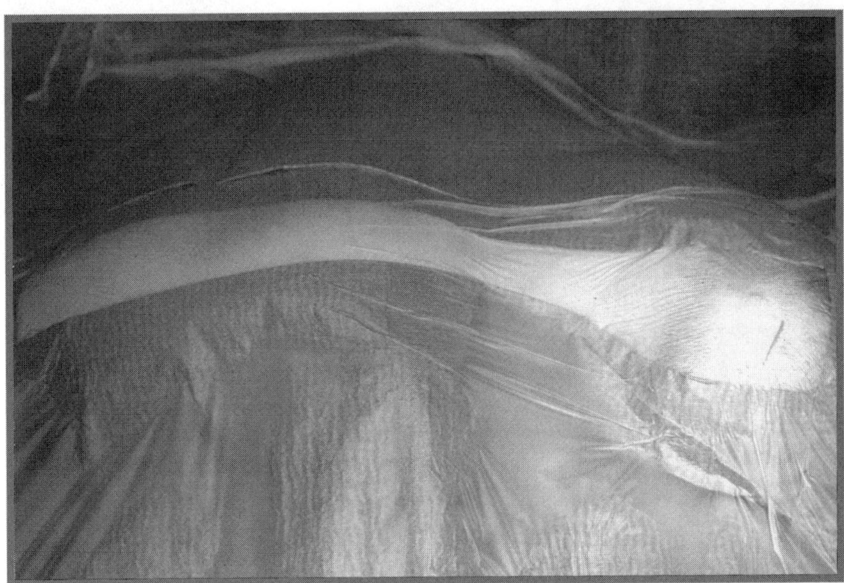

FIGURE 6-5
A complete shaving of the hair is not necessary. In any case, shaving or clipping must be done immediately prior to shunt insertion. Except for a small band of skin protected with a transparent plastic drape, the patient and the operative table are meticulously covered with disposable adhesive drapes.

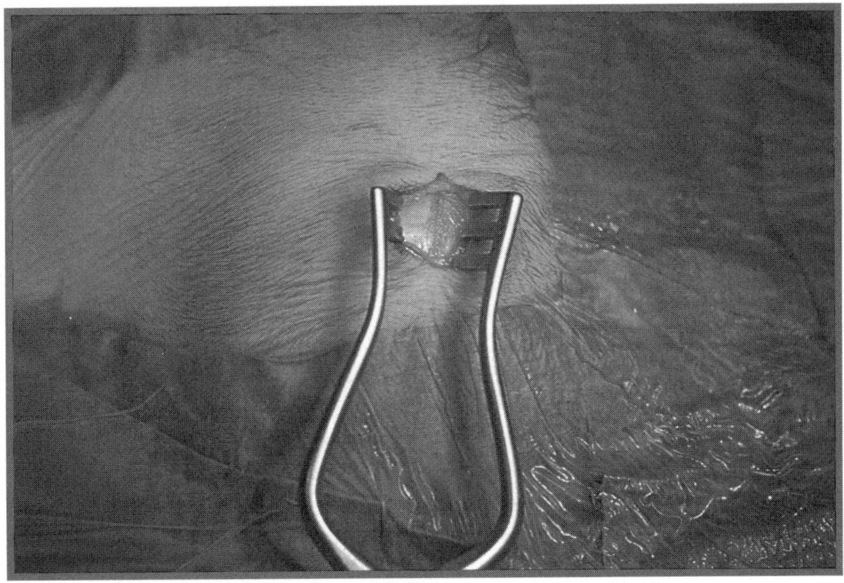

FIGURE 6-6
A short parieto-occipital incision, kept open with autostatic retractors, is commonly used for posterior insertion.

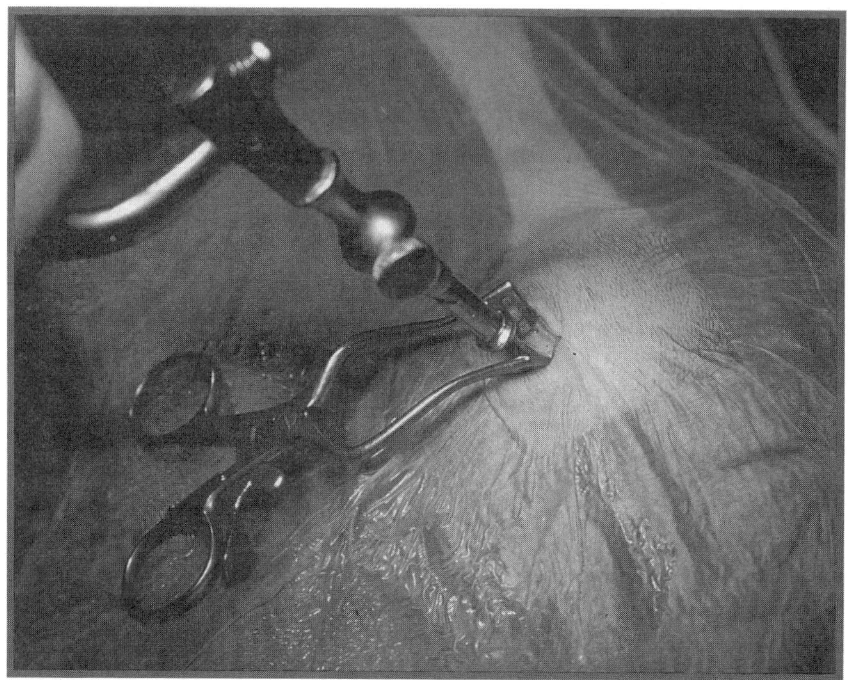

FIGURE 6-7
A burr hole 4 mm in diameter is made carefully to avoid injury of the dura.

ment (2) the tip of the ventricular catheter can be placed in the occipital horn, which is usually the more dilated part of the ventricular system, especially in newborns and children (21). The position of a frontal burr hole is at the point where the parasagittal line passing through the pupil crosses the coronal suture. The position of a posterior burr hole is at the point where the line joining the external orbital rim and the upper limit of the ear pavilion crosses the lambdoid suture, approximately 2.5 cm from the midline. It must be remembered that in some pathologies, like Dandy-Walker malformation or huge arachnoid cysts of the posterior fossa, the transverse sinus can be placed much higher than in normal subjects; in these patients, the position of the transverse sinus should be identified preoperatively by MRI and the placement of the burr hole should be modified according to the results of this exam.

The size of the burr hole depends upon the configuration of the shunt, the thickness of the calvaria, and the age of the patient. If the surgeon uses a shunt including a reservoir with burr hole configuration, then the diameter of the burr hole must allow the easy placement of the reservoir. In children, if a free ventricular catheter is used, the size of the burr hole must simply allow a punctiform coagulation of the dura and the introduction of the ventricular catheter. The author usually uses a 4-mm trephine (Figure 6-7). In newborns, a burr hole is not necessary--for anterior insertion, the catheter can be introduced through the external angle of the anterior fontanel, and for posterior insertion the

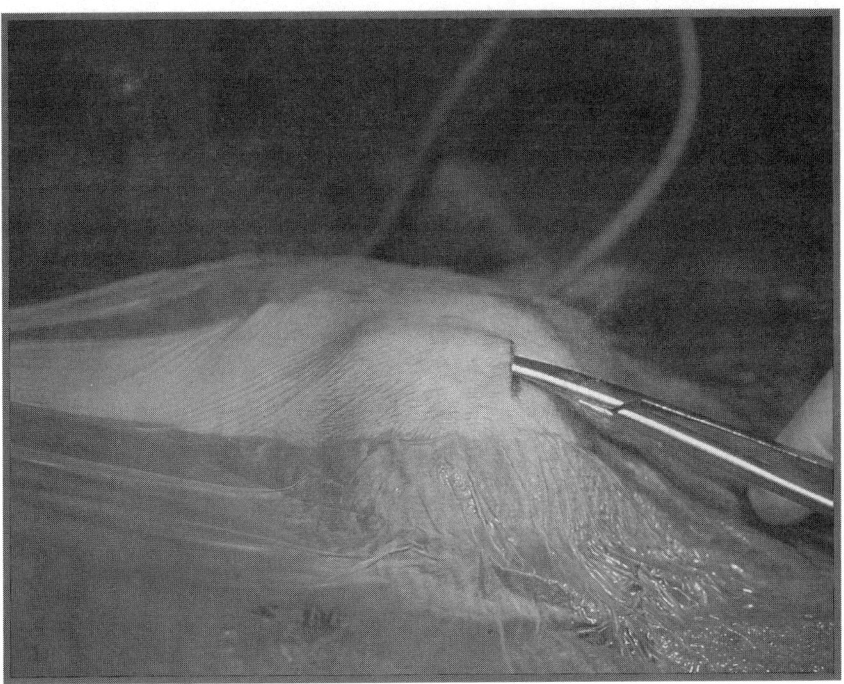

FIGURE 6-8
Using smooth scissors or forceps, a subgaleal pocket is created. The extent of subgaleal dissection, not too small, not too extensive, must be correlated with the size of the valve system, including accessories (reservoir or others).

catheter can be introduced through the lambdoid suture, which is usually large enough. In adults, with thick calvaria and small ventricles, the burr hole must be large enough to modify the direction of the ventricular catheter if the ventricle is not found at the first attempt.

SUBCUTANEOUS DISSECTION

The creation of a small subgaleal pocket to allow easy placement of the valve and appropriate skin closure is of primary importance. An inadequate subcutaneous dissection will require excessive traction on the distal catheter, or multiple manipulations of the material in case of a too small dissection, or will favor occurrence of subcutaneous hematomas, pouches of CSF, and shunt migration if it is too extensive. Dissection in the subcutaneous tissue and not under the galea will make impossible a skin closure in two layers. The author prefers to create a small subcutaneous pocket with scissors, three centimeters long and two centimeters large. The skin autostatic retractor, previously used, is temporarily removed. The scissors are introduced closed to the desired distance from the incision and pulled out opened (Figure 6-8). One single movement is usually sufficient: the repetition of the same movement unecessarily traumatizes the tissues.

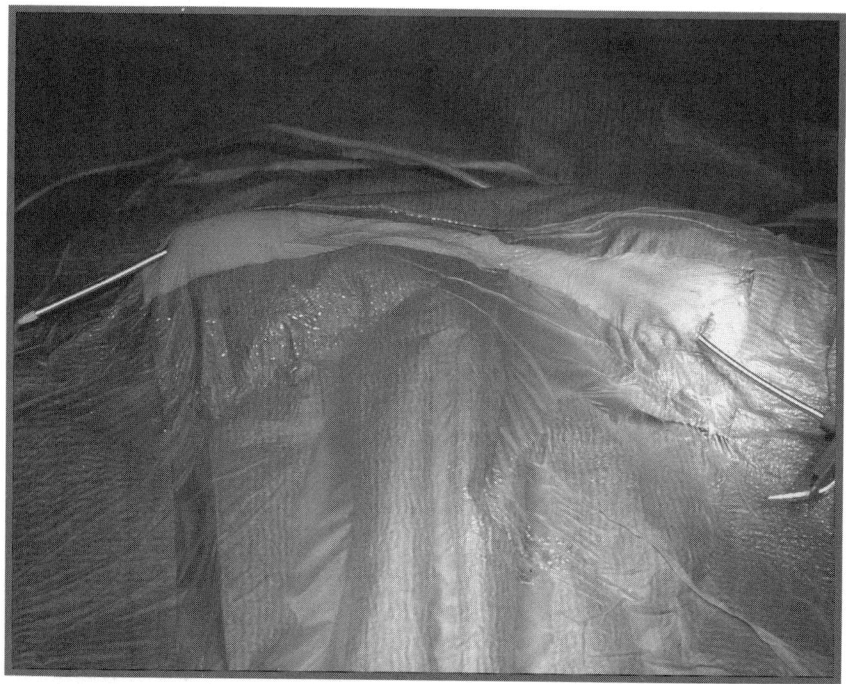

FIGURE 6-9
A tunneling device of a length and stiffness appropriate to the patient is passed from the cranial incision to the paraumbilical incision.

SHUNT PASSING

In ventriculoperitoneal shunt insertion, the stiffness and the length of the shunt tunneler is adapted to the patient. The author prefers disposable malleable tunnellers, either a very malleable 45-cm long tunneler in patients under one year of age or a stiffer 65-cm long tunneler for others. It is of primary importance to introduce the shunt passer into the same space of dissection previously created. When passing from above downward, care should be taken at the level of the neck and of the clavicle in order to avoid vascular injuries or pleural perforation. An optimal positioning of the patient preoperatively will facilitate this phase. One hand is pushing on the tunneler not too far from the scalp incision while the direction is controlled with the other hand through the skin covered with an adhesive plastic sheet. The track of the shunt passer must never become too superficial. This will reduce the risk of skin perforation and probably the risk of delayed tubing calcification. When the tip of the tunneler arrives at the appropriate abdominal location in the paraumbilical region, a punctiform incision of the skin with a scalpel is performed to push it out (Figure 6-9). Integral valve and peritoneal catheters can only be passed from above downward if the passer handle can be disassembled so that the tubular portion can be drawn out through the lower end. When the peritoneum is opened via a minilaparotomy, the tunneler is usually passed from below upward with the same precautions.

The fibrous muscular septae at the skull base may be quite tough, requiring firm but judicious force.

In particular circumstances, it can be impossible to rotate the head for adequate positioning of the patient (e.g., upper spine fusion, cranioskeletal anomalies etc.) or too risky to place the shunt anteriorly (e.g., tracheotomy, jugular central line, and so forth). In these cases, the shunt can be placed in the back. It is not recommended to use this route as a first choice because the mechanical specifications of the tubing are more important in this condition, leading to more calcification, fracture or disconnection or an unsightly fibrous band.

In ventriculoatrial insertion, the tunnelization is stopped at the medium part of the neck, on the anterior edge of the sternocleidal mastoidal muscle.

The shunt package is opened at this stage by the surgeon and not before. Many surgeons recommend soaking the shunt in an antiseptic solution. Some surgeons try to check the hydrodynamic characteristics of the valve in the operating room prior to inserting it, although the only thing that can be tested seriously is the patency of the system. In addition, these manipulations are probably the cause of some shunts contamination. Well-known manufacturers go to considerable effort to pretest the shunt systems so that intraoperative testing is probably unneccessary

The distal tubing is then connected to the plastic wire of the tunneller and pulled into it. The tunneler is then removed by pulling it from the abdominal incision, leaving in place the distal tubing of the shunt under the skin. In case of frontal burr hole, an additional incision behind the ear is always necessary, and placing the distal tubing under the skin is a two-step tunnelization.

OPENING OF THE DURA

With the autostatic retractor back in place, the dura opening is performed by a blind coagulation using a monopolar or a bipolar cautery. The opening must be smaller than the outer diameter of the ventricular catheter so as to ensure a tight dural catheter seal, especially in newborns with huge ventricular dilatation and a thin cortical mantle. This is mandatory to reduce the risks of CSF leakage around the catheter with high opening pressure or high resistance systems. A larger coagulation of the dura or a cruciform incision, described by several authors, probably does not give any advantage over the above-mentioned technique aside from the security of avoiding visualizing surface vessels.

VENTRICULAR CATHETER PLACEMENT

The controversy about the ideal placement of the ventricular tip is too complex to be discussed, butsome concepts must be emphasized. It seems appropriate to the authors to follow one of two strategies. One is to locate the tip of the ventricular catheter in the more dilated part of the ventricle to reduce the risks of malposition and to leave the tip in what remains as the largest portion of the ventricular system (normally the occipital horn) avoiding contact with the choroid plexus and ventricular wall. The other strategy is to place the ventricular catheter tip in the frontal horn, in front of the choroid plexus, from the

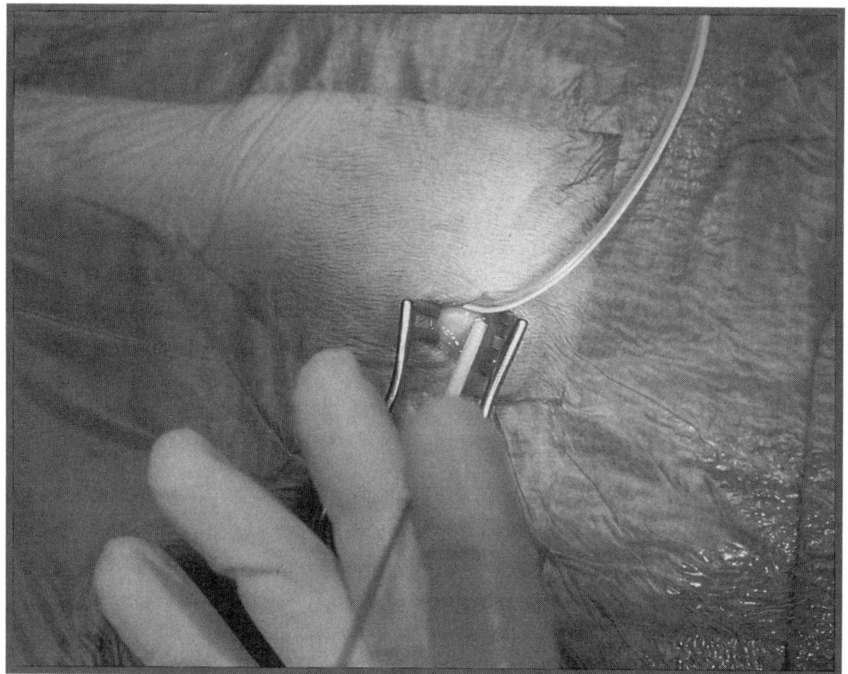

Figure 6-10
The ventricle is tapped with the ventricular catheter stiffened by its stylet. The stylet is removed as soon as the ventricle is entered.

occipital route. The length of the catheter from the outer table to the ventricular target can easily be estimated from the preoperative CT or MRI. The catheter is taken between the second and the third finger with the thumb on the back of the stylet. It is introduced into the brain parenchyma, stiffened by its stylet, through the punctiform coagulation of the dura previously done, and aimed at the center of the forehead (Figure 6-10). The surgeon realizes that the ventricle is entered because of the kinesthetic sensation offered by the perforation of the ependyma and because CSF will start to drop at the posterior extremity of the catheter. At this time, the stylet may be removed and the catheter gently pushed into the ventricle with a smooth forceps. The catheter will enter the ventricle smoothly, and its tip will follow the direction originally given and not perforate the opposite ventricular wall. When aiming for the frontal horn from the occipital route, the stylet must be left in place until nearly in the frontal horn, as early removal may allow the floppy catheter to be advanced into the temporal horn. The classical stylet can be advantageously replaced by an optic fiber of an endoscope. There may be slight advantagea to a right-angled catheter since there is a small risk of upward migration with a straight ventricular catheter just bent at the burr hole level. This is particularly the case when the cortical mantle is thin. In these conditions, after decrease of the ventricular size, the tip of the catheter will enter in contact with the ependyma and may penetrate the adjacent brain

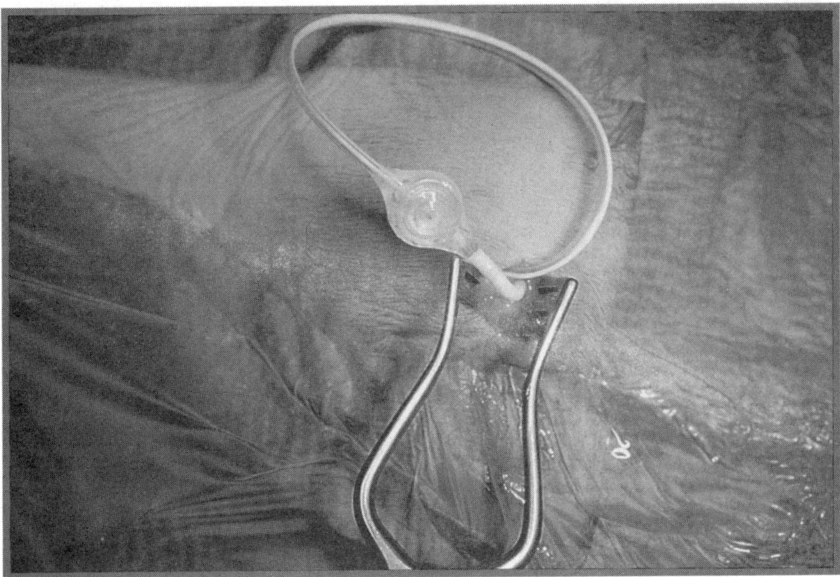

FIGURE 6-11
After connection of the ventricular catheter to the valve, the shunt system is cleaned of the debris that it may contain by gentle aspiration from the end of the distal tubing. If visual inspection shows clots or debris entrapped in the valve, the system must be replaced by a new one.

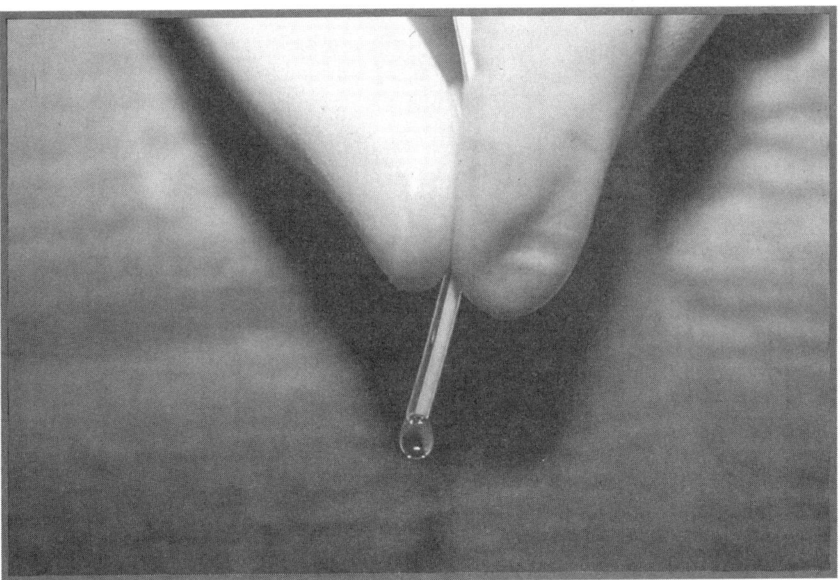

FIGURE 6-12
The valve and the ventricular catheter being in place under the skin, evidence of CSF flow from the distal end is mandatory prior to inserting the distal catheter in the drainage cavity.

parenchyma. Right-angled guides avoid the same problem when used with the straight catheter, but may erode the skin in premature infants.

CLEANING THE SHUNT SYSTEM AND CHECKING ITS FUNCTION

Before connecting the catheter to the valve, the authors prefer to allow the issue of a small amount of CSF (2 to 3 cc). This allows a routine sample of CSF for culture and cell count and clears the catheter of the debris produced by its insertion in the ventricle, which would otherwise flow through the valve, increasing the risks of valve obstruction. After connecting the catheter to the valve, some CSF should be gently aspirated from the distal end, and the absence of residual debris in the valve should be checked (Figure 6-11). Valves with a siphon-reducing device are an exception to this, as aspirating from below closes the membrane. These valves must be prefilled from above. The valve is then inserted under the scalp by gently pulling the distal catheter with one hand while the other hand is controlling its progression in the subgaleal pocket through the skin. The valve should usually be secured at the junction with the ventricular catheter. At this stage, it is mandatory to confirm that the shunt is functional. Cerebrospinal fluid must flow freely from the distal end of the tubing prior to its insertion into the peritoneal cavity (Figure 6-12). The shunt function may be encouraged by lowering its distal end slightly in order to increase the differential pressure applied to the drainage system or by pumping an existing reservoir.

DISTAL INSERTION

Ventriculoperitoneal shunt: The distal catheter may be introduced into the peritoneal cavity by trochar puncture or by minilaparotomy. Trochars are faster but increase the risk of viscus or vascular puncture and are not advised in case of previous abdominal surgery, such as shunt revision. In these cases a minilaparotomy is safest.

Ventriculoatrial shunt: In case of ventriculoatrial shunt, a percutaneous method is preferred in older patients. The jugular vein is tapped and catheterized with the Seldinger technique. The needle is then replaced by a peel-away introducer. Under radioscopy, the appropriate length of catheterization to reach the right atrium is determined with the distal portion of the distal tubing (this length is approximately equal to the distance between the neck incision and the teat on the same side minus 2 cm). The catheter is then removed and cut at this predetermined length. It can then be introduced in the right place without any connection and the peel-away catheter withdrawn.

SKIN CLOSURE

Skin closure is important, and it must be "perfect." Closure is carried out in two layers at the scalp incision with a thin ligature, using absorbable suture for the galea, absorbable or not for the skin. Skin staples are acceptable in older children as long as they will not contact or penetrate the shunt equipment. Three to four stitches are enough if the scalp incision is of the appropriate length

(Figure 6-13). The scar is then protected with a loose adhesive surgical dressing.

As already stated, what has been described is only an example of surgical procedure for shunt insertion. There are probably many other possibilities. But what seems important is for the surgeon to be convinced that shunt surgery is the major cause of shunt complications. The surgeon must be able to justify reasonably any of his or her choices at each step of the procedure.

POSTOPERATIVE MANAGEMENT

The immediate postoperative period is critical. Special care must be paid in two directions: prevention of skin problems leading to shunt contamination and assessment of shunt function and detection of early shunt complications.

The best way to avoid skin problems is a perfect skin closure. In addition, any pressure over the valve system, even for a short period, must be avoided. This is of particular interest in the youngest or debilitated patients. Parents and nurses must be aware of the mechanism of these complications, their risk, and their prevention.

For most of the available shunts, no special positioning is required after shunting. However, surgeons used to leave patients treated with a standard shunt, and at risk for occurrence of subdural collections, in a lying position for one or two days after surgery. When using a high resistance device in patients who are not able to function normally (e.g., infants and comatose patients), it is important to artificially increase the differential pressure applied to the shunt by slightly elevating the patient (Figure 6-14). This maneuver increases the flow through the shunt, helping to reduce the risk of subcutaneous CSF leak around the ventricular catheter, where it tends to accumulate. When the creation of a subcutaneous pouch of CSF is initiated, it is very difficult to cure because it allows free movement of the ventricular tubing, which favors further CSF leakage. Infants who have loose skin, large ventricles, a very thin cortical mantle in the occipital region, and relatively low ICP, are particularly at risk for this complication. If the goal is to drain these patients and to prevent occurrence of secondary chronic overdrainage complications (e.g., slit ventricles and craniostenosis), with one surgery, some kind of compromise, for example, patient positioning, has to be accepted. Some surgeons recommend treating these infants with an initial low-resistance, low opening pressure shunt and scheduling a shunt replacement when they are older. This type of management is questionable for two reasons: either this second operation is not done, increasing the probability of delayed chronic overdrainage complications, or the patient has to run the potential risks of two operations.

After a plain x-ray of the inserted material and clinical evidence of the effectiveness of normal function of the shunt, the patient can usually be discharged from the hospital after a few days. The parents, or the patient if old enough, must be provided with all pertinent information about shunts and shunt surgery. An appointement is set for 3 months postoperatively, with a CT scan or MRI.

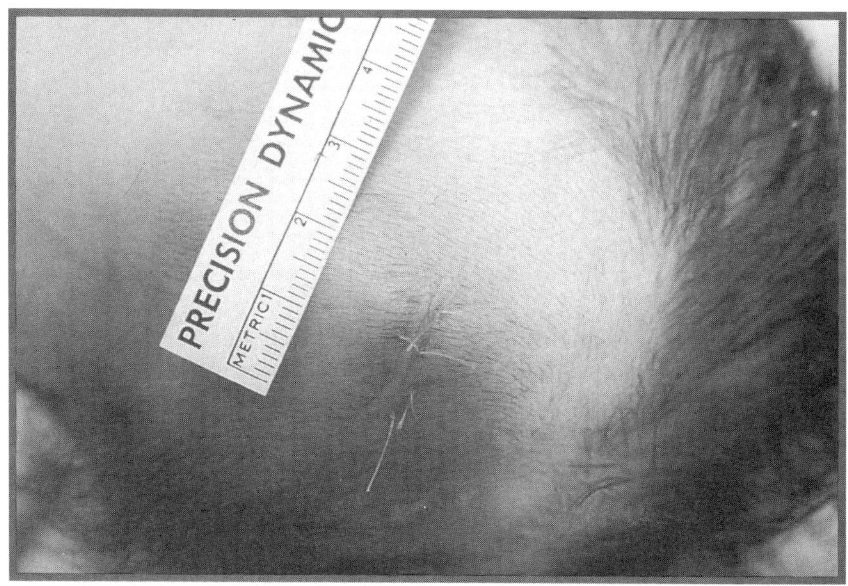

FIGURE 6-13
Closure of the short skin incisions in two layers must be perfect.

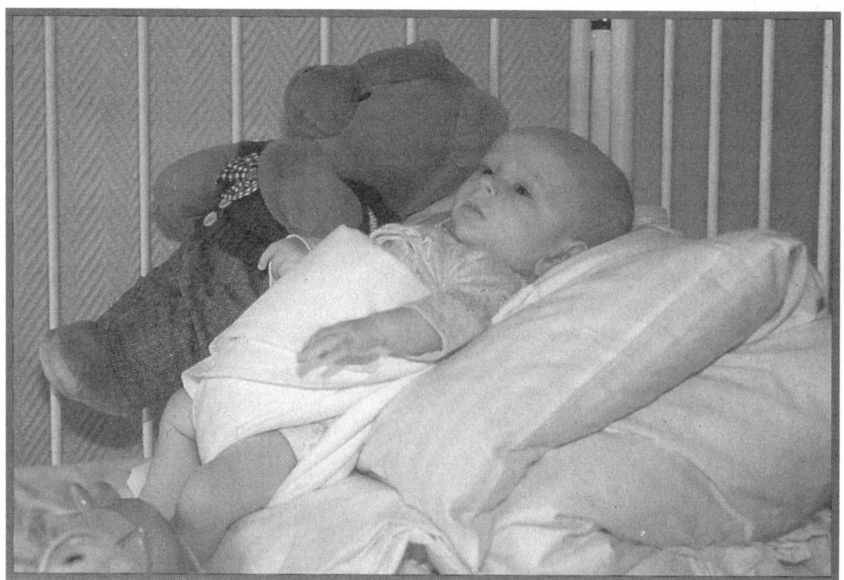

FIGURE 6-14
In some particular cases, patient positioning is necessary to artificially increase the flow through the shunt and thus prevent occurrence of a subcutaneous fluid collection.

HOW TO REVISE A SHUNT

The causes of shunt revision are so numerous that it is impossible to describe all the possible situations. However, some guidelines has to be kept in mind to avoid complications that can be serious.

It is mandatory to identify and suppress the cause of the first failure. It is interesting to note that, in most of the reported series, occurrence of a shunt complication is highly correlated with occurrence of a subsequent one. For instance, a simple reconnection of a calcified distal tubing disconnected from the valve will inevitably result in another disconnection or fracture if the distal tubing is not entirely replaced.

In case of very small ventricles, replacement of the ventricular catheter can be a frightening experience. The author recommends perfectly dissecting the catheter at the burr hole level in order to clearly identify the orifice through which it penetrates the cranium. The obstructed catheter is removed and immediately replaced by the new one without its stylet. It is mandatory to prevent CSF leak, which can further decrease the size of this already small ventricle. This new catheter is gently pushed through the tract of the old one in the ventricles using smooth forceps. In case of problems, instead of multiple taps, which carry a risk of bleeding, it seems safer to go for some aids, for example, the use of the optic fiber of an endoscope as a catheter stylet, ultrasound, a digitizer, or even stereotactic insertion of the ventricular catheter.

Pulling on a catheter attached to the choroid plexus can lead to a severe ventricular hemorrhage. When there is some resistance to retrieving the catheter from the ventricle, it is safer to catheterize the ventricular catheter down to its tip with a coagulation wire (generally used for endoscopic procedure) and coagulate while a gentle traction is exerted on the tubing. An alternative is to approach the catheter tip from a second burr hole with an endoscope and dissect free the cathether.

The function of the system, after final positioning of the ventricular catheter and the valve, has to be checked prior to the introduction of the distal tubing in the drainage cavity.

IN CONCLUSION

The rate of shunt failure occurring within the first few months after surgery, and likely related to the surgical technique, is unacceptably high in most of the reported series. Major progress will be accomplished in the treatment of hydrocephalus when every neurosurgeon is convinced that shunt surgery is as important as any other type of neurosurgery and requires all of our efforts for prevention.

REFERENCES

1. Sainte-Rose C. Third Ventriculostomy. In: Manwaring KH, Crone KR, eds. Neuroendoscopy. Volume 1. New York: Mary Ann Liebert,1992:47-62.

2. Epstein F, Murali R. Pediatric posterior fossa tumors : Hazards of the "pre-operative" shunt. Neurosurgery 1978;3:348-350.

3. Gurtner P, Bass T, Gudeman SK, Penix JO, Philput CB, Schinco FP. Surgical management of posthemorrhagic hydrocephalus in 22 low-birth-weight infants. Child's Nerv Syst 1992;8:198-202.

4. Pezzotta S, Locatelli D, Bonfanti N. Shunt in high-risk newborns. Child's Nerv Syst 1987;3:114-116.

5. Post EM. Currently Available Shunt Systems: A review. Neurosurgery 1985;6:257-260.

6. Choux M. Shunts and problems in shunt. Basel, New York: Karger, 1982:1-6

7. Epstein, F. : How to keep shunts functioning, or "The Impossible Dream. " Clin Neurosurg 1984;32:608-631.8. Griebel R, Khan M, Tan L. CSF shunt complications: an analysis of contributory factors. Child's Nerv Syst 1985;1:77-80.

9. Sainte-Rose C, Piatt JH, Renier D, Pierre-Kahn A, Hirsch JF, Hoffman HJ, Humpreys RP, Hendrick EB. Mechanical complications in shunts. Pediatr Neurosurg 1991-92;17:2-9.

10. Echizenya K, Satoh M, Mural H. Mineralization and biodegradation of CSF shunting systems. J Neurosurg 1987;67:584-591.

11. Giuffrè R. Choroidal and ependymal reactions. J Neurosurg Sci 1976;20:123-129.

12. Gower DJ, Lewis JC, Kelly DL. Sterile shunt malfunction. A scanning electron microscopic perspective. J. Neurosurg 1984;61:1079-1084.

13. Haase J, Weeth R. Multiflanged ventricular catheter for hydrocephalic shunts. Acta Neurochir (Wien) 1976;33:213-218.

14. Portnoy H D, Schulte R R, Fox J L, et al. Anti-siphon and reversible occlusion vaLves for shunting in hydrocephalus and preventing postshunt subdural hematomas. J Neurosurg 1973;38:729-738.

15. Sainte-Rose C. Shunt obstruction: a preventable complication? Pediatr Neurosurg 1993;19:156-164.

16. Chapman P H, Griebel R, Cosman E R, et al. Telemetric ICP measurement in normal and shunted, hydrocephalic patients. In: Chapman, PH, ed. Concepts in pediatric neurosurgery. Volume 6. Basel, New York: Kager, 1985:15-132.

17. Haase J, Bang F, Tange M. Danish experience with the one-piece shunt. A long-term follow-up. Child's Nerv Syst 1987;3:93-96.

18. Choux M, Genitori L, Lang D, Lena G. Shunt implantation: reducing the incidence of shunt infection. J Neurosurg 1992;77:875-880.

19. Albright AL, Haines SJ, Taylor FH. Function of parietal and frontal shunts in childhood hydrocephalus. J Neurosurg 1988;69:883-886.

20. Bierbrauer KS, Storrs BB, McLone DG, Tomita T, Dauser R. A prospective, randomized study of shunt function and infections as a function of shunt placement. Pediatr Neurosurg 1990-91;16:287-291.

21. Reeder J D, Kaude J V, Setzer E S. The occipital horn of the lateral ventricles in premature infants. An ultrasonographic study. Eur. J. Radiol 1983;3:148-150.

INDEX

D

N

O

P